VISION
AND
GOAL-DIRECTED MOVEMENT

NEUROBEHAVIORAL PERSPECTIVES

EDITORS

DIGBY ELLIOTT, PhD

LIVERPOOL JOHN MOORES UNIVERSITY

MICHAEL A. KHAN, PhD

BANGOR UNIVERSITY

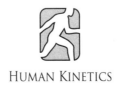

HUMAN KINETICS

Library of Congress Cataloging-in-Publication Data

Vision and goal-directed movement : neurobehavioral perspectives / Digby Elliott, Michael A. Khan, editors.

    p. cm.

Includes bibliographical references and index.

ISBN-13: 978-0-7360-7475-9 (print)

ISBN-10: 0-7360-7475-9 (print)

  1. Perceptual-motor processes. 2. Motion perception (Vision) 3. Visual perception. I. Elliott, Digby, 1950- II. Khan, Michael A., 1966-

  [DNLM: 1. Motor Activity--physiology. 2. Goals. 3. Intention.

4. Psychomotor Performance--physiology. 5. Visual Perception--physiology.

WE 103 V831 2010]

  BF295.V567 2010

  152.3'5--dc22

                                        2009036255

ISBN-10: 0-7360-7475-9 (print)

ISBN-13: 978-0-7360-7475-9 (print)

The Web addresses cited in this text were current as of June 2009, unless otherwise noted.

Acquisitions Editor: Judy Patterson Wright, PhD and Myles Schrag; **Managing Editor:** Melissa J. Zavala; **Assistant Editor:** Casey A. Gentis; **Copyeditor:** Jocelyn Engman; **Indexer:** Nancy Gerth; **Permission Manager:** Dalene Reeder; **Graphic Designer:** Bob Reuther; **Graphic Artist:** Denise Lowry; **Cover Designer:** Bob Reuther; **Photographer (interior):** © Human Kinetics, unless otherwise noted; **Photo Asset Manager:** Jason Allen; **Art Manager:** Kelly Hendren; **Associate Art Manager:** Alan L. Wilborn; **Illustrator:** Tammy Page; **Printer:** Sheridan Books

Printed in the United States of America   10 9 8 7 6 5 4 3 2 1

The paper in this book is certified under a sustainable forestry program.

Human Kinetics

Web site: www.HumanKinetics.com

United States: Human Kinetics, P.O. Box 5076, Champaign, IL 61825-5076
800-747-4457
e-mail: humank@hkusa.com

Canada: Human Kinetics, 475 Devonshire Road Unit 100, Windsor, ON N8Y 2L5
800-465-7301 (in Canada only)
e-mail: info@hkcanada.com

Europe: Human Kinetics, 107 Bradford Road
Stanningley, Leeds LS28 6AT, United Kingdom
+44 (0) 113 255 5665
e-mail: hk@hkeurope.com

Australia: Human Kinetics, 57A Price Avenue, Lower Mitcham, South Australia 5062
08 8372 0999
e-mail: info@hkaustralia.com

New Zealand: Human Kinetics, P.O. Box 80, Torrens Park, South Australia 5062
0800 222 062
e-mail: info@hknewzealand.com

E4488

CONTENTS

PART III: Learning, Development, and Application   279

CHAPTER 18 | OPTIMIZING PERFORMANCE
THROUGH WORK SPACE DESIGN **341**

James L. Lyons

CONTRIBUTORS

J. GREG ANSON
School of Physical Education, University of Otago

GRAHAM R. BARNES
Faculty of Life Sciences, The University of Manchester

SIMON J. BENNETT
School of Sport and Exercise Sciences, Liverpool John Moores University

GORDON BINSTED
Faculty of Health and Social Development, University of British Columbia

KYLE BROWNELL
College of Kinesiology, University of Saskatchewan

RACHEL BURGESS
School of Physical Education, University of Otago

DAVID P. CAREY
School of Psychology, University of Aberdeen

DIGBY ELLIOTT
School of Sport and Exercise Sciences, Liverpool John Moores University

PETER FEYS
*Department of Biomedical Kinesiology, Katholieke Universiteit Leuven
& REVAL, University College Hasselt and BIOMED, Hasselt University*

IAN M. FRANKS
School of Human Kinetics, University of British Columbia

LAWRENCE E.M. GRIERSON
Toronto Rehabilitation Institute, University of Toronto

STEVE HANSEN
School of Sport and Exercise Sciences, Liverpool John Moores University

SPENCER HAYES
School of Sport and Exercise Sciences, Liverpool John Moores University

MATTHEW HEATH
School of Kinesiology, The University of Western Ontario

WERNER F. HELSEN
Department of Biomedical Kinesiology, Katholieke Universiteit Leuven

ELKE HEREMANS
Department of Biomedical Kinesiology, Katholieke Universiteit Leuven

NICOLA J. HODGES
School of Human Kinetics, University of British Columbia

ROBERT R. HORN
Department of Exercise Science and Physical Education, Montclair State University

MICHAEL A. KHAN
School of Sport, Health and Exercise Sciences, Bangor University

OLAV KRIGOLSON
Department of Psychology, University of British Columbia

ANN LAVRYSEN
Departments of Biomedical Kinesiology and Psychology, Katholieke Universiteit Leuven

JAMES L. LYONS
Department of Kinesiology, McMaster University

DANA MASLOVAT
School of Human Kinetics, University of British Columbia

KRISTINA A. NEELY
School of Kinesiology, The University of Western Ontario

TYLER ROLHEISER
Department of Human Physiology, University of Oregon

ROBERT L. SAINBURG
Departments of Kinesiology and Neurology, Pennsylvania State University

GEERT J.P. SAVELSBERGH
Research Institute MOVE, Faculty of Human Movement Sciences, VU University Amsterdam
Institute for Biomedical Research into Human Movement and Health, Manchester Metropolitan University

REBEKAH L. SCOTT
School of Physical Education, University of Otago

LUC TREMBLAY
Faculty of Physical Education and Health, University of Toronto

JOHN VAN DER KAMP
Research Institute MOVE, Faculty of Human Movement Sciences, VU University Amsterdam
Institute of Human Performance, University of Hong Kong

Margot van Wermeskerken
Research Institute MOVE, Faculty of Human Movement Sciences, VU University Amsterdam

Daniel J. Weeks
Department of Psychology, University of Lethbridge

Timothy N. Welsh
Faculty of Physical Education and Health, University of Toronto

David A. Westwood
School of Health and Human Performance, Dalhousie University

PREFACE

Throughout the last 15 years, there has been an upsurge of interest in the role that vision plays in the control of goal-directed movement. This interest has been driven in part by the new prominence the study of action has found in the contemporary psychological literature. In order to interact with a complex environment, humans must code and store spatial information and then translate it into the appropriate motor commands needed to achieve the task goal. Researchers interested in perception and attention have realized more and more that people perceive and pay attention to objects and events in the visual environment so they can interact with them. As a consequence, a number of action-based accounts of various cognitive processes have emerged. The premise of much of this work is that visual perception, attention, and memory are intimately linked to movement preparation and execution.

The control of visually directed movement has been a topic of tremendous interest in the neuroscience literature. Much of this work has followed from years of behavioral research aimed at understanding the processes underlying the relationship between movement speed and accuracy. Technical advancements in neuroimaging and magnetic brain stimulation have led to a much better understanding of the neural foundation for goal-directed action. Neuroscientists and psychologists have taken their lead from movement scientists and have started to use three-dimensional movement analysis techniques to try to understand the complex interactions between movement planning processes and the rapid online regulation of goal-directed movement through the use of vision and other sources of feedback. It has become clear that the human visuomotor system is extremely flexible, and the regulation of movement depends on the learning and developmental history of the performer.

In this edited volume, we bring together some of the most active researchers in our field to review the latest developments in our understanding of vision, action, and the control of goal-directed movement. Section I features chapters that take a behavioral and process-oriented approach. Chapter 1 reviews the classic work of R.S. Woodworth (1899), "The Accuracy of

eBook
available at
HumanKinetics.com

Voluntary Movement," and then traces the effects his ideas had on related research throughout the next century. The chapter also discusses the models of speed–accuracy relationships and upper-limb control that guide current research. Chapter 2 continues along these lines by presenting new ideas about speed–accuracy relationships that take into account the performer's trial-to-trial strategic behavior as well as the role of learning and energy expenditure in optimal performance. This chapter also provides an account of specific kinematic techniques that have been developed to uncover the neural and behavioral processes associated with the online regulation of goal-directed actions.

Chapter 3 reviews the latest theoretical developments in the psychological literature on visual selective attention and the role of action in directing attentional processes. Chapter 4 builds on chapter 3 by establishing the links that bind attentional and movement planning processes in humans and other primates. In chapter 5, we see how the psychological and movement science literatures have merged in an attempt to understand how people represent the world in their memory in order to act on it. This chapter sets the stages for chapters 12 and 13 in section II, which discuss the neural basis for representations of perceptions and actions in greater detail.

The next two chapters in section I examine goal-directed reaching and aiming behaviors under situations that challenge the limits of the visuomotor system. Chapter 6 deals with multielement movements by bringing together ideas on movement preparation and the processes occurring during movement execution. Sometimes we can determine the capabilities of a system only by perturbing it and examining how it adapts to change in environmental or task circumstances. Chapter 7 reviews the empirical work that has taken this approach and explores how this research has contributed to our understanding of basic visuomotor processes. As the final chapter in section I, chapter 8 provides a precursor to the systems-oriented approach characterizing section II. The role of central and peripheral vision in limb control is examined along with a body of recent research that indicates that there may be differences in the way the lower and upper visual fields process movement-related information.

Although all the chapters in this volume deal with human motor behavior, the chapters in section II also explore the sensory and neural foundations of goal-directed action. Chapters 9 and 10 deal with pursuit eye movements and saccadic eye movements, respectively. The topics addressed in these chapters include optimizing the pickup of movement-relevant information, eye–hand coordination, and the influence of retinal and extraretinal ocular information on precision limb control. Chapter 11 provides additional insights into eye–hand coordination and also examines how it breaks down as a result of pathology.

Chapters 12 through 14 are concerned with the specialization of various cortical systems for the regulation of movement. In chapter 12, the most recent work on cerebral specialization and the neural foundation for performance differences between the left and right hands is discussed. Chapters 13 and 14 review the large body of recent work on the specialization of the ventral and dorsal visual streams for perception and action, respectively. Chapter 13 deals with issues such as the representation of visual space and the influence of context on perception and action in persons with normal function, while chapter 14 provides insights into the dissociation between perception and action in persons with specific brain injuries.

Section III of this volume contains four chapters that move the theoretical work presented in sections I and II into a broader context. Chapters 15 and 16 review recent research on how and why limb control changes with practice and development. This work has important implications for both skill instruction and rehabilitation. Although the study of observational learning has a long history in the movement sciences, recent developments in neuroimaging and movement analysis have allowed researchers to understand this type of motor learning on a whole new level. Chapter 17 reviews these new developments. Finally, chapter 18 extends the research on vision and goal-directed movement from the laboratory to the workplace. After providing an excellent overview of the development of human factors research, the chapter reviews approaches to work space design that maximize precision, efficiency, and safety.

Our primary goal in soliciting this collection of works was to provide a comprehensive account of the current state of affairs in vision and goal-directed movement. The contributors are all active researchers who are not committed to a single way of thinking. They are at the forefront of their fields partly because their ideas are evolving and constantly put to the empirical test. Thus the work presented here also provides a taste of the direction of research concerned with vision and the control of goal-directed action over the next decade. In fact, at the end of each chapter the authors speculate on the future directions of research in their area.

This volume was created as a resource for motor control and learning researchers already working in the field. It also provides a handbook for students, educators, and clinicians interested in goal-directed action. In this context, the volume is suitable for senior undergraduate and graduate special topics courses on vision and motor control. As editors of this volume, it has been a joy to compile, read, and organize this outstanding collection of papers written by our colleagues and friends.

PART I

A BEHAVIORAL APPROACH TO VISION AND GOAL-DIRECTED MOVEMENT

More than 100 years ago R.S. Woodworth (1899) published an influential monogram in which he reported the results of a number of studies examining the perceptual, cognitive, and motor processes associated with performing precise, goal-directed action. In this classic paper, Woodworth presented a theoretical model of goal-directed action to explain the well-known relationship between movement speed and movement accuracy and the variables mediating this relationship. Vision was fundamental to Woodworth's two-component account of limb control. It was deemed important for both planning and feedback-based control during movement execution. In addition to making his theoretical contribution, Woodworth introduced many of the methods for studying goal-directed limb control that we still use today. For these reasons, Woodworth's 1899 paper provides the starting point for this volume.

Part I begins with a review of Woodworth's groundbreaking findings and traces the effects his contributions have had on related research throughout and beyond the next century. In chapter 1, Elliott,Hansen, and Grierson review the models of speed and accuracy that were developed over the 20th century to build on the foundation provided by Woodworth. The chapter extends on ideas about movement preparation and limb control presented by Elliott, Helsen, and Chua in a 2001 *Psychological Bulletin* paper and presents a 21st-century version of the two-component approach to limb control.

In chapter 2, Elliott, Hansen, and Khan follow up on the ideas presented in chapter 1 by highlighting the flexibility with which the human performer uses vision and other sources of information to optimize goal-directed performance. Fundamental to understanding the strategic behavior people adopt to maximize speed, accuracy, and energy expenditure are the data acquisition, reduction, and analysis techniques used to examine both the microstructure of single movements and the trial-to-trial variation in limb trajectories. In this latter context, chapter 2 builds on work recently published by Khan and colleagues (2006) in *Neuroscience and Biobehavioral Reviews*. Together, chapters 1 and 2 establish an empirical and theoretical framework for the remainder of Part I.

Chapters 3, 4, and 5 each deal with specific processes essential to goal-directed limb control. About 15 or 20 years ago, topics such as selective attention were exclusive to the psychological literature. Moreover, there was little interest in the role of attention in movement planning or execution. In chapter 3, Welsh and Weeks provide a historical account of the new prominence of action in the visual selective attention literature. Using the work of Tipper, Lortie, and Baylis (1992), they show how action-based models of selective attention have been derived in order to account for the function of excitatory and inhibitory processes involved in movement planning and execution.

In chapter 3, Welsh and Weeks distinguish between automatic attention-capturing processes and volitional attention. It is the volitional, controlled aspect of attention that is intimately related to the topic of vision and movement planning that Anson, Burgess, and Scott explore in chapter 4. After outlining the cognitive and neural systems thought to be important for movement planning, Anson and colleagues explore the many chronometric and neurophysiological techniques that have been used to examine the role of vision in the planning process. By establishing the importance of visual and other frames of reference to action planning and by introducing the connection between movement planning and memory processes, chapter 4 provides an excellent link between chapter 3 on selective attention and chapter 5 on memory-guided limb control.

Under many circumstances, a person does not have access to full sensory information at the time of movement execution, and thus either the movement goal or the plan to achieve that goal must be represented in memory for some length of time. In chapter 5, Heath, Neely, Krigolson, and Binsted examine the ways in which visual information about the movement environment might be represented as well as look at the neural systems that support different types of information coding. The chapter extends on

Anson and colleagues' ideas about the role of the dorsal and ventral visual systems in movement planning by discussing the specialization of these systems for remembering (or not remembering) different sources of visual information. Like chapter 4, chapter 5 explores the importance of the visual frame of reference in goal-directed limb control. Some of these same issues are revisited under a different theoretical context in Part II of this volume (see chapters 13 and 14).

Chapters 6 and 7 explore issues surrounding the interface between movement planning and execution. Chapter 6 deals with complex goal-directed actions that involve more than one component. In these multiple-target situations, there is often temporal overlap between the processes involved in executing one task component and the processes involved in planning another. In this chapter Khan, Helsen, and Franks examine how advance information, physical task demands, and strategy influence the interdependence between processes preceding response initiation and processes occurring during movement execution.

The actions that we plan do not always unfold in the ways we intended. Sometimes the movement goal or environment changes while an action is in progress (e.g., the wind moves a tree branch as we reach for it). In chapter 7, Hansen, Grierson, Khan, and Elliott examine the ability of the visuomotor system to adapt to unexpected perturbations to either the movement environment or the task demands. In general, this chapter reviews research that explores the relative importance of movement planning and online control processes in precision movement by introducing events that systematically alter the effectiveness of the initial movement plan. Once again, detailed kinematic analysis of the movement trajectory is necessary to determine the time required for corrective processes to unfold.

The final chapter in Part I builds a bridge between the predominantly behavioral focus and the more systems-oriented approach in Part II. In chapter 8, Khan and Binsted give a systematic review of the literature exploring the functional roles of peripheral and central vision in target aiming. They then turn their attention to asymmetries between the upper and lower visual fields in the visual control of action.

Taken together, the eight chapters in Part I comprehensively cover the current behavior-based literature on the visual control of goal-directed action. Although by necessity there is some discussion of the specific sensory and neural systems involved in movement planning and execution, it is primarily Part II that explores the relationship between behavior and the neurophysiological systems supporting behavior.

CHAPTER 1

The Legacy of R.S. Woodworth: The Two-Component Model Revisited

DIGBY ELLIOTT, STEVE HANSEN, AND LAWRENCE E.M. GRIERSON

More than a century ago R.S. Woodworth (1899) published what has become a seminal monograph titled "The Accuracy of Voluntary Movement." The paper made important empirical and theoretical contributions in diverse areas such as speed–accuracy trade-offs, manual asymmetries in motor control, coordination, movement perception, and motor learning. Woodworth's two-component model of goal-directed action has probably had the greatest influence on contemporary accounts of motor control and learning. In this chapter, we review Woodworth's empirical work on the topic and his conclusions about the control of upper-limb movements. We then trace where his ideas have taken us throughout the last 109 years as well as identify where his ideas need to be reconsidered.

The Early Two-Component Model

Woodworth (1899) examined goal-directed action using a simple aiming procedure in which participants used a pencil to execute horizontal sliding movements between target lines separated by a fixed distance. Target lines were drawn on paper that was secured to a drum that rotated at a constant speed. This setup allowed Woodworth to measure not only the accuracy and consistency of the movement reversal points around the target line but also the spatial and temporal characteristics of the movement trajectories. By using a metronome to control the tempo at which participants moved and therefore control the participants' movement time (MT), Woodworth made the accuracy and consistency of the end point his primary measured outcome.

With respect to the characteristics of the movement trajectory, Woodworth found that all but the very fastest movements are made up of two components. The initial portion of each aiming attempt is relatively rapid and stereotyped; Woodworth termed this portion of the movement the *initial adjustment*. In recent years, researchers have used the terms *ballistic phase* or *initial impulse* to identify this portion of the movement. Woodworth's idea was that this initial stereotyped component of the aiming movement brings the limb into the vicinity of the target.

Woodworth also found that as the pencil approaches the target line, movement speed typically decreases and the number of bumps or discontinuities in the time–displacement tracing increases. This part of the movement varies to a greater degree with each aiming attempt. Woodworth hypothesized that during this phase of the movement the performer adjusts the movement in order to hit or come close to the target line. That is, participants add "little extra movements" (Woodworth, 1899, p. 54) to the initial impulse, or there is "a subtraction or inhibition of the movement, making it shorter than it otherwise might have been" (p. 58). Woodworth referred to this latter portion of the movement as the *current control phase*. It has also been referred to as the *homing phase*. The idea is that during this portion of the movement the performer uses visual and other forms of feedback to reduce aiming error inherent in the initial impulse.

Woodworth (1899) had participants perform aiming movements at different metronome speeds in order to examine the relationship between movement speed and movement accuracy and the possible contribution of the current control phase to the latter. Thus, as metronome tempo increased, the average MT for a series of aiming attempts decreased. Participants also performed under two different afferent conditions. In one condition they were allowed to keep their eyes open and thus had full visual information about the position of their limb and the target lines, while in a second condition they performed the same series of aiming movements with their eyes closed. Interestingly, the difference in the aiming error between these two conditions decreased as average MT decreased. This trend continued until there was no difference in error between the eyes-open condition and eyes-closed condition, an outcome that occurred at an MT of approximately 450 ms. Woodworth (1899) interpreted this pattern of results as a reflection of the temporal limitations associated with the current control phase of movement. The idea is that when MT is 450 ms or less, participants have insufficient time to use the visual feedback available in the eyes-open condition to engage in current control. Thus, at this MT accuracy is associated with the precision of the initial adjustment or impulse. For movements of a longer duration, end-point accuracy is dependent on the time the performer has available for current control.

Alternative Explanations of Speed–Accuracy Relationships

Although Woodworth's (1899) description of how limb movements are controlled held up well, his estimate of the time required for visual processing was challenged by Keele and Posner (1968) in the late 1960s. They reasoned that because Woodworth used reciprocal aiming movements in his protocol, his MT included not only the time needed to travel between the two target lines but also the time needed to reverse the direction of the sliding movement at each of the target locations. Thus his reciprocal procedure was overestimating the visual processing time.[1]

Keele and Posner (1968) conducted an influential aiming study using a discrete aiming procedure. Before the experiment, participants practiced making aiming movements from a home position to a small target at specific movement durations (150, 250, 350, and 450 ms). Participants were then asked to perform at these specific MTs under conditions of full vision and no vision. The full-vision condition was like the practice condition in that participants were able to see their limb and the target throughout the whole course of the movement. For the no-vision condition, the room lights were extinguished upon movement initiation. Thus for no-vision trials the performers could see their limb and the target during movement preparation but not during movement execution. Keele and Posner used what is now termed a *random feedback* procedure. This means that full-vision (50% of the trials) and no-vision (50% of the trials) conditions were randomly intermixed so that on any given trial the participant did not know whether the lights would be extinguished or not. The short MT in their study turned out to be a little longer than the MT used in practice (i.e., 190 rather 150 ms and 260 rather than 250 ms). The primary dependent measure was the proportion of times the participant hit the small target in each of the two vision conditions by the four MT conditions. Of interest was the finding that participants exhibited greater accuracy when they had vision available at all MT conditions except 190 ms. The results of their study left Keele and Posner with an estimate of visual processing time of somewhere between 190 and 260 ms. This figure was reasonably consistent with a visual two-choice reaction time (RT) and was widely accepted for the next 15 years.

In the same year he published his influential empirical work with Michael Posner, Steve Keele (Keele, 1968) published an important theoretical paper that extended Woodworth's ideas about movement planning and current control. Building on previous ideas presented by Crossman and Goodeve (1963/1983), Keele (1968) proposed an alternative to Woodworth's two-component explanation of speed–accuracy relationships that has come to be known as the *iterative correction model.* Fundamental to the iterative correction model is the notion of a motor program. Keele (1968) formalized the concept of the motor program by defining it as "a set of muscle commands that are structured before a movement sequence begins, that allow the entire sequence to be carried out uninfluenced by peripheral feedback" (p. 387).

Like Woodworth, Keele proposed that the initial portion of a goal-directed movement is under the control of a prestructured set of muscle commands. The unfolding movement is under the control of this motor program for approximately the first 200 ms of the movement until the central nervous system has time to process visual and proprioceptive feedback (Keele & Posner, 1968). According to the iterative correction model, feedback is then used to structure a second submovement designed to correct the error in the first submovement. The second submovement is controlled by a new motor program and, if time permits, feedback is used once again to engage the same type of corrective process.

According to the iterative correction model, an aiming movement is made up of a series of submovements, each of which is ballistic and organized according to the feedback available from the previous submovement. Thus, accuracy depends on the number of corrective submovements. In this model, more time means more submovements and therefore greater accuracy. Although the iterative correction model did a good job of mathematically explaining the relationship between MT and end-point error (Fitts & Peterson, 1964), kinematic data that became available over the next decade were not consistent with the idea of multiple corrective submovements (Carlton, 1979; Langolf, Chaffin, & Foulke, 1976).

More in line with Woodworth's (1899) two-component model was the single-correction model forwarded by Beggs and Howarth (1970, 1972; Howarth, Beggs, & Bowden, 1971) in the early 1970s. Like Woodworth, these researchers held that a single ballistic movement brings the limb into the vicinity of the target. Time permitting, a single corrective movement is made based on visual feedback about the relative positions of the limb and the target. Their notion was that a minimum amount of time is required for a single correction to be completed and thus the correction occurs at a fixed temporal interval before contact with the target area. In their empirical work, Beggs and Howarth (1972) found that occluding vision 290 ms before movement termination had little effect on movement accuracy. Thus they proposed that the single correction takes place approximately 300 ms before target acquisition. Accuracy depends on the precision of the single correction. In turn, the precision of the correction relates to the proximity of the limb and target at the time the correction is initiated. A longer MT allows the limb to be closer to the target when the correction is initiated. For movements of 290 ms or less, a correction is not possible. Apart from the estimate of the visual processing time, the main difference between the two-component model and the single-correction model is the nature of the corrective process (Elliott, Helsen, & Chua, 2001). For the former, the corrective process involves a graded homing in on the target, while for the latter it involves a single ballistic correction (c.f., iterative correction model).

Although the two-component model, the iterative correction model, and the single-correction model vary in their hypothesized processes, fundamental to each of these explanations of the speed–accuracy relationship is the role of visual feedback in determining end-point accuracy and between-trial end-point variability. In the late 1970s, Richard Schmidt and his students introduced a very different approach to the understanding of speed–accuracy relationships (Schmidt, Zelaznik, & Frank, 1978; Schmidt, Zelaznik, Hawkins, Frank, & Quinn, 1979). The premise of what has come to be known as the *impulse variability model* is that, independent of feedback processing, end-point variability in goal-directed aiming is related to the muscular forces required to accelerate, and presumably decelerate, the limb movement. Faster movements (i.e., movements with a shorter MT) and movements of greater amplitude require more muscular force. Variability in generating a specific target force increases proportionally with the absolute force required to move the limb. Of course, greater trial-to-trial variability in force production results in greater variability in end-point accuracy regardless of whether visual feedback is available. In many ways the impulse variability model of movement execution is similar to Weber's law for perception. Weber's law holds that a performer's ability to detect a difference between two sensory events is proportional to the absolute magnitude of the stimulation. Although the impulse variability model does a good job of predicting the relationship between MT and effective target width (i.e., variable error) for very rapid movements (Schmidt et al., 1979) and movements made without visual input (Wallace & Newell, 1983), the model begins to break down for visually directed movements of greater than 200 ms. Presumably for movements of this duration participants have an opportunity to correct errors associated with inaccuracies in force specification. While the impulse variability model turned out to be limited in its predictive scope, it did provide a platform for the optimized submovement model (Meyer, Abrams, Kornblum, Wright, & Smith, 1988), which also incorporates aspects of the two-component model and iterative correction model.

The Optimized Submovement Model

Woodworth (1899) and Keele and Posner (1968) used procedures in which they constrained the temporal characteristics of movement (i.e., MT) and measured end-point variability (Woodworth, 1899; see also Schmidt et al., 1979) or end-point accuracy (Keele & Posner, 1968).[2] Meyer and colleagues' optimized submovement model was developed to explain speed–accuracy relationships in spatially constrained goal-directed movements or the classic Fitts' aiming task (Fitts, 1954; Fitts & Peterson, 1964). In this type of task, performers must make movements of a specific amplitude toward targets of a specific size, and they must terminate their movements within the target boundary while minimizing MT. For spatially constrained actions, MT is the dependent variable of interest, and mean MT has been shown to increase linearly with the accuracy requirements of the movement as specified by Fitts' equation:

Mean MT = $a + b \log_2$(2movement amplitude / target width),

where a and b are empirically derived constants that depend on specific participant, task, and environmental variables.

The optimized submovement model incorporates components of both the impulse variability model and the dual-process models that recognize the importance of feedback-based corrective processes. The idea is that goal-directed aiming movements comprise submovements that maximize movement speed while taking into consideration a noisy neuromotor system. On a given aiming trial, an initial submovement is directed at the center of the target. The expected error associated with this submovement, and thus variability over a number of trials, increases proportionally with the speed or muscular force associated with accelerating and decelerating the limb. If MT remains similar across a series of aiming attempts, the result is a normal distribution of movement end points around the center of the target. The spread of this distribution is greater for faster, more forceful movements. When a given movement falls into one of the tails of the normal distribution (i.e., when the performer overshoots or undershoots the target boundaries), the movement needs to be corrected with a second submovement. Once again, there is variability associated with this second movement, so subsequent submovements may be required to eventually hit the target. The task of the performer is to strike a compromise between the movement speed and the need for time-consuming corrective submovements. That is, forceful movements get the limb to the target area more quickly but need to be corrected more often. Like the submovements of the iterative correction model, the corrective submovements of the optimized submovement model are organized according to visual and proprioceptive feedback acquired during the preceding submovement.

Unlike the impulse variability model, the optimized submovement model is able to explain the relationship between speed and accuracy in both short-duration and long-duration movements. This is because the optimized submovement model acknowledges the important role feedback plays in the corrective process. Mathematically, the optimized submovement model is more sophisticated than the earlier dual-process models of limb control, and it does a good job of predicting not only the performance outcome but also the temporal substructure of the kinematic events that compose the entire aiming movement. One weakness of the model is that it assumes a spatial symmetry in the movement error around the center of the target. This latter assumption is not consistent with the kinematics of most types of aiming movements.

Kinematic Evidence for Current Control

The specific characteristics of any goal-directed aiming movement depend, at least to a certain extent, on the physical constraints associated with the task. The Woodworth experiments, which provided the empirical evidence associated with the two-component model of limb control, involved sliding movements with a stylus on a moving surface. The classic Fitts experiments involved three-dimensional movements made with a handheld stylus aimed toward physical targets on a tabletop (Fitts, 1954; Fitts & Peterson, 1964). Since that time Fitts' paradigm has been adapted to include computerized aiming movements in which the displacement of a mouse or joystick propels a cursor toward a target displayed on a computer screen. Meyer and colleagues (1988), for example, had participants make wrist rotations to produce the one-dimensional movement of a cursor toward a target on an oscilloscope. In terms of the final portion of the trajectory, the kinematics can be quite different for this type of movement, which must be self-terminated. Like Woodworth's movements, computer-based movements of the limb that require self-termination are characterized by a slow, graded deceleration that occurs as the cursor or effector approaches the target (Chua & Elliott, 1993). Movements that are terminated by impact of a stylus on a tabletop sometimes involve an actual increase in velocity just before target acquisition (Carlton, 1979). As Elliott and coworkers (2001, p. 347) point out, "this strategy allows the performer to maximize movement speed during the final approach to the target while minimizing the energy requirements for braking the movement."

Contrary to the predictions of the optimized submovement model, an abundance of evidence indicates that the end point of the first submovement is centered short of the target center whether the aiming movement is computer based or made in real space. Specifically, the initial submovement hits the target or undershoots the target (Carlton, 1979; Elliott, Carson, Goodman, & Chua, 1991; Elliott, Binsted, & Heath, 1999; Elliott, Hansen, Mendoza, & Tremblay, 2004; Engelbrecht, Berthier, & O'Sullivan, 2003; Guiard, 1993). Very rarely do overshoots occur (Oliveira, Elliott, & Goodman, 2005). This makes sense in terms of the main tenet of Meyer and colleagues' model, which proposes that participants try to strike a compromise between the movement speed and the time necessary for a corrective submovement. Undershoots are favored because target misses do not all have the same cost; in terms of both time and energy, correcting target overshoots costs more than correcting target undershoots (Elliott et al., 2004). This is because in a target overshoot the limb must travel further and then overcome the inertia of a zero-velocity situation at the point of reversal. Moreover, limb reversals typically require a change in the roles played by the agonist and antagonist muscle groups, and this may require additional attentional resources during online control (Brebner, 1968; Elliott et al., 2004).

The relative cost of a second acceleration compared with a reversal depends on the physical constraints associated with the effector and the task environment. Fox example, Lyons, Hansen, Hurding, and Elliott (2006) had participants make three-dimensional aiming movements from a central home position to targets that were either farther away from or closer to the body and to targets that were either above or below the home position. Although the initial submovement undershot the target in all four conditions, the greatest degree of undershooting occurred with the targets located below the home position. According to Lyons and coworkers, this result is observed because the cost of a target overshoot is greatest in this condition, since a limb reversal in this situation occurs against gravity and therefore requires more time and energy. Presumably the relative cost of overshooting and undershooting also varies with the mass of the effector and the physical resistance associated with the movement environment (e.g., underwater or under reduced or increased gravitational pull). It would seem that in any given aiming situation, performers plan for the worst-case scenario. If a target overshoot is costly to correct, the performer is careful to avoid overshooting the target. This means that over a number of trials, a greater number will involve undershooting with the primary submovement. Planning for the worst-case scenario also applies to situations in which there is uncertainty about the afferent information that will be available during movement execution. Hansen, Glazebrook, Anson, Weeks, and Elliott (2006) have shown that when performers know that visual feedback will be available during movement execution for online regulation, they take less time to prepare the aiming movement. In addition, the velocity profiles are asymmetric, with a greater proportion of the total MT being spent after peak velocity rather than before peak velocity. In this situation participants adopt a strategy of getting to the target area quickly, so that more real time is available for current or feedback-based control. In contrast, when the performers know that visual feedback will be eliminated at movement initiation, they take more time to plan the movement, and they exhibit more symmetric velocity profiles. Peak velocity is also lower. The participants adopt a more feed-forward strategy of limb control because they know there will not be an opportunity for visual regulation late in the movement. Interestingly, when performers plan for the worst-case scenario under conditions of feedback uncertainty (i.e., randomly arranged trials of either vision or no vision), their RT and limb trajectories resemble the no-vision condition. This conservative approach to avoiding costly movement errors may be more pronounced in the elderly (Welsh, Higgins, & Elliott, 2007) and in special populations with particular perceptual and motor difficulties (Hodges, Cunningham, Lyons, Kerr, & Elliott, 1995).

It is clear that having advance knowledge about the availability of afferent information, the physical constraints associated with the aiming task, and the temporal and energy costs associated with a target miss affects how the current control phase of a movement is realized. However, Woodworth's ideas about feedback-based control late in the movement are correct in general. Moreover, it appears that Woodworth (1899) greatly overestimated the minimum time necessary for current control based on vision. Recent estimates of the minimum visual processing time associated with current control are closer to 100 ms than to 450 ms (Carlton, 1992; Elliott & Allard, 1985; Zelaznik, Hawkins, Kisselburgh, 1983; see also chapter 7).

How Ballistic Is the Initial Adjustment?

Although there is little argument that discrete feedback-based control contributes to limb regulation late in a movement, throughout the last 20 years it has become clear that a more continuous form of online control exists. This form of regulation begins to operate very early in most goal-directed aiming movements (Elliott et al., 1991; Elliott, Binsted, Heath, 1999; Hansen, Tremblay, & Elliott, 2005; Proteau & Masson, 1997) and probably depends more on feed-forward processes than on late regulation. As Helsen, Elliott, Starkes, and Ricker (2000) have demonstrated, this type of early control greatly reduces the spatial variability associated with the effector between the peak velocity and the end of the primary submovement (see figure 1.1). Thus Woodworth's (1899) initial adjustment does not appear to be as ballistic as previously thought.

One line of evidence for early feedback-based regulation comes from research using within-participant correlation procedures to study how well early kinematic events predict later events in the same movement. For example, Elliott and colleagues (1999; see also Heath, 2005) had participants

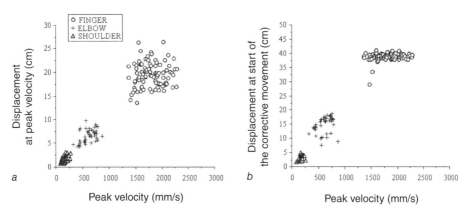

▶ **Figure 1.1**   Displacement at the shoulder, elbow, and finger (*a*) at peak velocity and (*b*) at the end of the primary submovement as a function of peak velocity.

Adapted, by permission, from W.F. Helsen et al., 2000, "Coupling of eye, finger, elbow and shoulder movements during manual aiming," *Journal of Motor Behavior* 32: 241-248.

make a series of discrete aiming movements both with and without vision and then examined how well the distance traveled between movement initiation and peak velocity predicted the distance traveled over the remainder of the movement. Under both the vision and the no-vision conditions, there was a negative correlation between these two amplitudes. However, the relationship was stronger when vision was available. Presumably, the performers truncated the latter portion of a movement to achieve something closer to the overall target amplitude if their limb had moved too far at peak velocity. The reverse was also true. This adjustment process was not evidenced by differences between the two vision conditions in the number of discontinuities near the termination of the aiming movements.

Trial-to-trial spatial variability and central tendency at specific kinematic markers under various feedback (Hansen, Elliott, & Tremblay, 2007; Khan, Chua, Elliott, Coull, & Lyons, 2002; Khan et al., 2006) and practice conditions (e.g., Hansen et al., 2005) also indicate that skilled performers can make very early modifications to their movement trajectories based on dynamic information about the limb's velocity and direction. For example, in a study in which participants were performing a computerized aiming task, Proteau and Masson (1997) introduced an unexpected moving background at movement initiation and found that the termination of the initial impulse (adjustment) was affected by the direction of the background movement. When the textured background moved in the same direction as the limb or cursor, participants terminated their movements later than usual. Presumably, they did so because the background movement caused the limb velocity to appear to be slower than it actually was and the participants made the appropriate adjustment to its speed and duration. Participants demonstrated the reverse misperception and subsequent adjustment when the background was moved in the direction opposite to the limb movement. In this situation, the limb appeared to be moving too fast and thus the participants terminated the movement early, causing an undershooting of the target position with the initial impulse.

In a series of experiments in which prismatic displacement was used to create a mismatch between the expected and the perceived direction of a planned movement, Hansen and colleagues (2007) found that the limb direction was modified early to match the perceived visual demands of the task. This early online control was evident particularly in female participants. This finding (see also Proteau & Masson, 1997) suggests that the ballistic phase of the movement is not as predetermined as originally thought (Beggs & Howarth, 1972; Woodworth, 1899). We have hypothesized that early, and perhaps more continuous (Elliott et al., 1991, 1999, 2001; Khan et al., 2006), limb control results from a comparison of early dynamic information from the limb with an internal model associated with either outflowing efferent information (von Holst, 1954) or expected sensory consequences associated with the movement planning process (Desmurget & Grafton, 2000; Wolpert & Ghahramani, 2000). This comparison process occurs very early and detects and corrects any discrepancies between the intended movement and the actual, unfolding movement. Because this type of control is not always accompanied by discontinuities in the movement trajectory (Elliott et al., 1999), it may be that early regulation is more continuous, comprising graded increases and decreases in muscle force driven by the dynamic properties of visual feedback and proprioceptive feedback from the limb. Alternatively, there may be "many overlapping discrete adjustments to the movement trajectory giving the movement the appearance of continuity" (Elliott et al., 1991, p. 415).

Two Types of Current Control

It is our contention that there are two types of visual regulation associated with goal-directed movement. Very early online control is associated with a comparison of dynamic information from the limb about velocity and direction with an internal representation of the expected sensory consequences of the movement. Ideally, this internal model guides the movement to a successful conclusion. However, when there is a mismatch between what is expected and what actually occurs, the discrepancy (error) drives corrective processes designed to reduce the difference to none. Because under normal circumstances the eyes fixate on the target before movement initiation (Binsted & Elliott, 1999), early control probably depends primarily on visual information from the periphery of the retina, which is designed for this type of dynamic information pickup (Paillard, 1982).

The second type of visual regulation occurs near movement termination and involves the use of foveal vision to compare the limb position with the target position. This is the type of regulation associated with Woodworth's original two-component model as well as its more recent variants (e.g., Elliott et al., 2004; Meyer et al., 1988). By its nature, this type of error-reducing regulation, which involves two afferent sources (visual and proprioceptive information from the limb and visual information from the target), is discrete and thus more likely to manifest as identifiable discontinuities in the trajectory.

In a series of recent experiments, we directly tested our ideas about early and late visual regulation by perturbing the movement environment in order to affect either one or both types of visual regulation. Our work was designed to discover the extent to which the two modes of online control operate independently or covary to determine not only the movement speed and accuracy but also the characteristics of the reaching or aiming trajectories (Grierson & Elliott, 2009). This was accomplished by introducing perturbations influencing the perceived position of the target and the perceived velocity of the limb. The idea was that the former manipulation affects late control while the latter influences early control.

Participants made rapid aiming movements away from the body and toward a small target that was defined by the intersection of three black lines. Depending on the experimental condition, perturbations were made (1) to the target, (2) to the visual background against which the aiming movement was performed, or (3) to both upon movement initiation. Following Mendoza, Hansen, Glazebrook, Keetch, and Elliott (2005) and Mendoza, Elliott, Meegan, Lyons, and Welsh (2006), we used the arrows associated with the Müller-Lyer illusion to affect perceived target position. Compared with the control condition, an arrows-in configuration introduced at movement initiation typically resulted in target undershooting, while a shift to an arrows-out configuration had the opposite effect (Mendoza et al., 2006). We also looked to see whether this Müller-Lyer type of perturbation resulted in a discrete adjustment to the limb movement late in the trajectory, which is the result consistent with the notion of late regulation based on limb and target information (e.g., Elliott et al., 2001; Woodworth, 1899); the results are discussed shortly.

Our second type of perturbation was adapted from the work by Proteau and Masson (1997) and involved introducing a moving background. Texture elements over which the limb traveled on its way to the target moved in either the same or the opposite direction of the moving limb. This manipulation made the limb appear to move more slowly or faster than intended and thus created a mismatch between the perceived velocity and the expected velocity (i.e., internal model) of the limb. These perturbations typically resulted in velocity adjustments that either extended or truncated the movement (Proteau & Masson, 1997). Of interest was whether these velocity adjustments, which are based on a comparison between current movement and feed-forward information about movement expectations, interact with adjustments based on late information about the relative positions of the limb and target.

The two types of perturbations had the expected effects when introduced alone. The Müller-Lyer type of perturbation influenced end-point error (resulted in relative undershooting for the arrows-in condition and overshooting for the arrows-out condition), and this bias was apparent only after peak deceleration, a finding indicating that late adjustments were made to the movement trajectory due to a misperception of target position. As noted in the work of Proteau and Masson (1997), the background manipulation was more robust when the background was moving in the opposite direction of the limb; participants terminated the movements early and demonstrated negative constant error relative to their performance during the other two background conditions. More importantly for our hypothesis about early regulation, this bias was already evident at peak deceleration.

These findings were also observed when the two types of perturbations were introduced together. Moreover, the condition for which the background moved in the same direction as the limb also elicited an effect. The kinematic analysis again indicated that the perturbation involving the moving background influenced early limb regulation more than it influenced late regulation, while the opposite was true for the conditions involving the Müller-Lyer illusion. Once again our findings supported the idea that there are two types of online limb control: (1) early continuous or pseudocontinuous regulation associated with dynamic information from the limb and (2) late discrete regulation tied to the perceived relative positions of the limb and target. Interesting for both performance and kinematic measures is the observation that the effects of our two manipulations were always additive and never interactive. This suggests at least some independence between these two modes of control (Sternberg, 1969).

The Two-Component Model Revisited

It appears that Woodworth's model has stood the test of time. It is certainly clear that goal-directed limb movement consists of two different phases— an initial movement phase that is more dependent on planning processes completed before the movement and a late phase that involves discrete feedback-based regulation. In contrast to Woodworth's original ideas and the more recent versions of the two-component model (e.g., Beggs & Howarth, 1970; Carlton, 1981; Elliott et al., 2004; Meyer et al., 1988), the initial movement phase appears to be susceptible to online regulation. That is, the initial impulse is not completely ballistic. Rather, the online regulation involves feed-forward processes, which are associated with the expected sensory consequence of the movement, as well as early dynamic information for the limb. When these two sources of information match, the movement unfolds as planned and can be viewed as ballistic. However, if there is a mismatch between what was planned and what was expected, graded adjustments can be made to the muscular forces used to propel and arrest the limb. These adjustments bring the central (i.e., feed-forward) and peripheral (i.e., feedback) sources of information into harmony.

Because this type of early control is driven by a movement representation that is formed well before movement initiation, there is very little time lag between the movement onset and the comparison processes that provide the basis for regulation. Thus this early control may explain the very short estimates of visual processing time required for the regulation of goal-directed aiming (e.g., Carlton, 1992; Elliott & Allard, 1985; Zelaznik et al., 1983; c.f., Woodworth, 1899; Keele & Posner, 1968). It may also explain why practice results in rather robust reductions in the end-point variability associated with the initial impulse (Elliott et al., 2004). As well, practice leads to early corrective processes that begin earlier (Hansen et al., 2005) and are more error reducing (Khan, Franks, & Goodman, 1998). At least some of the changes associated with practice could be due to the development of a more stable and precise representation of the movement being performed (Proteau, 1992). Alternatively, the comparison process could become more streamlined (Elliott, Chua, Pollock, & Lyons, 1995; Elliott et al., 2001). Issues associated with practice and online control are dealt with in more detail in chapters 2 and 15.

Future Directions

In our current work, we are exploring online control by introducing perturbations that create behavioral dissociations between early and late regulatory processes. As well as using visual illusions to affect the perceived velocity of the limb and the position of the target, we are physically perturbing the velocity of the limb, the movement of the target, or both (Grierson & Elliott, 2008). Once again, movement kinematics provides us with information about where in the unfolding movement these hypothesized control processes operate.

In addition to perturbing the movement environment, it is possible to disrupt the neural systems responsible for online control by using techniques such as transcranial magnetic stimulation (TMS). Following Desmurget and colleagues (1999), we expect the late (target-associated) correction to be sensitive to superior parietal stimulation, while we expect the internal model of anticipated feedback (against which actual feedback is compared) to be susceptible to premotor simulation of the left hemisphere at, or even before, movement initiation. Certainly some careful pilot work is needed to isolate the specific cortical areas and time course for magnetic stimulation.

Another way to study limb regulation processes is to examine groups of people who have difficultly with some aspect of limb control. Our research group has a long history of examining atypical goal-directed behavior in children and adults with Down syndrome (Elliott, Welsh, Lyons, Hansen, & Wu, 2006; Hodges et al., 1995). Following our recent work on anticipatory awareness of goal-directed action in adults with Down syndrome (Obhi et al., 2007), we have suggested that some of the clumsiness associated with perceptual–motor performance in this group may be the result of an inability to form or maintain an internal representation of goal-directed behavior against which to compare feedback. This makes persons with Down syndrome overly dependent on late afferent sources of information for limb control. If this is the case, the aiming behavior of persons with Down syndrome should be affected by perturbations that affect late but not early visual regulation. The challenge in this work is identifying methods of motor skill instruction and practice that minimize the effect of these deficiencies in information processing.

ENDNOTES

1. As Carlton (1992, p. 7) points out, Woodworth (1899) measured movement accuracy at only one end of the reciprocal aiming cycle. "If subjects only used visual feedback from the forward stroke, and if movements back and forth were made at equal rates, Woodworth's visual processing estimate of 450 ms could be halved to around 225 ms!"

2. For time-constrained movements such as those examined by Woodworth (1899; see also Meyer, Smith, & Wright, 1982), the relationship between MT and variable error (i.e., spatial variability at the end of the movement) is reasonably linear. For accuracy-constrained movements such as those associated with the Fitts' procedure (e.g., Fitts & Peterson, 1964), a logarithmic relationship between index of difficulty and MT is extremely robust and has in fact come to be known as *Fitts' law.* Carlton (1994) has suggested that the difference between the time-constrained and the accuracy-constrained relationships may be due to the former condition's added cognitive demand of producing a movement of a fixed time.

CHAPTER 2

The Optimization of Speed, Accuracy, and Energy in Goal-Directed Aiming

DIGBY ELLIOTT, STEVE HANSEN, AND MICHAEL A. KHAN

Many of the traditional models of speed–accuracy relationships and limb control are steady-state models (see chapter 1). They explain the relationship between speed and accuracy and sometimes energy expenditure by detailing sets of perceptual–motor processes that lead to particular movement outcomes. Most models fail to consider the learning history and strategic approach a performer brings to the task environment.

When people face a particular set of task demands for the first time, they experience at least some uncertainty associated with how to approach the task to best achieve the movement goal. For example, if a performer is told to move as fast as he can while still hitting the target, he must figure out just how quickly he can move while still achieving the accuracy required by the task instructions. Optimal performance is not achieved on the first trial and perhaps even after hundreds of trials. In this chapter we review the most recent research on how performers adjust their behavior to optimize the speed and accuracy of performance while simultaneously minimizing energy expenditure. We also examine how the costs and benefits of different movement outcomes as well as the expectancy and sensory conditions affect the strategic behavior of the performer. Of special interest is how differences in strategy affect the kinematics of goal-directed reaching or aiming trajectories. This chapter also examines how various methodological approaches contribute to our understanding of the strategic behavior and the resulting perceptual–motor processes associated with the optimization of speed, accuracy, and energy expenditure.

Practice and Goal-Directed Aiming

Even for very simple goal-directed aiming movements, practice allows people to get faster at aiming while still maintaining the accuracy requirements imposed by the experimenter (Elliott, Hansen, Mendoza, & Tremblay, 2004; Khan, Franks, & Goodman, 1998; Proteau, Marteniuk, Girouard, & Dugas, 1987). For many years, it was assumed that performance improved because of a shift from closed-loop to open-loop control following practice of a closed skill such as aiming (Pew, 1966; Schmidt & McCabe, 1976). The idea was that after multiple repetitions, the performer developed a central representation for the action (Keele, 1968). This representation was able to drive the movement with less dependence on response-produced feedback. Consistent with many of the models of speed–accuracy relationships reviewed in chapter 1, the notion was that feedback processing is time consuming. Thus, central control is more efficient after practice because it does not depend on feedback. Although it is beyond the scope of this chapter to delve deeply into specific models of motor learning (but see chapter 15), it is fair to say that the optimization of movement speed and accuracy depends on improvement in both efferent and afferent processes (Khan et al., 1998). That is, with practice the performer not only develops a more robust central representation for the goal behavior but also learns to process the movement-associated sensory feedback more rapidly and efficiently. Researchers have sought to describe and quantify these practice-based improvements by examining the spatial and temporal characteristics of individual movements and how those trajectories change with practice. Researchers have also studied how spatial variability unfolds over a movement trajectory during multiple attempts to achieve the same movement outcome. Of interest is how this variability fluctuates with expectancy, sensory condition, and experience (see Khan et al., 2006 for a review). As well, researchers have examined the sensory and practice conditions under which the characteristics of the early limb trajectory predict or do not predict movement outcome. In the next several sections of this chapter, we examine how these different approaches to movement analysis shed light on the cognitive and neural processes associated with the optimization of goal-directed reaching or aiming.

Individual Aiming Trajectories

More than 100 years ago Woodworth (1899) used a rotating drum to obtain time–displacement profiles of individual aiming movements. However, it was not until the advent of high-speed film (Langolf, Chaffin, & Foulke, 1976) and high-frequency graphics tablets (Chua & Elliott, 1993) and optoelectric systems (Elliott, Carson, Goodman, & Chua, 1991) that researchers began to take a detailed look at the spatial and temporal characteristics of individual movement trajectories. Typically this is done by differentiating profiles of displacement versus time in individual movement axes or resultant displacement to obtain instantaneous velocity. Velocity profiles are subjected to a second differentiation to obtain acceleration. In some cases a third differentiation is performed to obtain jerk. Symmetry of the velocity and acceleration profile, as well as discontinuities in the profile, provides important information about how a movement is planned and controlled. Movement initiation time and the characteristics of the early trajectory are taken to reflect the movement planning process. Later portions of the movement trajectory and discontinuities in the trajectory are more often associated with online control processes.

Figure 2.1 depicts displacement, velocity, and acceleration profiles for four different, but still typical, goal-directed trajectories in the primary axis of the movement. Figure 2.1*a* depicts a trajectory in which the primary acceleration and deceleration achieve the movement goal. Following Meyer, Abrams, Kornblum, Wright, and Smith's (1988) optimized submovement model (see chapter 1), this type of trajectory reflects a movement with only a primary submovement and no corrective submovements. In the trajectory in figure 2.1*b*, the initial acceleration and deceleration phase of the movement, or the primary submovement (see Meyer et al., 1988), overshoots the target goal. The negative velocity observed at the end of the movement reflects a reversal in direction that brings the limb back to the target position. Figure 2.1*c* is a more frequently observed trajectory (see chapter 1 and Elliott et al., 2004). Here the primary movement undershoots the target and a second acceleration in the direction of the movement is required to achieve the target position. Figure 2.1*d* is similar to figure 2.1*c* except that the correction to the initial trajectory occurs earlier, before primary deceleration is complete. In figures 2.1, *b* through *d*, we have indicated where the primary submovement ends and the corrective process begins according to most movement phasing protocols (e.g., Walker, Philbin, Worden, & Smelcer, 1997).

Discontinuities in the movement trajectory can be useful in identifying the onset of feedback-based regulation during movement execution. However, the absence of discontinuities does not mean that the movement was controlled completely off-line in an open-loop fashion. From a technical point of view, a discontinuity in velocity or acceleration must meet specific criteria in order for an investigator to label it as a correction or use it to identify the end of the primary submovement (see Chua & Elliott, 1993; van Donkelaar & Franks, 1991). This is necessary to separate true corrections from noise in the data acquisition system that is magnified by the differentiation process (Hansen, Elliott, & Khan, 2007; Franks, Sanderson, & van Donkelaar, 1990). Usually a discontinuity must meet both a temporal criterion and an amplitude criterion. For example, the change in acceleration or deceleration must be a minimum percentage of the peak values (e.g.,

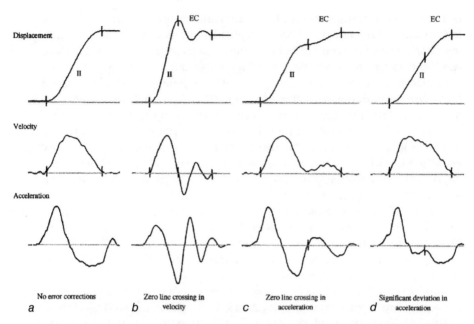

▶ **Figure 2.1** Sample position, velocity, and acceleration profiles showing the initial impulse (IT) and error correction (EC) phases of goal-directed movements. *(a)* The primary movement achieves the target goal. *(b)* The primary movement overshoots the target goal. *(c)* The primary movement undershoots the target goal. *(d)* The primary movement undershoots the target goal, and correction begins before primary deceleration ends.

Adapted, by permission, from M.A. Khan, I.M. Franks, and D. Goodman, 1998, "The effect of practice on the control of rapid aiming movements: Evidence for an interdependence between programming and feedback processing," *Quarterly Journal of Experimental Psychology* 51(a): 425-444. www.informaworld.com

10%) and last a minimum length of time (e.g., more than 70 ms; see Chua & Elliott, 1993). Because researchers generally are conservative when trying to separate corrective behaviors from noise in the data acquisition and reduction system, some discrete adjustments to the movement trajectory undoubtedly are missed. As well, given the research reviewed in chapter 1, it is now clear that the portion of the trajectory termed the *initial adjustment* (Woodworth, 1899) or *primary submovement* (Meyer et al., 1988) is not as ballistic as previously thought. Thus some researchers prefer to use the symmetry of the velocity and acceleration profile to make inferences about the relative importance of advance planning and online control. Specifically, trajectories with symmetric acceleration and deceleration are often associated with open-loop control. As the time of movement deceleration compared with movement acceleration becomes longer and longer, the performer is assumed to be engaging in greater closed-loop control.

Although certainly there are limitations associated with making inferences based on the characteristics of individual movement trajectories, these types of data have provided many insights into how the aiming behavior of a performer changes with practice, expectancy, and task demands. For example, the characteristics of aiming movements performed with and without visual feedback during movement execution clearly differ, particularly when the accuracy requirements of the movement are high. When vision is available for online control, the performer spends a greater proportion of the MT decelerating rather than accelerating (Carson, Goodman, Chua, & Elliott, 1993; Chua & Elliott, 1993; Elliott, Chua, Pollock, & Lyons, 1995). Given that error is greater under conditions of no vision, it is assumed that this extra time is spent processing and effectively using response-produced visual feedback in the vicinity of the target. Interestingly, the performer must know that visual feedback will be available for online control in advance of movement onset. When the availability of vision for online control is uncertain, the performer appears to prepare for the worst-case scenario. That is, the performer spends more time preparing the movement (i.e., longer RT) and exhibits a more symmetric velocity and acceleration profile (Hansen, Glazebrook, Anson, Weeks, & Elliott, 2006). Thus even when vision is available for online control, under conditions of uncertainty, the characteristics of the trajectory resemble those of a no-vision situation rather than those for conditions in which the performer is 100% confident that vision will be available for online control.

Differences in trajectory symmetry between vision and no-vision conditions are quite robust. However, studies comparing the number of trajectory discontinuities under vision and no-vision conditions have yielded conflicting results. Although discontinuities in the trajectory certainly become more prevalent as the precision requirements of the movement increase (Jagacinski, Repperger, Moran, Ward, & Glass, 1980), some investigators have reported that there are more discontinuities when vision is available (Chua & Elliott, 1993; Khan & Franks, 2000), while others have not (Elliott, Binsted & Heath, 1999; Meyer et al., 1988). Some of these discrepancies could be due to the rules used to identify discontinuities in the profile and the associated filtering procedures. Just as likely, however, are between-task differences in the salience and use of proprioceptive feedback for online limb control.

For the purposes of this chapter, perhaps more interesting than the kinematic differences in performance between various sensory and expectancy conditions is the manner in which, as practice progresses, participants change their aiming strategy to optimize performance. One consistent finding is that when vision is available, performers adopt a strategy in which the limb achieves a higher peak velocity earlier in the movement (Elliott et al., 1995; Elliott, Lyons, & Dyson, 1997; Khan & Franks, 2000; Khan et al., 1998). In spite of the fact that higher peak velocities are associated with greater spatial variability (e.g., Schmidt, Zelaznik, Hawkins, Frank, & Quinn, 1979), this strategy allows performers to achieve shorter and shorter MTs while still maintaining their aiming accuracy. The strategy works because it moves the limb into the target area quickly, providing greater real time for visual guidance when it will be most effective, which is when the limb is near the target (see chapter 10).

Several other findings may be related to the strategy of getting to the target area quickly. For example, while the primary submovement often undershoots the target even after extended practice (Khan et al., 1998), the distance traveled increases with practice (Pratt & Abrams, 1996). This allows corrections to be less time consuming (Abrams & Pratt, 1993) and more error reducing (Khan et al., 1998). The strategies that participants adopt depend on what sensory information is available during practice. While participants increase the velocity of the primary impulse to get to the target area more quickly when vision is available, the velocity of the initial impulse is lower when vision is not available (Khan & Franks, 2000). It seems that when vision is not available, participants rely more on movement planning to achieve optimal accuracy. Khan and colleagues (1998) have shown that participants undershoot the target in the initial impulse phase when visual feedback is available but that initial impulse end points are not biased when participants practice without vision. On this basis, these researchers proposed an interdependency between movement planning and sensory information processing. On one side, improved movement programming reduces the extent to which discrete error corrections are needed. On the other side, the ability to utilize sensory information to perform effective error corrections influences how movements are planned. When vision is available, participants plan movements to optimize its use and hence remain reliant on visual information after extensive practice. When vision is not available, participants rely more heavily on movement planning in an attempt to minimize the need for discrete error corrections.

Elliott and coworkers (2004) also demonstrated that with practice the primary submovement travels a greater distance toward the target, both reducing the need for corrective submovements and making the submovements that do occur more efficient (because they are closer to the target). These researchers have proposed that the degree of primary movement undershooting early and late in practice is tied strategically to the variability associated with the primary submovement end points (see also Khan et al., 1998; Worringham, 1991). The idea is that target overshoots are more costly than target undershoots in terms of both time and energy (see also Engelbrecht, Berthier, & O'Sullivan, 2003). Through trial and error, performers discover the degree of spatial variability associated with a series of aiming trials and then strategically center the distribution short of the target so that only a small percentage of movements will overshoot the target and need to be corrected with a reversal. With continued practice, however, performers are able to reduce the variability associated with the distribution, and thus they begin to center their distribution of primary submovement end points closer and closer to the target. This strategy is captured in figure 2.2, which illustrates that early in practice, the number

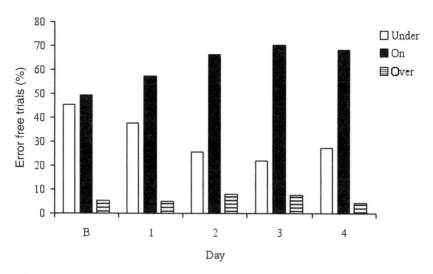

▶ **Figure 2.2** Percentage of trials for which the initial submovement undershoots, hits, and overshoots the target area as a function of day (B = baseline for which no MT feedback was provided).

Adapted, by permission, from D. Elliott et al., 2004, "Learning to optimize speed, accuracy, and energy expenditure: A framework for understanding speed-accuracy relations in goal-directed aiming," *Journal of Motor Behavior* 36: 339-351.

of undershoots and target hits are close to equal, while the percentage of overshoots is small. Then, throughout 4 days of practice, the number of undershoots decreases and the number of hits increases, while the number of overshoots stays approximately the same. Thus, as participants reduce the variability of the primary movement end points, they learn to sneak up on the target with their primary submovements.[1] In the study by Elliott and coworkers (2004), this strategy allowed participants to reduce their average MT from 380 ms to 310 ms during the 4 days of practice.[2] The reduction in primary submovement variability can be associated with more precise movement planning (Khan et al., 1998), with early continuous online regulation during the primary submovement (Elliott et al., 1991), or with both. The latter proposal is consistent with some of the ideas regarding internal models for feed-forward control and early online regulation discussed in chapter 1 (see also Desmurget & Grafton, 2000).

Within-Performer Spatial Variability

In the previous section, we reviewed evidence suggesting that the spatial variability associated with the primary submovement end point dictates the strategic behavior an individual adopts for optimizing limb control and ultimately performance. If spatial variability at one point in the trajectory can provide information about speed, accuracy, and energy expenditure in goal-directed aiming, then spatial variability throughout the trajectory should give us even broader insights into the planning and online regulation of goal-directed aiming. In this regard, Khan and colleagues proposed that the contribution of visual feedback to movement planning and to error correction during movement execution can be inferred by comparing variability in the limb trajectory between vision and no-vision conditions (see Khan et al., 2006). The reasoning is that an error occurring in the initial movement command sent to the limb, whether due to noise in the neuromotor system or inappropriate specification of movement parameters, results in a spatial error early in the limb trajectory. The resulting spatial error is magnified as the limb progresses unless a correction is implemented. If we assume a random variation in error throughout a series of trials, the spatial variability of the trajectory of the limb (i.e., within-subject standard deviation of spatial position) should increase, according to a lawful function, as the movement progresses. If the limb trajectory is corrected during movement execution, then the resulting variability profile should deviate from that representing movement that is programmed in advance and not modified online.

The benefit of analyzing spatial variability to elucidate the contributions of visual feedback in movement planning and online control was demonstrated by Khan, Lawrence, Fourkas, Franks, Elliott, and Pembroke (2003). These researchers required participants to perform a video aiming task in which movement of a pen on a digitizing tablet was translated to movement of a cursor on a monitor. Movement of the pen was constrained along a single dimension in the right to left direction. The aiming task was performed over a range of MTs (225 to 450 ms), and the cursor was visible either throughout the movement (so that participants had full vision) or at the starting position (so that participants had no vision during movement execution). The within-participant standard deviation in the position of the pen was calculated at peak acceleration, peak velocity, and peak deceleration and at the end of the movement. Analysis of the variability profiles revealed that when MT was relatively short, the magnitude of the variability profile was greater in the no-vision compared with the full-vision condition (see figure 2.3). However, the ratio in variability between visual conditions at each kinematic marker did not change as the movement progressed. Hence, though the variability profiles differed in magnitude, they were similar in form between the vision and no-vision conditions. Thus the benefit of having visual feedback was due to off-line processing and not corrections made during movement execution. That is, participants used visual feedback from a completed trial as a form of knowledge of results to improve the programming on subsequent trials. In contrast, when MT was longer, the ratio in variability between vision and no-vision conditions decreased as the movement progressed. More

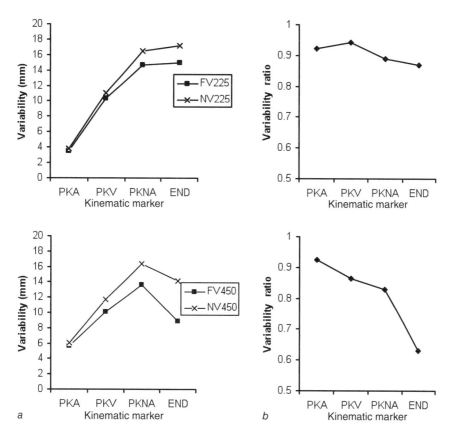

▶ **Figure 2.3** *(a)* Variability in distance traveled and *(b)* ratios in variability between full-vision (FV) and no-vision (NV) conditions at peak acceleration (PKA), peak velocity (PKV), peak negative acceleration (PKNA), and movement end (END) in the 225 and 450 ms MT conditions.

Adapted, by permission, from M.A. Khan et al., 2003a, "Online versus offline processing of visual feedback in the production of movement distance," *Acta Psychologica* 113: 83-97.

specifically, there was a relatively larger reduction in variability from peak deceleration to the end of the movement in the vision compared with the no-vision condition. This implies that during the later stages of the movement, visually based modifications occurred and subsequently altered the shape of the variability profile.

Analysis of spatial variability can be adapted to investigate visual control processes used in the control of movement direction. In tasks with a direction requirement but no amplitude constraint, participants are required to move through the target in a manner similar to that of striking a ball (Abahnini, Proteau, & Temprado, 1997; Bard, Hay, & Fleury, 1985; Bard, Paillard, Fleury, Hay, & Larue, 1990). Since these movements do not have a well-defined acceleration and deceleration phase, Khan, Lawrence, Franks, and Elliott

(2003) adapted the variability analysis by calculating the deviation from the longitudinal axis at 25%, 50%, 75%, and 100% of the distance between the home position and the target. Spatial variability was then defined as the within-participant standard deviation of these directional errors.

By analyzing variability in movement direction, Khan and colleagues (2003b) demonstrated that variability increases linearly in both vision and no-vision conditions when MT is short (150 ms; see figure 2.4). However, when MT is long (450 ms), the form of the variability profiles for the vision condition deviates from that of the no-vision condition. While the variability for the no-vision condition increases linearly, the variability for the vision condition levels off at about 75% of the movement, revealing a significant quadratic component. Hence, the form of the variability profile is modi-

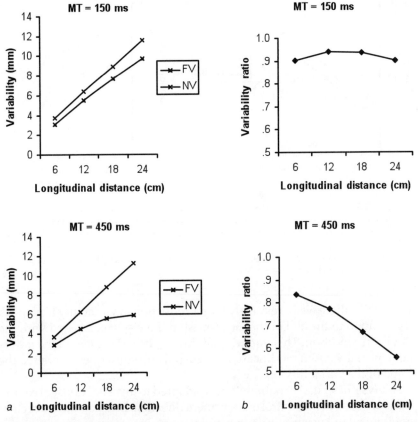

▶ **Figure 2.4** *(a)* Variability in direction and *(b)* ratios in variability between full-vision (FV) and no-vision (NV) conditions at longitudinal distances of 6, 12, 18, and 24 cm in the 150 and 450 ms MT conditions.

Adapted from M.A. Khan et al., 2003b, "The utilization of visual feedback in the control of movement direction. Evidence from a video aiming task," *Motor Control* 7: 290-303.

fied by adjustments that are based on visual feedback and made during movement execution.

One important difference between the two studies just discussed is that the work concerned with amplitude variability (Khan, Lawrence, Fourkas, et al., 2003) examined spatial variability at specific kinematic markers (peak acceleration, peak velocity, peak deceleration, and the end of the movement), while the work concerned with direction (Khan, Lawrence, Franks, et al., 2003) examined variability at percentages of the movement trajectory (25%, 50%, 75%, and 100%).[3] Although the former approach is appropriate for one-dimensional aiming movements in which the limb and the task environment are unperturbed, the latter approach has distinct advantages for three-dimensional movements and movements in which the performer must adjust the trajectory to a perturbation. This is because it cannot be assumed that adjustments to the limb trajectory and therefore variability are constrained to the primary direction of the movement. Moreover, even if resultant kinematic markers are identified, an adjustment to the trajectory can elicit peaks with a greater amplitude than the peaks associated with primary submovement. This artificially increases the spatial variability associated with that kinematic event. In this context, Hansen, Elliott and Khan (2008) introduced a three-dimensional approach to the study of spatial variability as a series of movements unfold.

Hansen and coworkers (2008) quantified the three-dimensional variability of rapid aiming movements by using the standard deviations of spatial position in the x, y, and z dimensions to create ellipsoids. They then used these ellipsoids to examine how limb control processes change with practice and visual conditions. More specifically, they calculated the average position of the finger in each of the three dimensions every 4% of the movement trajectory following data filtering and the determination of the movement duration. The percentage of the trajectory used to create the ellipsoids was arbitrary. A within-condition standard deviation of the average position was calculated for each of the three dimensions. The standard deviations were then employed as the radii of an ellipsoid in order to calculate the volume of spatial variability. This method provides the volume of the ellipsoids as a dependent variable to employ during initial analyses, the standard deviations in each dimension to employ during subsequent multiple analyses of variance, and the data to graphically display the within-condition variability trajectories (with the aid of computer software such as Matlab).

Three-dimensional variability differences were evident during the execution of movements under conditions of full vision compared with conditions of no vision (Hansen et al., 2008). Variability in the secondary and tertiary axes of movement, as well as overall variability, was reduced with practice (Hansen et al., 2008). The analysis demonstrated increased consistency in the secondary and tertiary axes of movement and more accurate indications of temporal changes in the variability profile when compared with methods in which the variability was measured in the primary axis of movement. The ellipsoid methodology has also been used to identify individual differences in movement execution (Hansen & Elliott, 2009). Quantitative differences in movement planning and execution can be investigated by employing the ellipsoid methodology and target perturbation paradigms. For example, movement execution can be observed as the position of the target is changed from a left location to a right location upon movement initiation. Comparisons can then be made between the condition in which the target remains unperturbed and the condition in which the target moves from the right to the left location (see figure 2.5). Again,

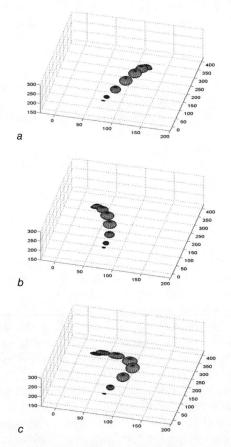

▶ **Figure 2.5**   Three-dimensional variability ellipsoids for experimental conditions in which the target *(a)* remained at the location on the right, *(b)* moved to the location on the left upon movement initiation, or *(c)* remained at the location on the left. Each ellipsoid represents the spatial variability every 12% of the movement within a condition and across the performance of 20 participants. Movements began proximally and moved distally.

reduced variability within a condition indicates more efficient sensorimotor processes that can be associated with concurrent visual–motor processing, or feed-forward control.

Do Early Events Predict Late Events?

Another way to examine the relative contributions of advance planning and online processes to goal-directed performance is to determine how well the early characteristics of the movement trajectory predict the later events, including end-point accuracy. In this context, Elliott and colleagues (1999) examined the relationship between the movement amplitude achieved at peak velocity and the distance traveled between the peak velocity and the end of the movement. They based their analysis on the assumption that the first part of the movement (i.e., the part up to peak velocity) is dependent on the movement planning process and the latter portion of the movement is regulated via response-produced feedback. Their notion was that under conditions permitting online regulation, early planning errors are corrected during the deceleration phase of the movement. This results in a negative relationship between the distance traveled before and the distance traveled after peak velocity. For example, if on a given trial the limb travels less than the optimal distance before peak velocity, then it must travel a greater distance after peak velocity and vice versa. Within-participant correlation coefficients computed across trials supported this line of reasoning. Moreover, Elliott and colleagues (1999) found a strong negative relationship between the amplitudes associated with these two portions of the movement in both a full-vision condition and a condition in which vision was eliminated upon movement initiation. However, the relationship was significantly more robust when vision was available.

Heath and colleagues (Heath, 2005; Heath, Neely, & Binsted, 2007) have adapted this general procedure and examined the relationship among the cumulative amplitudes achieved at progressive kinematic markers (e.g., peak acceleration, peak velocity, peak deceleration, and the end of the movement). They reasoned that amplitudes achieved early can positively predict amplitudes achieved late only when there is no online regulation to correct amplitude error. As is the case with variability (e.g., Khan et al., 1998), any early bias (e.g., moving too far at peak acceleration) should become more and more exaggerated as the movement unfolds (e.g., overshooting the target at the end of the movement). For this correlational protocol, a reduction in the Pearson r or r^2 values toward 0 between early and late cumulative amplitudes indicates online regulation between the two kinematic events at which the amplitudes are measured. Thus by conducting these within-participant correlational analyses at different points in the trajectory, Heath (2005) has not only identified the sensory and memory conditions (see chapter 5) under which online regulation is important but also gained an understanding of where in the trajectory amplitude errors are most often amended. Like Elliott and coworkers (1999), Heath and colleagues (Heath, 2005; Heath et al., 2007) found that vision of both the limb and the target is important for online limb regulation. In the context of this chapter, however, it would be interesting to see how variables such as expectancy (Hansen et al., 2006) and practice (Elliott et al., 2004; Khan et al., 1998) affect the relationships between early and late kinematic events.

Lessons From the Serial Reaction Time Literature

Although mean performance and within-performer variability provide us with a number of insights into the information processing strategies and constraints associated with rapid goal-directed movement, dependent variables that are based on a number of trials, even trials performed by the same person, do not provide a window into the trial-to-trial strategic behavior of individual performers. More than 25 years ago, Patrick Rabbitt (1981) tried to identify the cause of perceptual–motor slowing associated with aging by using a serial RT paradigm. In this type of protocol, participants are asked to respond with the right index finger to a signal in right space and with the left index finger to a signal in left space. They are told to respond as quickly as possible but not to make a mistake (i.e., lift the right index finger when the left index finger should be used to respond). Each participant completes hundreds of consecutive trials with an equal probability of making a left or right response. Rabbitt (1981) suggested that rather than thinking about the specific information processing events that must occur to complete this task (e.g., stimulus identification, response selection, response execution), it is more appropriate to consider the strategic behavior the participants engage in to meet the experimenter-imposed task demands. Since his participants had never been in a lab situation, Rabbitt reasoned that they must first explore the task boundaries to determine how fast they are able to react to the experimental stimuli without making an error. Most participants start out with long RTs and then, as trials progress, gradually respond faster and faster until they make an error. The trial after an error generally is correct but quite long. Then the performer begins to speed up again, trying to discover what Rabbitt called the *safe fast zone*. Once performers discover this zone, they attempt to track it (i.e., stay within it), because responding below this zone is associated with a higher probability of error and responding above this zone results in a long RT. Although a goal-directed reaching or aiming task is more complex than performing simple finger lifts in a two-choice RT task, both involve some of the same types of strategic behavior. For both tasks, a performer must discover how fast to go without missing the target. Given that online corrections are possible but time consuming, performers must discover what types of errors are more or less costly and then plan their movements accordingly.

In an attempt to apply Rabbitt's (1981) ideas to goal-directed movement, Elliott and colleagues (2004) identified trials in their aiming experiment in which a participant missed the target and then examined the characteristics of the trials that preceded and followed the error. Errors were classified as aiming attempts undershooting or overshooting the target. Interestingly, while undershooting errors involved reasonably fast movements, overshooting errors were characterized by an MT that was longer than the average. Perhaps this should not be surprising because aiming attempts that overshoot a target must cover a greater distance. Contrary to their expectations, Elliott and coworkers (2004) found that trials after an error were not longer than other trials (c.f., Rabbitt, 1981). What was revealing was that the trials just before an overshoot were quite fast. It may be that a fast but successful movement results in a more forceful movement on the next trial—a movement that, at least in some cases, overshoots the target. Elliott and coworkers also examined the rare cases in which two errors occurred in a row. While in some cases both these errors were undershoots, more often the error on trial $n + 1$ was the reverse of trial n (an overshoot was followed by an undershoot or vice versa). However, consistent with the idea that participants plan for the worst-case scenario, in several thousand trials there was not one case in which a participant committed two overshoots in a row.

Like Rabbitt (1981), Elliott and colleagues (2004) focused on trials that followed an explicit error. However, when compared with simple finger lifts associated with a serial RT task, outcomes from a manual aiming attempt can be classified with greater precision. Rather than examining trial-to-trial differences around an aiming attempt that completely misses the target, it might be more revealing to examine the probability of primary submovement hits, undershoots, and overshoots following like or different trials. It would be expected, for example, that following a primary submovement hit, the performer would attempt to repeat the same type of movement. Following a target undershoot or overshoot, the performer would attempt to extend or shorten the primary movement amplitude. If it is the movement planning process that requires adjustment following a suboptimal movement, perhaps any trial-to-trial effect will be most apparent in early kinematic markers.

Optimizing Energy Expenditure and the Cost of an Error

Thus far in this chapter, we have considered the strategic behavior and visual–motor processes that minimize MT while achieving the accuracy required by the task demands. In most cases, movement trajectories that minimize MT are energy efficient. For example, movements that hit or initially undershoot a target are faster than movement overshoots because the limb travels less distance. Moving a fixed mass (e.g., the arm) a short distance consumes less energy than moving it a greater distance. As Lyons, Hansen, Hurding, and Elliott (2006) have demonstrated, participants especially avoid target overshoots, for which a corrective submovement must be made against gravity (see chapter 1). A correction made against gravity is more time and energy consuming than corrective submovements made in other planes.

Although MT and energy expenditure typically covary in reaching and aiming tasks, human performers do tend to minimize energy expenditure even when energy expenditure is independent of time. One line of evidence for this principle of energy minimization is a study on ballistic target aiming by Oliveira, Elliott, and Goodman (2005), in which participants propelled a small disk down a track to achieve a specific target distance. In an unassisted situation, applying greater force meant achieving greater distance. In a second situation, however, participants used a rubber tube to propel the disk down the track. For this assisted condition, participants needed to apply a force against the assistive force of the rubber band to prevent the disk from traveling too far. Thus, applying more force against the band meant the disk traveled less distance. As is evident in figure 2.6, participants initially adopted an energy minimization strategy in which they undershot the target in the unassisted condition and overshot the target in the assisted condition. Just as in other types of aiming (e.g., Elliott et al., 2004), participants were able to sneak up on the target distance as

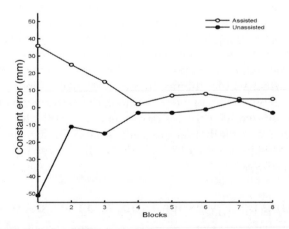

▶ **Figure 2.6**   Constant error as a function of trial block in the assisted and unassisted conditions.

Adapted, by permission, from F.T.P. Oliveira, D. Elliott, and D. Goodman, 2005, "The energy minimization bias: Compensating for intrinsic influence of energy minimization mechanisms," *Motor Control* 9: 101-114.

they started to lower the variability of their aiming attempts. Interestingly, even for tasks in which overshooting appeared to have advantages over undershooting (e.g., basketball shooting where an overshoot might bounce off the backboard and go into the basket), even skilled performers adopted a strategy minimizing energy expenditure under conditions in which sensory information is degraded (de Oliveira, Huys, Oudejans, van de Langenberg, & Beek, 2007).

It may be that energy minimization is linked to a biological imperative that has contributed to our survival as a species (Sparrow & Newell, 1998). Certainly, energy minimization should increase in importance as both the energy requirements of the task and fatigue increase. With respect to target undershooting in the reaching and aiming tasks that we have been discussing, there may also be a safety principle involved that has an evolutionary or at least a learned strategic link. For example, in attempting to retrieve a cooking pot from a fire, it is much safer to undershoot the pot handle than plunge the hand into either the pot or the fire. Eating with a fork, working with a circular saw, and reaching for a glass of very old whiskey are all activities in which an undershoot causes fewer problems than those caused by an overshoot (i.e., please don't spill the single malt).

Conclusions and Future Directions

It is clear from this review of the literature that there is no definitive relationship among speed, accuracy, and energy expenditure in goal-directed behavior. Rather, the relationship among these three variables is dynamic. It changes not only with practice but also with specific task demands and the costs and benefits associated with particular movement outcomes. Throughout the last few years there have been a number of new approaches to kinematic data analysis. Some of these approaches examine central tendency and variability associated with different aspects of the movement trajectory. These techniques, which require us to pool data over a number of trials, can provide insight into how goal-directed performance is optimized under different task conditions and with practice. Changes in performance that contribute to within-participant variability, however, probably occur on a trial-to-trial basis as performers attempt to repeat what they have just done or improve upon their previous performance. Certainly as our data acquisition systems become more and more precise, we are better able to explore the trial-to-trial discovery process associated with improving goal-directed performance. Although undoubtedly there are principles of optimization that apply to most people, future research should also focus on individual and group differences in goal-directed action. For example, we have recently applied our thinking on the optimization of performance with practice to the problem of age-associated perceptual–motor slowing (Welsh,

Higgins, & Elliott, 2007). As well, data from our lab have made it apparent that male and female performers often achieve similar movement outcomes in different ways. Females often adopt a more feedback-based strategy to limb control, while males are more likely to rely on feed-forward processes to optimize speed and accuracy (e.g., Hansen et al., 2007). Insight into the foundation for these gender differences might be gleaned by manipulating the costs and benefits associated with particular movement outcomes and examining trial-to-trial changes in behavior. In the context of individual differences associated with age, gender, and disability, it makes sense that the optimization process differs depending on the specific information processing strengths and weaknesses a person brings to the task. We now have the data acquisition and analysis techniques to explore these individual differences in a systematic way.

ENDNOTES

1. Trommershauser, Gepshtein, Maloney, Landy, and Banks (2005) have demonstrated that performers shift their mean aiming performance to compensate for increased variability even when that variability is created artificially by randomly perturbing visual feedback about the position of the effector.

2. Consistent with the idea that target overshoots take more time than target undershoots to correct, throughout the 4 days of practice Elliott and coworkers (2004) reported a mean MT of 370 ms for undershoots, 330 ms for primary submovement hits, and 440 ms for overshoots.

3. For the study involving directional accuracy, participants were able to accelerate through the target area. Thus the trajectories did not have the typically ordered sequence of kinematic events.

CHAPTER 3

Visual Selective Attention and Action

TIMOTHY N. WELSH AND DANIEL J. WEEKS

The rapid manual aiming movement has been an extremely useful task for studying the programming and control of goal-directed actions and the neural substrates underlying aiming processes in both average and special populations. The research reviewed throughout this book is a testament to the effectiveness and scope of manual aiming studies. Although the research on manual aiming movements has been illuminating, the majority of it has been conducted in limited task environments. While such sparse environments are vital to isolating the processes of interest, the vast majority of environments in which people execute aiming movements in daily life are rich and complex. Objects appear, disappear, and move from one location to another. Even relatively stable environments, such as work desks, car dashboards, or elevator control panels, present multiple stable objects that afford a wide variety of responses. In order to operate effectively in such complex environments, humans must selectively attend to a specific subset of the available information and select the most appropriate response from the available options. In this chapter, we explore the processes of selective attention and the reciprocal influences that action and selective attention have on one another.

Attention

A basic assumption of cognitive or reductionist models of performance is that humans have a limited capacity for information processing. That is, we are able to interpret, evaluate, and plan responses to only a very small subset of the massive amount of sensory information we receive at any given moment. Because of our limited capacity to process information, we must be able to select the subset of information that is vital to the task we are performing while filtering out the information that is not essential. This process of selecting and filtering, known as *selective attention,* consists of both automatic and controlled processes. Before describing the individual processes of attention, a review of the general characteristics of attention is necessary in order to provide the context for discussing these processes and their implications for motor control.

Characteristics of Attention

As just noted, a fundamental characteristic of our information processing system is that it has a limited capacity. It can process only a certain amount of information at any given moment in time. While most people implicitly understand this principle (as evidenced by our parents' or teachers' frequent scolding for us to "pay attention"), Cherry (1953) provided a useful analogy that succinctly demonstrates it and the other two characteristics of attention: the cocktail party.

Recall the last time you attended a busy party or a poster session at a major conference. Dozens, if not hundreds, of conversations were going on simultaneously, beer bottles and wine glasses were clinking, people were shuffling from one place to another, and many interesting pieces of art or posters were hanging on the walls. Such an environment is very rich and complex, and though you might be interested in joining as many conversations or viewing as many posters as possible, you can engage efficiently in only one conversation or poster at one time. Indeed, you often have to choose between listening to the presenter describing an experiment or reading the poster to figure out what was done. It is difficult to both read and listen, and even when you focus on the visuals, it is not efficient to examine more than a single figure at a time. This inability to interpret all the information desired reveals the limited capacity that humans have to actively engage and process information at any given moment.

The second thing to note from these situations is that you can change the focus of your limited capacity for information processing (attention) from one sensory system to another and from one visual object to another. That is, you can shift your attention around the environment. These attention shifts allow you to process a wide variety of information over a given length of time and may be voluntary or involuntary. Voluntary (also known as *top-down, or endogenous)* shifts of attention are controlled in that you purposely move the focus of your attention from one stimulus to another based on your goals. For example, you can voluntarily move your attention from figure to figure on a poster, or you can shift your attention to a conversation developing behind you (particularly when the new conversation is more interesting than the one you are having). In contrast, involuntary (also known as *bottom-up, reflexive, or exogenous)* shifts of attention occur because of a sudden change in the environment that captures your attention in a way that is outside of your control. These reflexive captures might be caused by new objects or people suddenly appearing in your vision or by your name being dropped unexpectedly in the conversation going on behind you. The distinction between voluntary and involuntary shifts of attention and the processes that influence reflexive attentional capture are described in greater detail in the following section.

The final property of attention is its divisibility. That is, it is possible to process and act on more than one piece of information at a time. For example, a person working diligently to interpret the graphs of a four-way interaction may be doing so at the cost of partially missing the information being described by the presenter. On the other hand, since humans are highly sensitive to the sudden appearance of new visual stimuli or to the announcement of our name, we are able to rapidly and accurately acquire and process that information (in an almost automatic fashion) at little cost to any other task we are simultaneously performing. The ability to divide attention and effectively process different pieces of information simultaneously, however, is bounded by the limited capacity of the processor. As highlighted in the cocktail party example, complex or novel stimuli that require controlled, attention-demanding processing take up a larger portion of the processing capacity, whereas simpler, automatically processed stimuli require a smaller portion of the attentional resource. Thus, the more automatically we can process a single piece of information, the more resources we have left over for processing other bits of information. On the other hand, when we attempt to decode a highly complex piece of information, we are left with few resources for the engagement of other information. The relevant point here is that even though we have a limited capacity for information processing, the system is not exclusively a serial system. Stimulus and response information can be processed in parallel as long as the sum of the processing does not require more resources than the system possesses. When resources are exceeded, the processing of at least one of the information sources suffers, and interference occurs. While interference can be measured in many ways, the two typical measures of interference are RT and errors. Thus, although we can divide our attention among a series of tasks, we need to be selective about the information to which we dedicate our limited capacity. The distinction between automatic and controlled processing, the relationship of these types of processing to attentional capture, and the consequences for these different types of processing all play a role in understanding the relationship between attention and motor control.

Selective Attention and Attentional Capture

The major consequence of our limited information processing is that we need to be able to focus on the information that is relevant to our goals and ignore the information that is irrelevant. The process through which we separate relevant and irrelevant information is broadly known as *selective attention*. Originally, selection was considered to be a process in which only the relevant information is focused upon. That is, it was believed that we have a filter system that allows target information to enter the information processing system but catches and subsequently decays nontarget information (e.g., Broadbent, 1958). However, more recent work suggests that selection also involves active inhibition of nontarget information (Tipper, 1985). This issue of active inhibition and its influence on motor control is addressed later in this chapter (see "Trajectories of Selective Reaching Movements"). First, we must discuss how information gets into attention and how attention is shifted from stimulus to stimulus.

As mentioned, shifts of attention from and to stimuli can be voluntary or involuntary. Voluntary, or endogenous, shifts of attention occur because the agent has decided that the information currently being attended to is no longer relevant or that other pieces of information or locations in space are more relevant. Studies of endogenous attention shifts usually employ symbolic cues (e.g., arrows or alphanumeric characters) to inform participants of the possible locations of upcoming targets. These studies have revealed that such attention shifts are not automatic (i.e., that people can ignore these cues) and are more demanding on the system. Because endogenous shifts are under voluntary control and require more resources, they take longer to develop (about 300 ms; Jonides, 1981). On the other hand, because they are controlled and driven by the individual, they can be maintained for longer durations (Cheal & Lyon, 1991; Müller & Rabbitt, 1989).

Reflexive, or exogenous, attention shifts are those that are driven by the stimuli. Attention is drawn to, or captured, by the stimulus in a way that is outside of cognitive control (Jonides, 1981; Posner, Nissen, & Odgen, 1978). Environmental changes such as the abrupt appearance (onset) or disappearance (offset) of a stimulus (Pratt & McAuliffe, 2001), the sudden change in the luminance or color of a stimulus (Folk, Remington, & Johnston, 1992; Posner et al., 1978; Posner & Cohen, 1984), the abrupt onset of object motion (Abrams & Chirst, 2003; Folk, Remington, & Wright, 1994), and the presentation of a color singleton (Treisman & Gelade, 1980) have all been shown to drive attentional capture. Because these shifts are driven by the stimulus, they involve little or no decision making, and they occur much more rapidly (about 100 ms; Cheal & Lyon, 1991; Müller & Rabbitt, 1989). Because reflexive shifts of attention are beyond the control of the individual, however, they can be elicited by stimuli that do not fit within the goals of the task, and thus they present a greater opportunity for interference.

Although originally it was thought that exogenous attention shifts are outside of intentional control (attentional capture by dynamic stimuli or singletons is not influenced by the goals of the task), Folk and colleagues (1992) demonstrated that this is not necessarily the case. In their study, these researchers asked participants to identify a stimulus that was presented in one of four possible locations. For some participants, the target stimulus was a color singleton (a red stimulus appeared at one location at the same time that white stimuli were presented at the other three locations). For the other participants, the target was a single stimulus of abrupt onset (the target appeared in one location and the other three locations remained empty). The key manipulation was that participants received cue information 150 ms before the target display. The cue was presented at one of the possible target locations and could be a single, abrupt-onset stimulus or a color singleton. Thus, the cue and target could be of the same identity (e.g., a color singleton cue followed by a color singleton target) or of a different identity (e.g., an abrupt-onset cue followed by a color singleton target). Across the set of experiments, the cue influenced RT only on trials in which the cue shared characteristics with the target. RT was uninfluenced by cues that were not the same as the target. Thus, dynamic changes or color singletons captured attention only when the participant was expecting and searching for a dynamic change or color singleton, respectively. Stated more succinctly, attentional capture was dependent on the expectations of the participant. Folk and colleagues proposed that the cue captured attention only when it shared characteristics with the target because people establish an attention set in which they form their expectations for the characteristics of the target stimulus. Stimuli meeting the attention set automatically capture attention, whereas stimuli that do not meet the set do not. Thus there may be no pure reflexive attentional capture because the characteristics of the stimuli that drive exogenous attentional capture are determined, at least in part, by the anticipated characteristics of the target. This phenomenon has come to be known as *contingent involuntary attentional capture.* Although subsequent work has revealed that the attentional set is relatively broad in that it can distinguish only between dynamic (e.g., abrupt-onset) and static (e.g., color singletons) stimulus characteristics (Folk et al., 1994; Gibson & Kelsey, 1998; Johnson, Hutchinson, & Neill, 2001), recent work has indicated that the motor system may also contribute to the development of the attentional set and work to specify the characteristics that capture attention. We address this issue in later sections.

Summary

The processes of selective attention have been studied extensively, and the preceding review is at best a light treatment of this vast literature. Nevertheless, the review provides the background concepts that are critical for understanding the role attention plays in shaping action. These concepts include the following: Attention is a limited resource. However, when information from multiple sources enters the limited information processor, it can be processed in parallel if the sum of the resources needed to decode the information does not exceed the limitations of the system. When more information enters than can be processed, the efficiency of the system decreases and the system slows down and becomes inaccurate. To prevent inefficiencies and errors from accumulating, humans have developed an elaborate set of mechanisms to pull the information that is relevant to the task out of the information that is irrelevant to the task. While attention is selective, it can be shifted from location to location and from object to object so that individuals may process a variety of information in a short length of time. Finally, the shifts of attention through the environment can be endogenously (performer) or exogenously (stimulus) driven, though exogenous captures of attention are under a certain degree of voluntary control. That is, stimuli that seem to capture attention involuntarily do so only when they fit with the goals and expectations of the observer.

Action-Centered Selective Attention

The research discussed thus far has been derived from more traditional cognitive sciences and has been driven by a model that treats perceptual processes (stimulus identification), cognitive processes (decision making), and motor processes (movement programming) as serial and sequential. As such, the experimenters typically were not concerned with output (response mode) and required participants to complete a simple or choice button-press task to identify the stimulus. Given that the main focus of the work was to investigate the processes leading up to the response, the response itself was not necessarily considered to be relevant to the processes under scrutiny. As Allport (1987) pointed out, however, the attention system evolved to identify stimuli for the purpose of organizing goal-directed actions rather than somewhat arbitrarily mapped button-press responses. From this simple observation came a research movement that studies attention by using more natural responses that require target engagement. While Rizzolatti, Riggio, and Sheliga (1987) and Rizzolatti, Riggio, Dascola, and Umilta (1994) were the first to suggest that the overlapping of attention and eye movement systems points to a tight coupling of attention and action, the first substantial behavioral study of attention in goal-directed aiming movements was reported by Tipper, Lortie, and Baylis (1992). The series of experiments conducted by Tipper and coworkers (1992) has become the foundation for the study of action-centered attention that is the focus of the remainder of this chapter.

Frames of Reference and Attentional Capture in Selective Reaching Tasks

The ingenuity of the experiments by Tipper and coworkers (1992), as well as the effect these studies have had on the field, cannot be overstated. The purposes of these experiments were to (1) determine whether interference effects observed in traditional key-press experiments are also observed when rapid goal-directed aiming movements are required and (2) assess the coordinate system or frame of reference that attention employs when performing goal-directed aiming movements. While the first purpose is straightforward, the second requires additional discussion.

A wide variety of studies have provided evidence that attention can work in retinotopic, allocentric, and egocentric coordinate systems. According to the retinotopic frame of reference, attention moves like a spotlight through the environment, with the fovea (central vision) as the focus of this beam. Following the work by Eriksen and colleagues (e.g., Eriksen & Eriksen, 1974), it was suggested that objects that are closer to the fovea receive attentional priority over those that are more distant. According to the allocentric (environmental) system, objects in the environment are coded with respect to their absolute position in space. In this way, objects closer to the absolute position of the target receive attentional priority. Finally, attention can be distributed egocentrically. Here, attentional resources are distributed throughout the environment such that the objects that are closer to the individual receive the attentional priority. Tipper and coworkers acknowledged that evidence exists in favor of each of these coordinate systems and subsequently suggested that the three alternatives are not necessarily mutually exclusive. They proposed that attention is a flexible resource and is distributed according to the action that is being performed. In this action-centered view of attention, attentional preference goes to the stimuli that are more salient to the task being completed.

To test these models, Tipper and coworkers (1992) asked participants to complete rapid aiming movements toward one of nine locations arranged in a 3 × 3 matrix on the surface of a board (see figure 3.1a). On a given trial, the target appeared at any one of the nine possible locations with or without a simultaneously presented distracting, nontarget stimulus appearing at one of the other eight locations. In experiment 1, the home position for all movements was a location at the bottom of the board between the target array and the person (the black box square in figure 3.1a). Although the location of the target and the location of the distractor (when present) were randomized, targets were presented in the middle row more often than they were presented in other rows, and only trials involving targets in the middle row were analyzed. The trials that had targets in the middle row were selected for analysis because it was on these trials that specific predictions for the different coordinate systems could be developed and tested.

If an environmental frame of reference is employed in the aiming tasks of experiment 1, then there should be a symmetrical pattern of interference in which the distractors appearing in the back, same, or front rows cause an equal amount of interference. A symmetrical pattern of interference is expected because a distractor presented in any row is equidistant from a target appearing in the middle row. If an egocentric frame of reference is employed, then an asymmetric pattern of interference is expected, with

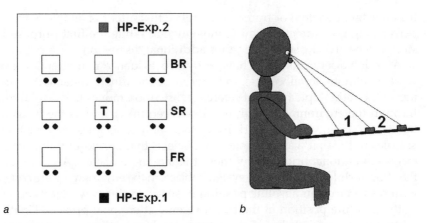

▶ **Figure 3.1**   *(a)* Diagram of the movement environment in the studies of Tipper and coworkers (1992). *(b)* Diagram of a participant in experiment 1 of Tipper and colleagues (1992). The hand is on the near-home position. Note that visual angle 1 is greater than visual angle 2, revealing that the retinal projections of the stimuli in the back row are closer to the projections of the stimuli in the middle row than are the projections of the stimuli in the front row.

Reprinted, by permission, from S.P. Tipper, C. Lortie, and G.C. Baylis, 1992, "Selective reaching: evidence for action-centered attention," *Journal of Experimental Psychology: Human Perception and Performance* 18: 891-905.

distractors in the front row causing more interference than that caused by the distractors in the back row. More interference is expected from distractors in the front row because stimuli closer to the body capture more attention than stimuli farther from the body are able to capture. If attention is distributed in a retinotopic system, then the opposite pattern of asymmetrical interference is expected: Interference is greater from a distractor in the back row compared with a distractor in the front row. This pattern of interference is predicted because, assuming participants fixate on the center button in the matrix (as they were instructed to do), the location of the back row on the retina is closer than the front row to the fovea (see figure 3.1*b*). Finally, if attention is flexible and distributed according to the stimuli that are most salient to the task being performed, then distractors in the front row should cause greater interference than that caused by distractors in the back row. Although this pattern of interference is the same as that predicted for the egocentric model, the prediction is based on different premises. Specifically, when a participant begins the aiming movement from the bottom of the board, a distractor in the front row causes greater interference because (1) the hand has to pass over the front row in order to get to the target and (2) stimuli requiring shorter movements, which are more efficient to organize and complete (Fitts, 1954; Fitts & Peterson, 1964), should be more salient than stimuli that afford longer movements that take more time and energy to perform.

    In short, experiment 1 revealed two important patterns of interference. First, distractors in the front row caused more interference than distractors in the back row—the proximity-to-hand effect. Second, distractors occupying the same side of space as the effector caused more interference than distractors appearing in the contralateral space—the ipsilateral effect. While these results immediately discount retinotopic and environmental frames of reference, they generally are consistent with predictions based on both egocentric and action-centered models. In order to differentiate between these two models, Tipper and coworkers shifted the starting location of the movements to the top of the board (the gray square in figure 3.1a). If an egocentric frame of reference is at work, then the same pattern of interference is expected because distractors in the front row are still closer to the body than are the distractors in the back row. However, if an action-centered frame of reference is being used, then back row distractors should generate greater interference than that generated by front row distractors because a distractor in the back row now lies between the home position and the target. In support of the action-centered model, a proximity-to-hand effect was observed, in that the distractors in the back row caused more interference when the starting position was moved to the top of the board.

Overall, Tipper and coworkers (1992) drew two main conclusions from their work. First, the distribution of attention is determined by the action to be performed. Second, there is a tight link between attention and action such that stimuli that are salient to the action being performed capture attention and automatically activate response-producing processes that allow the individual to interact with the stimuli (see also Meegan & Tipper, 1999). While the latter conclusion about the intimate link between attention and action perhaps is the contribution most relevant to the present chapter, a review and update of the notion of the frame of reference used in selective reaching actions are warranted.

Spatial Arrangement of Target and Distractors   While the discovery of the proximity-to-hand effect was a fundamental first step in the development of action-centered models of attention, more recent work has tested the generalizability of the proximity-to-hand effect and thereby expanded our understanding of the frames of reference used during selective reaching tasks. This more recent work does not contradict the proximity-to-hand effect or the general conclusion that attention is captured by the most salient stimuli in the environment. This more recent work does, however, suggest that the proximity-to-hand effect may be a special case in which the environment affords such a pattern of results.

A series of studies conducted by Keulen, Adam, Fischer, Kuipers, and Jolles (2002, 2003) clarified the role that the spatial relationship between target and distractor plays in determining the pattern of interference. These researchers noted that the distance between the possible locations of the target and the distractor was relatively large in the studies by Tipper and coworkers (1992) and questioned whether the distance between target and nontarget objects influences the use of a specific coordinate system. The possible influence of the distance between target and distractor was based on the two-component model of aiming movements (Woodworth, 1899). As reviewed extensively in chapter 1, the two-component model of goal-directed action is based on the idea that aiming movements consist of an initial ballistic, programmed phase that gets the limb to the area of the target and a secondary corrective phase that uses feedback to ensure accurate completion of the movement. There is some evidence suggesting that each of these processes utilizes different coordinate and neural systems (see chapters 1 and 4).

To determine if the separation between target and distractor influences coordinate system use, Keulen and colleagues (2002) analyzed the pattern of interference that emerged when participants made aiming movements to targets in environments in which distractors were presented close (2 mm) to the target or relatively far away (20 mm) from the target. These researchers hypothesized that the larger distances influence the programming phase more than they influence the current control phase because it is in the initial programming phase that the individual decides where in space the movement will terminate. Because the discrepancy between target location and distractor location is much greater in environments with large distances between target and distractor, the authors hypothesized that an action-centered frame of reference is used in such environments and thus predicted an asymmetrical proximity-to-hand pattern of interference. In addition, large distances between target and distractor should have little influence on the corrective phase because once the decision is made to go to a specific target, the target is quite isolated from the distractor and so the distractor has little influence on the control of movement. In contrast, because the decision about where to move in space is not very demanding when targets and distractors are close together, Keulen and colleagues suggested that distractors close to the target have very little influence on programming and interfere more with the current control phase. As such, the authors hypothesized that the performers would treat near and far distractors with similar priority (an environmental coordinate system) and that a symmetrical pattern of interference would emerge, with equal amounts of interference caused by distractors closer to and farther away from the home position.

In a finding consistent with the hypothesized shift in coordinate systems, Keulen and colleagues (2002) observed that distractor interference is symmetrical when the separation between target and distractor is small but is asymmetrical when the separation is large, with near distractors causing more interference than that caused by far distractors (see also Keulen et al., 2003). The main temporal interference effects were found in the time required to execute the movement (i.e., MT; see also Pratt & Abrams, 1994). However, in the initial studies (e.g., Tipper et al., 1992), only total time (RT + MT) was analyzed. As the predicted pattern of symmetrical and asymmetrical interference is based on conditions that influence either the programming phase or the current control phase, Keulen, Adam, Fischer, Kuipers, and Jolles (2004) sought to replicate and extend their initial work by examining the kinematics of aiming movements in order to determine whether the spatial arrangement of target and distractor influences these stages separately. In this follow-up study, these researchers divided MT into the time leading up to peak velocity and the time after peak velocity (which are conventional indexes of the efficiency of motor programming and control, respectively; see Khan et al., 2006 and chapter 2). Consistent with these researchers' hypotheses, a large separation between target and distractor increased the time leading to peak velocity, whereas a small separation increased the time after peak velocity.

In sum, the studies of Keulen and colleagues (2002) clarify the important role that the spatial relationship between the target and the distractor plays in determining the interference a specific nontarget location can have on goal-directed aiming movements. At first glance, the finding that a distractor that is farther away from the home position than the target is can cause interference when it is close to the target seems to contradict the proximity-to-hand effect. However, this finding actually reveals that distractors can affect the different stages of response organization and execution. As such, the results of these studies are consistent with the idea that attentional distribution is flexible and is determined by the context of the action.

Spatial Location Versus Response Efficiency   The studies reviewed thus far were designed to determine the coordinate system employed by the attention system during selective reaching movements. The search for a dominant coordinate system, however, might be a misguided pursuit considering Tipper and coworkers' (1992) two original proposals regarding action-centered attention: (1) Attentional distribution is flexible (i.e., not stable or consistent) and is dependent on the task to be performed. Because the distribution of attention and attentional capture may differ across tasks (Welsh & Pratt, 2008; see the following section for more detail) and within the various stages of a single task (Keulen et al., 2002), it might be unreasonable to pursue a single, or even dominant, coordinate system for goal-directed selective action. (2) The capture of attention by a particular stimulus automatically activates response-producing processes that allow the individual to interact with that stimulus. Interference effects arise because of limitations and conflict in the response selection stage of the information processing system. Interference in a particular task does not occur because people are employing a specific coordinate system that determines the relative saliency of the spatial location of a particular stimulus. Instead, interference develops when target and nontarget responses compete for activation in the limited processing system. Thus, it is the relative efficiencies with which individual responses to the target and distractors are organized that determines the presence and magnitude of interference. If the response to the distractor is organized more quickly than the response to the target is organized, then it will be active in the response selection stage and require more time and effort to inhibit so that the target response can emerge. In such instances, an interference effect is observed. On the other hand, if the response to the target is organized more quickly than the response to the distractor is organized, then little to no time and effort are required to inhibit the nontarget response and no interference is detected. The process of selection in a goal-directed aiming task can thus be conceived of as a horse race for activation, with each horse representing each activated response and the speed of each horse representing the efficiency of each response-producing process (see also Welsh, Elliott, & Weeks, 1999; Welsh & Elliott, 2004a).

The horse race analogy can readily account for the ipsilateral effect observed by Tipper and coworkers (1992) because movements into ipsilateral space are more efficient to organize and complete than are movements into contralateral space (e.g., Fisk & Goodale, 1985). Similarly, the analogy can explain the proximity-to-hand effect because movements of shorter amplitude are more efficiently organized and completed than are movements of greater amplitude (Fitts, 1954; Fitts & Petersen, 1964). Although the race model can account for the ipsilateral and proximity-to-hand effects, it is a useful model only if it successfully predicts new patterns of interference. Indeed, the strongest evidence in favor of a race model over a coordinate system comes from situations in which the proximity-to-hand and ipsilateral effects are eliminated or altered by environments set up in such a way that ipsilateral and close distractors targets afford responses that are less efficient than responses to distractors that are in contralateral space or are farther from the home position than the target is. Two recent studies have provided such evidence.

Support for the response efficiency or race model conceptualization of interference came from a study by Tipper, Meegan, and Howard (2002). Their method for decreasing the efficiency with which a response to a particular target is organized and completed was to put a small translucent barrier in front of one target button. This barrier did not prevent the participants from seeing or engaging the target, but it did provide an obstacle that the performers had to reach around. Thus the barricaded response was more complex and less efficient than any of the responses lacking a barrier. As in the experiments of Tipper and coworkers (1992), targets and distractors appeared at any of the potential locations, including the location behind the barrier. The researchers predicted that if response efficiency determines the degree of competition, and thus interference, observed RT effects should be smaller when the distractor is behind the barrier compared with when it is not behind the barrier. The results were consistent with this prediction because the barrier significantly decreased the magnitude of the negative priming effect. The negative priming effect is an increase in the RT to targets on trial n that are presented in a location where a distractor appeared on trial $n - 1$. Negative priming is thought to occur because selection on trial $n - 1$ involves active inhibition of the nontarget response, and inhibition left over from the selection on trial $n - 1$ hinders the generation of that response on trial n. Thus, the decrease in negative priming for targets behind barriers suggests that less inhibition was required to stop that response on trial $n - 1$. Less inhibition was required to stop the response to the distractor appearing behind the barrier on trial $n - 1$ because the nontarget response was less efficiently organized and did not reach a level of activation sufficient to require inhibition.

While Tipper and coworkers (2002) provided indirect evidence for the role of response efficiency in selective reaching tasks, Welsh and Zbinden (2009) directly tested the role of response efficiency. Recall that the proximity-to-hand effect is the finding that distractors between the home position and the target cause more interference than that caused by distractors located farther from the home position (Tipper et al., 1992). It was suggested that this pattern of interference is due to the fact that, with reference to Fitts' law (Fitts, 1954; Fitts & Petersen, 1964), shorter movements are more efficient to program and execute than are movements of larger amplitudes. However, note that the size of each potential target location in the study of Tipper and coworkers (1992) was identical. According to Fitts' law, movement efficiency is determined by both the movement amplitude and the width of the target: $ID = \log_2(2A / W)$, where ID is the index of difficulty, A is the amplitude of the movement, and W is the target width. Thus, by varying only the movement amplitude, Tipper and coworkers were looking at only one component affecting movement efficiency, and the proximity-to-hand effect might be a product of an environment in which target width is constant.

To test this idea, Welsh and Zbinden (2009) varied both the amplitude and the width of the distractors to determine if greater interference is caused by all distractors that are located closer to home regardless of their size (the proximity-to-hand effect) or only by distractors that afford more efficiently executed actions regardless of their location (a response efficiency interpretation). In this study, there were two potential target locations (20 and 40 cm from the home position). The size of the target (a green circle) changed depending on the location of presentation so that the target ID was kept at 3.3 bits of information for all targets. The distractor (a red circle) was presented in the other potential location on 75% of the trials. The size of the distractor was varied such that it afforded a movement of more $(ID = 4.3 \text{ bits})$, equal $(ID = 3.3 \text{ bits})$, or less $(ID = 2.3 \text{ bits})$ efficiency. Consistent with the race model, interference was observed only when the ID of the distractor was less than that of the target. Importantly, the greatest interference was observed when the distractor that had a lower ID was farther from home than the target was. Although this interference effect is opposite to the proximity-to-hand effect, it does not contradict the latter effect because both can be accounted for by the horse race perspective, in which the efficiency of response-producing processes determines interference. Thus, like the results of Keulen and colleagues (2002, 2003), the results of Welsh and Zbinden (2009) are consistent with the notion of action-centered attention.

Properties of the Target and Distracting Stimuli   In the previous section, we introduced a horse race model for explaining interference effects in selective reaching tasks. Interference occurs when responses to target and nontarget stimuli compete for activation. The presence and magnitude of the interference are related to the competitiveness of the race. We now turn to the question of how individual responses get entered into the race.

According to both premotor (Rizzolatti et al., 1994) and action-centered models of attention (Tipper et al., 1992), response codes are evoked automatically (and entered into the race for activation) whenever an object is attended. Given the overlapping cortical networks of attention and motor systems (particularly in the posterior parietal cortex; Rizzolatti et al., 1994), the activation of responses with attentional capture should not come as a surprise. What should be equally apparent from this anatomical arrangement, but is considered much less often, is the upstream influence that motor systems may have on attentional capture.

As reviewed earlier, the involuntary capture of attention can be influenced by expectations about the target characteristics (e.g., an abrupt-onset cue captures attention only when the expected target is a single abrupt onset; Folk et al., 1992). To recap, contingent involuntary capture of attention is based on the idea that an individual approaches a task with an attentional set in which the expected characteristics of the target are maintained. Stimuli that match the properties in the attentional set capture attention, while those that do not match do not capture attention. It has been shown that this attentional set is tuned broadly in that it is able to distinguish between dynamic discontinuities, such as abrupt onsets, offsets, and motion stimuli, and more static stimuli, such as color singletons. However, in consideration of the tenets of action-centered attention, a few researchers have started to ask if the motor system can also influence the attentional set and attentional capture. This line of inquiry began with the idea that stimuli have different meanings for the motor system in different action contexts. For example, the sudden onset of a yellow or red light at an intersection may be very relevant to the driver because that individual has to apply the brakes, but the same light changes might go unnoticed by a passenger.

The methodology across the few studies on this topic is fairly straightforward—ask participants to perform a selection task with one type of response (e.g., a rapid aiming movement). Then have the participants or another group of participants complete the same task with another type of response (e.g., a reach-to-grasp or a key-press response) and determine whether there are differences in the patterns of interference. One of the first studies to look at this issue was conducted by Bekkering and Neggers (2002). In this study, participants were presented with an array of bars and were required to either point to and touch the target bar or reach to and grasp the target bar. The individual bars in the array were either green or orange and were oriented at a 45° or a 135° angle. The target bar for a given trial was identified by its color and orientation (e.g., green bar at a 135° angle), and distractors differed from the target in terms of color, orientation, or both. Bekkering and Neggers were interested in determining whether the selectivity of the attention system differed between the pointing and the grasping tasks. Their measure of selection errors was the number of trials on which the first saccade (an overt shift of attention) was directed toward a distractor that differed from the target in color or orientation. They hypothesized that if attentional selectivity is modified by task, then color errors should be similar across pointing and reaching tasks because the color of an object is no more relevant to a pointing movement than it is to a grasping movement. However, because the orientation of the object is much more relevant for grasping than it is for pointing, the attention system should become more highly tuned to orientation on grasping tasks, and fewer orientation errors should be made on grasping trials than are made on pointing trials. In support of these predictions, during the grasping task fewer saccades were made to distractors with the incorrect orientation, whereas color errors were consistent across both types of tasks. Thus, the attention system became more highly tuned and selective for a stimulus dimension that was most relevant to the task at hand. Similar action-dependent increases in perceptual sensitivity have been observed by Fagioli, Hommel, and Schubotz (2007; Fagoli, Ferlazzo, & Hommel, 2007), who found that changes in the size of an object are more easily detected when a grasping action is prepared, while changes in object location are more readily detected when a pointing action is prepared.

While the studies of Bekkering and Neggers (2002) and Fagioli and colleagues (2007) revealed that differences in end-point engagement alter perceptual and attentional sensitivity to specific dimensions, Welsh and Pratt (2008; see also Higgins & Welsh, in progress, 2009) found that the action to be performed alters attentional capture in more a conventional interference paradigm. Here, the authors were interested in taking a more direct look at the possible influence that the motor system has on the formation of the attentional set. Recall that it has been suggested that the attentional set is formed by the perceptual expectations of the performer and that it can be tuned only broadly, such that it can distinguish between static and dynamic stimulus properties. In this way, all dynamic discontinuities capture attention when any kind of dynamic discontinuity is expected (Folk et al., 1994; Gibson & Kelsey, 1998; Johnson et al., 2001).

The studies of attentional capture, however, typically are conducted with key-press responses. Given the relatively arbitrary mapping, in some cases, between targets and responses, all that is required to complete this task is to identify the stimulus and match it to one of a series of possible responses. In such key-press tasks, a constant and stable source of information is not required for successful completion. In support of this idea is the finding that in these types of tasks onset and offset stimuli capture attention to a similar degree (Pratt & Arnott, 2008; Pratt & McAuliffe, 2001). Onset and offset stimuli, however, provide very different action opportunities when a manual aiming response is required. To maximize movement accuracy, aiming responses need a constant and stable source of visual information regarding the target location, and movement accuracy decreases when the target is removed from the environment (see chapter 5). Welsh and Pratt (2008) sought to determine if this difference in action affordance influences the attentional set and subsequently affects the effectiveness with which a particular stimulus captures attention. For this study, participants had to complete either a choice key-press response or an aiming movement to a target presented in one of four locations. For a given block of trials, the target was an onset or offset stimulus. On 75% of the trials, the target was presented with a simultaneously occurring offset or onset distractor, respectively. Onset and offset stimuli were paired with each other because they are relative extremes in that they afford similar responses in a detection key-press task but drastically different responses in an aiming task. Because the action system needs a constant and stable source of information to complete aiming movements, an onset stimulus affords a specific response and action goal while an offset stimulus affords an unspecific response or no response at all. The findings of Welsh and Pratt (2008) were indeed consistent with the hypothesis that the action system can influence the attentional set: Onset distractors caused interference in both key-press and aiming tasks, whereas offset stimuli caused interference in only key-press tasks.

The results of Welsh and Pratt (2008) are also consistent with the horse race model of interference in selective reaching tasks. Recall that the central tenets of the model are that (1) all stimuli that capture attention evoke response-producing processes that allow the individual to interact with the stimuli and (2) interference is observed because of a conflict in response selection. If targets and distractors do not both capture attention, there are no competing response codes and thus there is no interference during response selection. In the aiming task of Welsh and Pratt (2008), the offset distractor did not cause an interference effect—because of its weak affordance properties, it did not capture attention, did not evoke response codes, and subsequently did not create a conflict in response selection.

Trajectories of Selective Reaching Movements

To this point, our discussion has revolved around interference effects observed in temporal measurements such as RT and MT. It has been argued that these interference effects are observed because response codes to both target and nontarget stimuli are activated in the motor system, and time and effort are required to inhibit the nontarget response and allow the target response to emerge. Recently, however, developments in the ability to analyze movement execution have provided interested researchers with the opportunity to take a more detailed look into how response processes are represented. One particularly revealing measure of response execution is the trajectory of the reaching movement early in execution. Studying early movement trajectories is preferred over studying late trajectories because early movement trajectories are a more pure and accurate reflection of the programmed component of the action at the moment of movement initiation. Markers late in the trajectory, such as end-point error, are the result of a number of other processes such as online correction and the continuing selection process. Thus, end-point location and similar late markers are a poor indication of bias in programming even in visual open-loop conditions that allow proprioception to be used to correct the initial motor plan (c.f., Fischer & Adam, 2001; Sailer, Eggert, Ditterich, & Straube, 2002).

In support of action-centered attention, research on early movement trajectories has shown that the trajectories of selective reaching movements veer toward (Welsh et al., 1999; Welsh & Elliott, 2004a, 2005) and away from (Howard & Tipper, 1997; Tipper, Howard, & Houghton, 1999; Welsh & Elliott, 2004a, 2004b) nontarget stimuli. As these deviations are present early in the movement path, they are thought to reflect the coding of the target and nontarget responses in the movement system at the moment of movement initiation. Since movement direction is coded by a series of directionally tuned neurons in primary and premotor cortex (Georgeopoulos, 1990), deviations that are observed when nontarget stimuli are present in the environment are caused by response codes to the nontarget stimuli being excited or inhibited. While there is general agreement that deviations toward or away from stimuli result from nontarget response codes that have raced for activation and from inhibitory mechanisms working to eliminate them, there is no consensus on the processes that lead to the response codes. There are two leading models that attempt to explain these deviations—the response vector model and the response activation model. As the response activation model proposed by Welsh and Elliott (2004a) was developed to address perceived shortcomings of the response vector model of Tipper, Houghton, and colleagues (Tipper et al., 1999), the two models have much in common.

First, each model is based on the idea that attention to an object automatically activates a response to interact with that object. Second, each model suggests that competing responses to target and nontarget stimuli race for activation and are represented simultaneously in the motor system. The suggestion that multiple responses can be activated simultaneously is not new (see Coles, Gratton, Bashore, Eriksen, & Donchin, 1985). Finally, each model proposes that the characteristics of the initial portion of the response reflect the summation of the activation levels of each competing response at the moment of movement initiation. Activation of nontarget response codes causes characteristics of the nontarget response to be incorporated into the response, the result of which is deviation toward the nontarget. Inhibition of the nontarget response causes characteristics opposite those of the nontarget response to be incorporated into the initial response and so the result is deviation away from the nontarget. The main differences between the two models revolve around the number and the timing of the inhibitory mechanisms that eliminate the nontarget response, and so the models differ in their explanations of how deviations toward and away from a stimulus develop.

According to the response vector model (Tipper et al., 1999), there are two inhibitory mechanisms that work to eliminate nontarget response codes. The activation of these two mechanisms depends on the salience (defined as action relevance) of the nontarget stimulus. Reactive inhibition is the main inhibitory mechanism, and it works to inhibit responses to stimuli of relatively high salience. The model suggests that this main inhibitory mechanism is very strong and quickly reduces the responses to salient nontarget stimuli to below baseline. Thus the neural activity associated with the nontarget response is below the baseline level at the moment of movement initiation. The secondary mechanism is the on-center, off-surround (oCoS) selection mechanism. It is weak and works to inhibit nontarget responses to stimuli of low salience. The oCoS selection mechanism is based on the discovery of an oCoS coding at the neural level of premotor and primary motor cortices. The oCoS coding works to hone the direction of movement by enhancing the activity of directionally tuned cells that are tuned for a similar direction while actively inhibiting cells that are tuned for movements in other directions (Georgeopoulos, 1995). It is proposed that this oCoS selection mechanism is weak and unable to completely eliminate the nontarget response. As such, some neural activity associated with the nontarget response lingers at the moment of movement initiation. Thus, the response vector model accounts for deviations toward nontarget stimuli by suggesting that they occur because of an ineffective oCoS mechanism being unable to eliminate the nontarget response of low salience. On the other hand, deviation away from a stimulus occurs because reactive inhibition completely eliminates the nontarget response to the highly salient stimulus and actually reduces the neural activity of that response to below baseline levels (see Tipper et al., 1999 for more details). In short, the salience of the stimulus determines the mechanism of selection and subsequently the direction of movement deviation.

The response activation model (Welsh & Elliott, 2004a) argues for a single selection mechanism that works to eliminate all nontarget responses, regardless of the salience of the stimuli that evoke these responses. According to the model, the oCoS mechanism plays a functional role in honing and specifying individual motor plans as opposed to participating in the selection process (c.f., Tipper et al., 1999). The response activation model relies heavily on a race approach to selection and accounts for deviations toward and away from a nontarget stimulus by suggesting that the inhibitory mechanism takes time to develop and eliminate nontarget responses. Thus, the results of the race depend on three factors: (1) the efficiency with which each response is produced (the speed of the runner), (2) the degree to which a particular response is preactivated or preinhibited (how close to or far from the finish line a runner begins), and (3) the time course and efficiency of inhibitory development. When a nontarget response is inhibited, because of preinhibition or because enough time has elapsed to allow the inhibitory mechanism to succeed, the movement deviates away from the location of the nontarget stimulus. When a nontarget response is active, either because not enough time has elapsed to allow the inhibitory mechanism to succeed or because the response was preactivated or very efficiently organized, the movements deviate toward the location of that nontarget stimulus. Salience plays a role in movement deviations by determining the level of preactivation or the efficiency of response processing but not the strength and type of inhibitory mechanism.

An extensive review of the evidence favoring or contradicting each model is beyond the scope of this chapter. Suffice it to say that there are experimental findings easily accounted for by each model and results that require some more creative interpretations. That said, a study by Welsh and Elliott (2005) did present substantial evidence to support the response activation model. This particular study examined the specific role that salience plays in determining the direction of movement deviation since it is in the predicted effect that salience has on response coding and inhibitory mechanisms that truly differentiates the two models. The response vector model holds that movements deviate toward distracting stimuli of low salience (because of incomplete oCoS selection) and away from distractors of high salience (because of complete nontarget response inhibition). In contrast, the response activation model predicts little or no movement deviation toward distractors of low salience (because of relatively inefficient nontarget response organization) and large movement deviation toward distractors of high salience (because of incomplete nontarget response inhibition). Welsh and Elliott (2005) manipulated salience by providing 75% valid precue information about the location of the target. They hypothesized that this validity manipulation would make the precued location highly salient relative to the uncued locations. Thus, the distractor that appeared at an uncued location on two-thirds of the valid trials would be of relatively low salience. On the remaining 25% of the trials, the target appeared at one of the uncued locations alone or with a distractor. Importantly, the distractor on invalid trials was always presented at the cued location (a highly salient location). The findings, which were consistent with the response activation model, showed that movements did not deviate toward or away from the distractor on valid trials, whereas movements deviated toward the distractor on invalid trials. In our opinion, this pattern is difficult to reconcile with the response vector model. It is clear, however, that more work is needed to understand the selection process and how it shapes action.

Summary and Future Directions

Throughout this chapter we have reviewed the recent work highlighting the important role attention has in shaping action and the way in which action alters how we attend to objects in the environment. This emphasis on the interaction between attention and the motor system is a component of a larger movement in cognitive psychology that is beginning to recognize the important role the motor system plays in what have been considered to be higher-order cognitive processes (such as perception; Grosjean, Shiffrar, & Knoblich, 2007; Proffitt, Stefanucci, Banton, & Epstein, 2003; Witt, Proffitt, & Epstein, 2005). Here, we have focused on the reciprocal relationship between action and attention with two goals in mind. First, we have aimed to further the position that studying selective attention in more natural reaching and grasping responses sheds new light on the complex processes involved in cognition (c.f., Allport, 1987). Based largely on the groundbreaking work by Tipper and colleagues, a growing wealth of evidence has revealed that selection is a dynamic process in which information and responses can be processed in parallel as they race for activation. Second, we have aimed to demonstrate how the incorporation of more complex responses such as aiming or grasping allows for a rich data set that can unearth new aspects of phenomena that initially were established with simple or choice key-press responses. This use of aiming and grasping movements in paradigms that typically employ key-press responses is not unique to attention, and this modification to conventional methodologies likely will have a wide-reaching influence on psychological phenomena. For example, recent studies have analyzed movement trajectories in paradigms such as the Simon effect (Beutti & Kersel, 2009), decision making (McKinstry, Dale, & Spivey, 2008), and unconscious processing of masked cue stimuli (Cressman, Franks, Enns, & Chua, 2007) to provide a deeper understanding of these processes and their influence on action. Thus, examining attention and cognition more broadly in the context of the motor performance demanded by the task at hand should prove to be a valuable research strategy in developing extant models of human behavior for use in human factors contexts (see Welsh, Weeks, Chua, & Goodman, 2007) and for understanding movement and cognitive disorders (Welsh, Ray, Weeks, Dewey, & Elliott, 2009; Welsh & Elliott, 2001). We expect this exciting trend to continue.

CHAPTER 4

Vision and Movement Planning

J. GREG ANSON, RACHEL BURGESS, AND REBEKAH L. SCOTT

If the old adage "seeing is believing" is true, the link between what we see and what we do should be relatively simple and straightforward: See then act! From a perspective of motor preparation, it is easier to explain seeing than it is to explain believing. Seeing can be ascribed to the neurophysiology underpinning the retinal response to light and the resultant changes in activity of neurons in the primary visual area (V1) or primary visual cortex (Schall, 2001). In contrast, believing defies a simple neurophysiological explanation. Believing does not depend on vision alone and is a consequence of the nature of the visual information, information from other sensory modalities and from memory, and the dynamic output of the brain associated with multiple behavioral phenomena including intent, planning, goal setting, and action. One view (Sober & Sabes, 2005) posits that the overall goal of motor planning is to minimize error—that is, the visual information and proprioceptive information simultaneously derived from the same external source are evaluated and weighted by a multisystem sensory apparatus and then integrated in advance of a planned response initiation. Although the emphasis of this chapter is on vision and movement planning, we offer a caveat up front: Movement planning is not an exclusive prerogative of the visuomotor system.

Understanding how the brain works remains one of the significant challenges for neuroscientists in the 21st century. Within the realm of goal-directed action, the debate over whether the central nervous system is host to internal models representing neural control parameters for motor control or movement planning is unlikely to subside (Latash, 2007; Morasso, 2007). Given this background, it is perhaps unsurprising that the role of vision in the planning of goal-directed action likewise remains a focus of contention. This chapter attempts to straddle the often implicit boundary between the neurobiological literature and the neurobehavioral literature on vision and movement planning. It includes brief comments on the relationship between the two visual systems and movement planning, the neurophysiology of planning and vision in human and nonhuman primates, and the behavioral aspects of vision and planning. In addition, this chapter describes the influence of the memory of the visual environment on real-time movement preparation.

Two Visual Systems

One risk in categorizing a system as having discrete functional components is that some behaviors may not fit into a category. While the real-time and memory-dependent forms of object-directed action have been elegantly portrayed as outcomes of the dorsal stream and the ventral stream visual pathways, respectively (Goodale & Milner, 1992; Goodale, Westwood, & Milner, 2003), these systems do not appear to accommodate control of saccadic eye movements—eye movements that are likely a part of any movement task in which the preparation includes fixating on a single point before movement initiation. The control of saccadic eye movement rests with subcortical structures, specifically the superior colliculus. The superior colliculus also receives descending input from cortical structures and directly from retinocollicular pathways that under conditions of visual fixation can alter RT for object recognition without the participants knowing that they have seen the stimulus (Gazzaniga, Ivry, & Mangun, 2002). Even if pathways are well described, caution is recommended in drawing strong associations between changes in brain state and behavior: "Brain states and behaviour can be as unpredictable as the weather" (Schall, 2001, p. 40). Nonetheless, researchers have attempted to investigate the unique functional properties of the components of the two visual systems and their contribution to movement planning. In this context we suggest a further caveat: The two visual systems do not represent the entire contribution of the visual system to the control of movement. Structurally and functionally, they probably are not divorced from the influence of other visual systems such as those involved in saccadic eye movement.

In an attempt to discern differences between planning (dorsal visual stream) and online control, Danckert, Sharif, Haffenden, Schiff, and Goodale (2002) conducted a temporal analysis of a grasping movement to measure size contrast on grasp aperture within the Ebbinghaus illusion. They concluded that object-directed grasping is not affected by pictorial illusion and proposed that planning uses a context-dependent visual representation while control is context independent and occurs online. In this same theoretical context, Binsted and Heath (2005) asked participants to perform discrete aiming movements to targets of various widths (the index of difficulty varied between 1.5 bits, which was easy, and 5.0 bits, which was more difficult). Vision was either available or unavailable during reaching.

The purpose of the study was to test the hypothesis that information in the lower visual field accesses the visuomotor system specifically by the dorsal (the where or how of action) visual pathway (Goodale et al., 2003). Binsted and Heath (2005) also proposed that the presence of vision during reaching facilitates online (feedback) control, whereas the absence of vision requires control to be based on central planning (feed-forward control). Although vision (and online control) did improve the reaching trajectory, there was no difference in MT or accuracy when participants fixated on the upper or lower visual field. Thus a preferential effect of the lower visual field and the dorsal visual system was not demonstrated. Taking a position consistent with a unified visual system and movement planning, Meegan and colleagues (2004) proposed a single visual representation for perception, motor planning, and motor control as opposed to the separate action (dorsal) and perception (ventral) functions put forth by the two–visual systems model. Meegan and colleagues used a Müller-Lyer illusion task in which participants, after a 10 ms or 3,000 ms delay, either judged (perceptual) or performed (action) an aiming movement to determine the length of a Müller-Lyer image (stimulus) presented for either 10 ms or 3,000 ms. Neither memory delay or stimulus duration influenced the illusory effect. Furthermore, the overall effect was not altered in the aiming movement when the hand was not visible despite a difference in movement accuracy. The authors concluded that the illusion had comparable effects on perceptual and motor tasks, which implies that the results are consistent with a common representation model. However, separation of functional attributes of the dorsal visual system for movement planning is not without support.

Recently, Prabhu, Lemon, and Haggard (2007) examined the effect of sustained versus brief illumination of a target followed by paired-pulse TMS on facilitation of activity in the agonist muscle performing a reach and grasp task. The relationship between TMS-induced motor evoked potentials (MEP) and preparatory muscle activity was reliable only in the condition in which the target remained illuminated throughout the trial. Prabhu and coworkers (2007) interpreted their results in favor of the properties of the dorsal visual stream because the preparatory muscle activity was apparent only when sustained vision was present and when real-time movement preparation was optimal. With respect to control of visually guided movement, it appears that the strength of the two–visual systems model in the arena of movement planning remains open to question.

Although many studies have investigated the extent to which the dorsal and ventral systems independently contribute to movement planning, fewer studies have focused on decision making. Perhaps this is because decision making per se is unlikely to be the sole prerogative of either the dorsal or the ventral system and is probably not even collectively limited to the dorsal and ventral visual systems. Nonetheless, at least one study (Heekeren, Marrett, Ruff, Bandettini, & Ungerleider, 2006) has attempted to assess vision and decision making by requiring different motor responses to a single stimulus source. Heekeren and colleagues (2006) required participants to respond with either a button press or a saccadic eye movement to a random-dot display varying in visual coherence. Although not part of the rationale for this study, it seems that the specific movement tasks (saccadic eye movement or button press) could provide a methodological way of determining the extent to which the two visual systems (dorsal and ventral) and the saccadic eye movement system have unique or general roles in vision and movement planning. In the study, the participants' task was to discriminate the direction of motion in the dot display. The study was conducted during a functional magnetic resonance imaging (fMRI) recording session, and the hypothesis was that high coherence in the stimulus display would lead to correct decisions about its movement direction, and that these decisions would be associated with increased fMRI. That is, increased neural activity, as reflected by the altered hemodynamic response within specific brain regions, should occur independently of whether the motor response was carried out by a saccade or a button press. The researchers noted that four areas appear to be identified with decision making: the left posterior dorsolateral prefrontal cortex (DLPFC), the left posterior cingulate cortex, the left inferior parietal lobule, and the fusiform or parahippocampal gyrus. The greatest change was seen in the DLPFC. The researchers argued that the DLPFC compares signals from sensory processing areas during perceptual decision making and that this functional activity transcends task and response specificity, linking sensory processing, decision making, and action. One limitation of this interpretation is that fMRI measurements lack temporal resolution. Thus robust descriptions of events that may be defined as much by the time course of processing as by the change in fMRI signal are, as of yet, difficult to substantiate. However, it is interesting that the left DLPFC has also been reported to be uniquely involved with motor preparation of either one-hand or two-hand speeded responses (Anson, Scott, & Hyland, 2007; Swinnen, 2002).

The two–visual systems model (with the dorsal system representing the how or where and the ventral representing the what) has provided significant opportunities to compartmentalize not only the functional attributes of vision and movement but also the extent to which movement planning is holistic versus system specific. What must be kept in mind was perhaps best summed up by Robert Porter, who stated that "the whole brain can be considered the organ of movement" (Porter, 1987, p. 4).

Vision and Movement Planning: Behavioral Perspectives

Behavioral perspectives associated with vision and planning include precuing, practice, feedback, and the influence of target location. Precuing refers to providing information in advance of an imperative signal to initiate a planned movement. Precued information can specify the direction, distance, and limb to be moved as well as the location of a visual target (Eversheim & Bock, 2002). It might also specify the nature of the available visual feedback (Hansen, Glazebrook, Anson, Weeks, & Elliott, 2006; Lawrence, Khan, Buckolz, & Oldham, 2006) and whether participants will be directed to use target-centered or hand-centered visual information (Chieffi, Allport, & Woodin, 1999). The nature of visual feedback and practice schedules have also been shown to influence ongoing movement planning and the development of optimal control strategies (Khan, Elliott, Coull, Chua, & Lyons, 2002; Proteau & Carnahan, 2001).

In their discussion of precuing and target location, Eversheim and Bock (2002) suggested that precues focus attention on a limited area of space and so, because they provide advance information about a visual target, speed up motor preparation (movement planning). This in turn leads to faster RT. The researchers noted that the effectiveness of a precue on movement planning is diminished when a secondary task is inserted after the precue but before the stimulus and so suggested that persistent attention to the precue (not just its presentation) is necessary to realize RT benefits. In an experiment manipulating precue information about target location and the persistence of visual feedback, Hansen and colleagues (2006) reported that RT (simple RT) and, by inference, movement planning are fastest when there is no uncertainty about the presence of visual feedback and the location of the target. Interestingly, the time taken to move a stylus to a target was longer in this condition. This condition was also associated with longer deceleration to the target and diminished errors, perhaps reflecting optimized preparation and performance. In contrast, when participants knew exactly which target to move to and that vision would be occluded, RT lengthened significantly, MT shortened, and radial error increased by 76%. Although the precue provided certainty with respect to target location, this information was not sufficient to optimize movement planning. Consistent with the conclusions of Eversheim and Bock (2002), Hansen and colleagues (2006) suggested that optimal performance is contingent on visual feedback that is sustained throughout the performance of the task. In a different experimental condition, Hansen and colleagues precued the target but set the probability that visual feedback would be available to 50%. In this situation the predicted worst-case scenario was no vision. Participants appeared to prepare in advance for this situation as the default because RT was shorter than it was when visual feedback was provided. It seemed that participants treated the provision of visual feedback as unexpected and so were required to amend the prepared movement plan. This resulted, perhaps not intuitively, in longer RT (simple RT). MT was unaffected by the .5 probability of visual feedback. Under choice RT conditions, RT was predictably longer because target location remained unknown until stimulus onset. Advance knowledge of the availability of visual feedback did not provide any temporal advantage in planning the response. Hansen and colleagues (2006) suggested that taken together, these results support a hierarchical model of motor preparation in which precuing target location (providing movement-specific information) is more important than knowing whether or not visual feedback will be provided.

Research on visual feedback and practice in limb control provides another perspective on vision and movement planning. For example, Proteau and Carnahan (2001) manipulated visual feedback such that in one condition vision of the arm and target was provided (egocentric reference frame) and in another condition vision of the arm was occluded (allocentric reference frame). Target aiming improved with practice in a modality-specific manner in each condition. Following practice in the allocentric condition, when vision of the arm was blocked, performance accuracy diminished. This finding indicates that effective movement planning requires vision of both arm and target. Similar results were reported by Chieffi and coworkers (1999), who investigated visuospatial memory in instructed hand-centered or target-centered pointing tasks. Hand-centered visuospatial instruction was associated with smaller error. In an experiment examining the detailed relationship between visual feedback and kinematic profiles of rapid aiming movements, Khan and colleagues (2002) noted that the kinematic profile changes when participants know that vision will be available during a trial: Preparation time was shorter, peak deceleration occurred earlier, and time needed to adjust limb trajectory after peak deceleration lengthened. Trajectory variability increased up to peak deceleration and then decreased to the end of movement. This outcome is consistent with a strategy of minimizing the time spent on preparation and movement initiation and relying on visual feedback for the terminal phase of the aiming movement. For movement planning in general, knowing that visual feedback is available appears to be less important than knowing the location of the target. However, visual feedback is a significant factor in minimizing movement end-point error, and its utility improves with extended practice, an observation implying an important interaction between practice and movement planning.

One challenge in determining the nature of vision and planning is isolating the role of vision. In most human studies, planning is facilitated by contributions from other sensory systems such as proprioception. Sometimes as a consequence of selective sensory loss through injury or disease, unique situations occur that provide an opportunity to study the influence of vision on movement planning (Darling & Rizzo, 2001; Ghez, Gordon, & Ghilardi, 1995). Darling and Rizzo described a case study of a young adult who had been born with bilateral lesions of the visual cortex (a missing right occipital lobe, a missing ventral portion of the left occipital lobe, and poor visual acuity of 3/400) but could still point to visually presented targets as quickly as control participants could. However, the movements, although fast, were characterized by greater end-point variability in the hand movement, greater curvature in the hand path (especially for movements made with the left hand), and large sensorimotor transformation errors (i.e., the mapping between limb coordinate systems and target location manifested in large errors that were dissociated for distance and direction). The researchers suggested that because this individual was capable of rapid pointing, the movement impairment was due not only to a visual defect but also to a defect in the development of neural mechanisms necessary for planning and control of reaching movements. These mechanisms develop in early life and require the visual cortex. Another study (Ghez et al., 1995) investigated aiming movements in a group of patients who had large-fiber sensory neuropathy and thus were deprived of proprioceptive feedback. Of interest were the effects that visual information had on the accuracy of moving a handheld cursor on a digitizing tablet (the work space) to targets that were displayed on a computer screen. The experiment manipulated the nature of the visual feedback (arm only, cursor only, or both arm and cursor) and the timing of the visual feedback (either during or preceding the task). Accuracy improved when concurrent visual feedback on both arm and cursor was provided. Viewing the cursor alone provided feedback relative to target accuracy; seeing the arm alone required a complex corrective action, as the target was not visible in the work space. Individuals who had vision of the limb before but not during the movement improved movement duration and diminished directional error. However, these effects were not retained for more than a few minutes unless vision of the arm was restored. Ghez and colleagues (1995) suggested that vision of the limb was used to update internal models of the movement by providing orientation of the limb at rest and dynamic information when the limb moved. Vision of the cursor provided information about the dynamic properties of the limb and its response to neural commands. In the absence of proprioceptive information, individuals relied on concurrent visual feedback for accurate reaching; visual feedback provided before the movement was insufficient to sustain improved performance. Although the absence or impairment of proprioception permits an opportunity to examine movement planning in an environment more dependent on vision, it is likely that planning efficacy is enhanced when all sensory modalities are intact.

Vision and Movement Planning in Nonhuman Primates

In experiments involving human participants, our understanding of the role of the visual system relies strongly on inferences from empirically derived hypotheses. In contrast, the study of vision and movement planning in nonhuman primates provides a rich source of information about the biological substrates underpinning the neural mechanisms of vision and the ways in which these mechanisms interconnect with neural mechanisms of movement preparation. An obvious caveat is that it is difficult to know how the results from thousands of practice trials on relatively simple (in human terms) tasks performed by monkeys equate to the performance of significantly fewer practice trials on relatively complex aiming tasks delivered by humans. Additionally, when human or monkey electrophysiological data are interpreted as representative of behavioral phenomena, significant challenges arise. What do deciding, choosing, and acting look like at the level of neurons and synapses? In an excellent review, Schall (2001) suggested that deciding, choosing, and acting are properties of the work of the brain and may involve several cerebral cortical areas and subcortical structures. In laying the groundwork for mapping neural action to behavior, Schall provided helpful operational definitions of *choice, decision*, and *action* which are all terms closely allied to the processes underlying movement planning or motor preparation. Schall's thesis is that in order for biologists and behaviorists to have meaningful discourse about motor preparation, they need to have a mutually acceptable understanding of important terms. *Choice* is defined as "an overt action performed in the context of alternatives for which explanations in terms of purposes can be given." *Decision*, specifically in terms of deciding to do something, is associated with "the preceding deliberation about the alternatives." Therefore, deciding in Schall's context comes before choosing. *Action*, when it is purposeful as opposed to incidental, is characterized by "reference to an intelligible plan" and goal direction (Schall, 2001, pp. 33-34).

The idea expressed by Robert Porter (1987) that the whole brain can be regarded as the organ of movement is exemplified by the diversity of brain regions associated with movement planning. Comment in this chapter is restricted to involvement of the visual system and limited to aiming tasks involving the upper limbs and tasks that involve saccadic eye movement. This task distinction is important as it appears that brain areas associated with saccadic eye movement may or may not be involved (or studied in parallel) in other aiming tasks. The now classic work on movement planning in monkeys conducted by Georgopoulos and colleagues (e.g., Georgopoulos, Ashe, Smyrnis, & Taira, 1992; Georgopoulos, Crutcher, & Schwartz, 1989; Georgopoulos, Kalaska, Caminiti, & Massey, 1982) demonstrated that single neurons in the arm area of the primary motor cortex show firing rates that are contingent on the direction of the planned movement. Upon examining the recordings from many cells, these researchers discovered that the aggregate firing rate results in a population vector representing the preferred direction for different groups of neurons. An important finding was that the neuronal population vector points in the direction of the movement to be initiated and thus clearly represents the outcome of movement planning. Given that the primary motor cortex is identified as the source of the final common pathway (Sherrington, 1947), it can be assumed that other brain regions projecting to the primary motor cortex may be involved in movement planning. For example, it has been reported, based on single-cell recordings in monkeys, that many neurons in the basal ganglia (specifically the putamen, caudate, and globus pallidus) are preferentially active during motor preparation in a precued reaching task and are time locked to movement initiation (Jaeger, Gilman, & Aldridge, 1993). Single-cell recordings have also defined a reach region in the parietal cortex (Gail & Andersen, 2006). Activity in neurons in prefrontal cortex frontal eye fields has been observed; this activity is related to visual input and specific to the delay between stimulus onset and movement initiation, although the association was described as weak (Sommer & Wurtz, 2001). In a visuospatial-delayed matching to sample go, no go task, single-cell recordings from the DLPFC indicated that 90% of the preferentially active neurons display a tuning function related to the specific location of the visual cue (Sawaguchi & Yamane, 1999). Compte and coworkers (2003) recorded activity from neurons in the DLPFC, obtaining recordings from 229 neurons in four macaque monkeys during performance of an oculomotor delayed-response task. Their results indicated that during the mnemonic delay the variability in the interspike interval is greater than it is during the fixation cue regardless of the remembered cue. These researchers (2003) suggested that highly irregular prefrontal activity is consistent with the dynamics of working memory.

This diversity in brain regions demonstrating visuomotor selective changes in activity supports the caveat regarding single-entity representation for visuomotor planning. Adding confusion to the debate is the observation that in the nonhuman primate literature studies on saccadic eye movement represent a unique area of research, and yet saccadic eye movement is not always controlled or accounted for in human studies of vision and planning. The extent to which planning or production of saccadic eye movements can be taken to represent motor preparation is unclear despite informative research proposing control of such movements as a model of neural control of voluntary movement (Hanes & Schall, 1996; Mazzoni, Bracewell, Barash, & Andersen, 1996). One reason for a lack of clarity is that the neural circuitry subserving saccadic eye movement may be different from and not dependent on the proposed circuitry underlying the two–visual systems hypothesis that has provided the rationale for many, primarily human, studies of visuomotor planning and motor preparation (Coles, 1997).

Generally, there appears to be a lack of agreement over which brain systems provide neural control of saccadic eye movements: Hanes and Schall (1996) base their model of the control of voluntary initiation of saccades in the neural circuits of the frontal eye fields in the frontal cortex, whereas Mazzoni and colleagues (1996) locate motor planning of intentional saccadic eye movement in the lateral intraparietal area and posterior parietal cortex (the latter is also part of the dorsal stream in the two–visual systems model). Abstract phenomena such as planning and preparation and—dare we say it—programming remain elusive in terms of identifying brain areas specific to their functional outcomes. According to Desmurget, Pelisson, Rossetti, and Prablanc (1998), a general theoretical model is unlikely to be forthcoming because the central nervous system can resort to numerous strategies for encoding target location and planning hand displacement. In contrast, identification of neuron-specific activity associated with specific movement parameters such as direction and force is unequivocal.

Vision, Movement Planning, and Memory

In one sense memory or memorization is an ubiquitous phenomenon associated with movement planning and with vision. When feedback is manipulated as part of the experimental design, the results of its withdrawal or elimination imply that performance outcomes are dependent on existing or advance knowledge of the task requirements. In turn, this knowledge is dependent on stored representation of the response or stored information about how the response should be executed. Furthermore, when a precue paradigm is used to provide the performer with selective, partial information, such as the direction or extent of the upcoming response, the performer must remember the precued information and link it with the remaining information specified in the stimulus in order to initiate the correct response. In some circumstances (which we discuss more fully toward the end of this chapter) a visual precue can contain the complete set of response parameters (e.g., the limb being moved and the direction and extent of the movement). Such circumstances create a simple RT (SRT) situation. In this situation the only uncertainty for the participant is the exact time at which the imperative stimulus will occur. However, consider the following scenario: Suppose the experimenter decides to manipulate the duration of the precue so that in one condition it remains illuminated for 500 ms followed by the remainder of the time preceding the imperative stimulus and in the other condition the precue remains available until the imperative stimulus occurs. Will there be any difference in the time required to initiate the response (i.e., the SRT)? Remember, whether it's presented continuously or for 500 ms, the precue contains all the information needed for preparation and planning of the visuomotor response, and therefore the precue provides the same information in both conditions. A reasonable prediction is that SRT is unaffected.

Memory-Guided Reaching

Digby Elliott and many of his colleagues (Binsted, Rolheiser, & Chua, 2006; Elliott & Calvert, 1990; Heath, 2005; Heath, Westwood, & Binsted, 2004; see also chapter 5) have extensively researched questions about vision and movement planning that frequently include memory-related issues. Elliott and Calvert (1990) questioned whether the representation of the movement to be performed includes the whole movement environment or just the position of the single target—the outcome goal of the response preparation process. In their study, they manipulated the target uncertainty and the amount of visual information provided before and during an aiming movement. They reported that under conditions in which vision was occluded, even presenting a brief visual representation of the target was sufficient to guide movement.

In examining the planning of reaching movements to visual targets, McIntyre, Stratta, and Lacquaniti (1998) hypothesized that such movements depend on short-term memory. To test their hypothesis, they had participants point to a target (a sphere 44 mm in diameter) with either the left or the right hand. The study included two lighting conditions (dim light or total darkness) and variable delay periods (0.5, 5.0, or 8.0 s). The researchers reported the outcome as a three-dimensional error score in terms of constant error and variable error. Error increased as a consequence of the increased delay and the lighting condition. In total darkness both magnitude and direction error increased with longer delays; in the dim light only magnitude error increased as the delay lengthened. McIntyre and coworkers concluded that distance information and direction information are stored separately in short-term memory and that separate reference frames serve the eyes and the effector (the arm in this case).

Heath and colleagues (2004) also investigated memory-guided reaching movements, paying particular attention to regression-based serial measures of the coefficient of determination (r^2) in determining the variance accounted for by changes in spatial position at peak velocity, peak acceleration, peak deceleration, and end-point accuracy. They concluded that errors in planning are not corrected during the course of the action, leaving open the question of whether stored target information is used to correct planning or whether there are errors in the stored target information that in turn are reflected in the memory-guided reaching movement. Krigolson and Heath (2004) focused on background visual cues in their study of memory-guided reaching. They illuminated the background to the target area with LEDs to highlight the allocentric reference frame. In the nonvisual background condition only the target was illuminated. Three target locations in the midline were located near, middle, and far, and the visual conditions included visually guided (target remained lit) and open-loop movements, with responses initiated at a delay of either 0 or 1 s. When the visual background was present, participants were more accurate and less variable, but their MT was longer, demonstrating increased time in the deceleration phase of the movement and possibly indicating online corrections to the trajectory. Furthermore, when visual feedback was accompanied by visual guidance to the target end-point, variability (variability within the target location) was diminished.

In a later follow-up experiment, Heath (2005) examined the role of vision of the limb, the target, or both in online control of memory-guided reaching. He proposed that visually guided reaching is characterized by performance structured to take advantage of visual information within the reaching environment. He predicted a longer time following peak velocity accompanied by more discrete movement corrections (implying an essential role for end-point vision) and hypothesized that vision of the limb is necessary for improving reaching accuracy. Heath (2005) also proposed that such online control of visually, memory-guided reaches is mediated by the dorsal visual pathway and that a real-time visuomotor mechanism could reside in the posterior parietal cortex. Whether this brain region is hemispherically specific was not indicated. Heath hypothesized that if the whole reaching movement is preplanned, then R^2 in the early (peak acceleration), middle (peak velocity), and later (peak deceleration) stages of the reach should be equally robust. Participants were instructed to make their responses as fast and accurately as possible under conditions in which vision of the limb was allowed or occluded. There was no difference in RT between the two conditions. A mean RT of 200 ms indicated that responses are likely prepared in advance; MT was slower for the vision condition than for the occluded vision condition. Heath inferred that the stored representation engages vision of the limb in completing the response. This inference was based in part on the observation that accuracy was significantly greater and variability was less when vision of the limb was available. When vision of the limb was occluded, constant error was significantly greater as reflected in undershooting.

Binsted and colleagues (2006) extended the question of visuomotor representation of manual aiming by examining performance in a reciprocal tapping task. They proposed that vision of both the limb and the environment (point-of-light targets) is necessary for accurate spatial performance and that both feed-forward and feedback mechanisms are involved, with vision being essential for updating the change in environment and for error handling during the continuous alternating movements. Participants were asked to perform 72 trials of reciprocal tapping of two targets 30 cm apart for 11 s. In each 11 s trial the point-of-light targets were illuminated for the initial 5 s. Thus subjects were required to maintain their tapping performance during seconds 6 through 11 although the targets were unlit. Average MT was 304 ms and end-point variability increased after the targets were removed. The increase in end-point variability occurred even though vision of the moving limb was unaffected, implying that continuation of accurate performance was dependent on visual information about the targets. One explanation for the loss of accuracy after removal of the targets is that removing the targets disrupted information available to the ventral visual stream.

In a novel experiment, Westwood, McEachern, and Roy (2001) studied grasping of a Müller-Lyer figure in order to elucidate the role of visual feedback and the effect of delaying visual feedback. Two forms of the Müller-Lyer illusion (arrows in or arrows out) were grasped under four vision conditions: full, open loop, brief delay, and 2,000 ms delay. The effect (estimation of object size) of the Müller-Lyer illusion was greater in the open-loop and delay conditions than it was in the closed-loop condition, but the former conditions did not differ from each other. This suggests that the absence of vision rather than the time without vision was the determining factor. A smaller effect was observed in the full-vision condition and illustrates the importance of online visual feedback. In a further exploration of the influence of visuomotor memory on reaching, Westwood, Heath, and Roy (2003) asked participants to reach for one of three possible targets. The study employed the four vision conditions described for the previous experiment but with modifications. In all conditions, participants saw the cued target for 2,000 ms. In the open-loop condition, vision was occluded at movement onset. In the brief delay condition, vision was occluded immediately following the cue and before the go signal. In the 500 ms delay condition, the target environment was displayed for 2,000 ms and occluded for 500 ms before the target cue and go signal. The 2,000 ms delay condition was the same as the 500 ms condition but featured a longer (2,000 ms) occlusion. Performance in the open-loop condition was characterized by overshoot errors, whereas performance in the delay conditions resulted in reduced error but greater end-point variability. No evidence of a speed–accuracy trade-off was reported. As in their previous study, Westwood and colleagues (2003) concluded that the visuomotor system operates in real time because under occlusion conditions, participants were unable to take advantage of the precued information specific to the target. Whether such effects are sensitive to the amount of practice or the specificity of the instructions given to participants was not broached.

Memory Mechanisms and Planning

How does a person remember the location of a target and how to move the limb to reach that target? What is the effect of the temporal delay between seeing what to do and subsequently doing it? It has been suggested (Heath & Westwood, 2003) that stored representations are useful only if the memory delay is minimal. This suggestion implies that the decay of information is not offset by rehearsal of the displayed task requirements. Heath and Westwood noted that diminished accuracy and increased variability are a consequence of increased memory delay. Lemay, Bertram, and Stelmach (2004) suggested that the memory coding (the storage mechanism) of target representations typical of pointing movements involves three sources of information: (1) egocentric references, or information from the body (including eye, shoulder, and hand references); (2) allocentric references, or visual cues from the surroundings independent of the body; and (3) both egocentric and allocentric references. They argued that an allocentric memory-coding mechanism is potentially more flexible, as it doesn't require the constancy implied in the relationships between body part location and target location. Lemay and colleagues investigated whether allocentric or egocentric references best serve memory coding by having participants localize, memorize, and reach to one of six target locations under three context conditions. The target was a fluorescent dowel that could be positioned at one of the six locations on a template. Context conditions included (1) no context (the target appeared alone in the dark), (2) stationary context (the target was surrounded by an illuminated square), and (3) moving context (the illuminated square moved between the initial view and the recall). Error was greatest in the no-context condition and similar for the stationary and moving contexts, both of which had strong allocentric representations. Thus Lemay and colleagues (2004) concluded that an allocentric reference serves as a preferred code source for memorizing pointing movements even when both egocentric and allocentric frames of reference are available. The notion of multiple frames of reference serving a memory mechanism for pointing to remembered targets was further reviewed by Lemay and Stelmach (2005). These researchers were interested in determining whether humans use a hand-centered egocentric frame, an eye-centered egocentric frame, or both to construct a memory representation of the target. The task was to locate, memorize, and point to a target in a dark environment. During the delay interval (before pointing to the remembered target), participants were instructed to move either their hand or their eyes in order to disrupt hand-centered and eye-centered memory of the target, respectively. The outcome measure was variability of movement amplitude and movement direction. Perturbing hand movement affected direction error while perturbing eye movement affected amplitude error, a finding that prompted the authors to conclude that pointing amplitude is represented via an eye-centered frame of reference while direction of pointing is associated with a hand-centered frame of reference. It is tempting to suggest that the latter conclusion is analogous to the cortical motor neuronal cell mapping of movement direction preference reported by Georgopoulos and colleagues (Georgopoulos et al., 1989; Georgopoulos et al., 1982), although doing so is perhaps reaching too far! Generalizing from motor cortex single-cell recordings in monkeys who have practiced hundreds (possibly thousands) of trials to humans who have performed one or two experimental sessions containing relatively few trials and often many conditions is tenuous.

From a slightly different perspective, Trommershäuser, Mattis, Maloney, and Landy (2006) probed the limits of human movement planning by varying the time at which visual feedback was provided during the task. They had observed that in tasks where the outcome results in reward or penalty, humans maximize gain by employing speed and accuracy strategies. The researchers noted that this strategy is also employed when reward (payoff) information is not provided before stimulus onset as long as the information is provided 200 to 400 ms before the end of the movement. This observation seems to rule out performance characterized by ballistic, completely preprogrammed responses. In their experiment, Trommershäuser and colleagues required participants to hit a target without hitting a penalty region surrounding the target. The penalty region was displayed 0, 200, or 400 ms after illumination of the target region (which was also the cue to initiate the response). RT (median RT = 200 ms) was unaffected when the delayed display of the penalty region occurred at 0 or 200 ms, and it was suggested that an optimal response planning strategy was maintained despite the unpredictable time of delivery of the visual feedback. When the penalty region was not displayed until 400 ms following the target region, performance was compromised, as was demonstrated by the migration of the mean movement end point closer to the penalty region. The authors concluded that as long as relevant visual feedback came between 200 and 400 ms before the end of movement it could contribute to the movement plan even though the movement had been initiated. This interpretation implies that the movement planning process is dynamic and can incorporate information that becomes available after the plan is hatched. This idea was supported independently by Vaziri, Diedrichsen, and Shadmehr (2006) in a study that examined why the brain predicts sensory consequences of oculomotor commands associated with the generation of saccadic eye movements. According to Vaziri and colleagues (2006), the brain generates a copy (an internal estimate generated by a process called *remapping)* of the new retinal location following a saccade to a target even though the target remains visible after the saccade. It is thought that the brain integrates information about target location from two sources—the remapping and the peripheral view of the target—and that this dual source of information reduces variability in the estimate of both the target location and the required trajectory of the saccade to reach the target. Thus relying on a dual source of information is more reliable than using a single information source.

Precuing, Memory, and Movement Planning

Even when participants know precisely what they are required to do before an imperative stimulus arrives, fast and accurate performance is not guaranteed. If such were the case, it would signal a victory for proponents of strong motor programming, who argue that the entire response is prepared in advance and unaltered by concurrent feedback. A wealth of studies reviewed in this chapter does not support this outcome. Even the start performance of a world-class sprinter (an example in which the only uncertainty is when the gun will sound) as measured in SRT to the stimulus is prone to error (Gleick, 1999)—not only do some sprinters jump the gun by overanticipating the arrival of the imperative stimulus but also correct performances vary by tens of milliseconds, which is enough to significantly affect the final outcome of a 100 m sprint. Although the sprinter has all the information about the start of the event except the exact arrival time of the stimulus, there is still a memory-related element inextricably associated with the movement planning process preceding the sound of the gun. The memory-related element underpins the rationale for practicing the start (or any motor skill for that matter). Why should an individual practice the start if there are no flow-on benefits from the practice? For practice to be beneficial, its effect must be able to be drawn on at some time in the future and thus it must be retained over time—it must be remembered. The nature of memory has occupied the thoughts and doings of scientists for centuries. In relatively modern times, Hebb (1949) advanced the theory of cell assemblies, collections of neurons whose synapses are modified with practice and whose synaptic efficacy represents remembered performance. This theory has persisted and continues to be researched in questions addressing long-term potentiation (LTP) and long-term depression (LTD), markers of structural and functional change (plasticity and metaplasticity) in the activity of single nerve cells and groups of nerve cells (see, for example, Abraham & Bear, 1996; Bliss & Collingridge, 1993; Reynolds, Hyland, & Wickens, 2001).

In the domain of movement planning, the brain mechanisms underlying motor preparation have remained elusive, although evidence supporting specific structural links includes the two–visual system notion (Goodale & Milner, 1992; Goodale et al., 2003) and direction-specific neuron activity in the primary motor cortex (Georgopoulos et al., 1992, 1989, 1982). In an intriguing experiment, Smyrnis, Taira, Ashe, and Georgopoulos (1992) recorded motor cortical activity from single neurons and measured RT in two monkeys performing a memorized delay task. In the delay task, a cue (300 ms) signalled the location of one of eight targets arranged in an octagonal display centered on the start position. The monkeys held a manipulandum over the start position, which was illuminated when the manipulandum was in the correct starting location. Following the cuing of a single target and a variable delay (450-1,050 ms), the start position light was extinguished and served as an imperative stimulus for the monkey to move the manipulandum to the cued target as quickly and accurately as possible in order to receive a juice reward. Memorization was manipulated such that in one condition the cued target remained lit until the monkey moved the manipulandum to it (a nonmemorized delay task) and in another condition the cued target was lit for 300 ms before the delay interval and the monkey was required to remember the location of the target until the imperative stimulus occurred (a memorized delay task). Given that the precue provided all the necessary information about the task except for the timing of the stimulus, it can be argued that both the nonmemorized and the memorized conditions are SRT tasks (just like the task of the sprinter in the blocks waiting for the gun). Therefore a difference in RT might not be expected. However, Smyrnis and coworkers (1992) reported that RT in the memorized delay condition was shorter than RT in the nonmemorized delay condition. During the memorized delay the change in the population vector of the cortical neurons occurred earlier accompanied by a larger magnitude of change in the vector associated with the target direction, a finding that supports the RT result. The results of this study appear to contradict many of the studies demonstrating a dependence on real-time visual feedback for optimal performance. However, in the majority of these studies performance measures (e.g., end-point error or variability) were outcome related rather than estimates of the speed of planning, as is inferred from RT measures. Nonetheless, a contradiction remains in that the results from Smyrnis and coworkers indicated that a monkey's performance was faster (better) under conditions in which vision of the target was not enhanced.

We were intrigued by the results of Smyrnis and colleagues (1992), particularly the RT results indicating that when memorization is required and presumably the brain has to work harder, preparation time and response initiation are faster. A similar study of age-matched subjects with and without Parkinson's disease reported no difference in RT between memorized and nonmemorized delay conditions of a three-target task (Labutta, Miles, Sanes, & Hallett, 1994). However, significant methodological differences between the studies hindered close comparison of the results with those of Smyrnis and colleagues (1992). In a series of studies (Jordan, Hyland, Wickens, & Anson, 2005; Mohagheghi, Anson, Hyland, Parr-Brownlie, & Wickens, 1998; Parr-Brownlie, Wickens, Anson, & Hyland, 1998) we attempted to replicate the results of Labutta and colleagues (1994) and Smyrnis and colleagues (1992) with experiments involving human subjects. Mohagheghi and coworkers (1998) required participants to use a forearm supination and pronation movement to position a pointer to one of four targets. The targets were arranged in an arc, with two targets to the left (pronation) and two to the right (supination) of a central LED. In an attempt to replicate the results of Labutta and colleagues, Mohagheghi and coworkers used a similar foreperiod schedule of 3, 5, and 9 s in one condition and a schedule of 1, 2, and 3 s (1 s being inclusive of the delay duration used by Smyrnis and colleagues) in a second condition. Both conditions included blocks of memorized and nonmemorized delay trials. There was no difference between the two memory delay conditions in either schedule. However, RT in the long schedule was significantly longer than RT in the short schedule. Furthermore, within each schedule, the RT to the shortest foreperiod (1 and 3 s for the shortest and longest schedules, respectively) was associated with a significantly longer RT. Perhaps as a consequence, RT to the 3 s foreperiod was 85 to 100 ms shorter when it was the longest foreperiod in the short schedule compared with being the shortest foreperiod in the long schedule. In terms of movement planning, these results indicate that a long (3-9 s) interval between the cue and the eventual stimulus onset may result in decay of the prepared motor response. This decay diminishes optimal preparation and, within a foreperiod schedule, RT to the shortest foreperiod is likely to be longer. This is not explained by a foreperiod aging factor, as RT to the middle and longest foreperiod in each schedule did not differ significantly. Another point to consider is that in this study even the shortest foreperiod (1 s) was close to the upper limit of the distribution of foreperiods used by Smyrnis and coworkers (1992). In a follow-up study Parr-Brownlie and colleagues (1998) used a similar task and replicated the foreperiod and memorization delay design used by Smyrnis and coworkers (1992). They found that RT in the nonmemorized delay task was significantly shorter than RT in the memorized delay task, a result opposite of that reported by Smyrnis and coworkers. In one sense the results have intuitive appeal; the nonmemorized delay task provided constant illumination of the cued target and likely enhanced the visual feedback of the movement environment. However, the experiment was a less-than-true replication of the Smyrnis and colleagues study because the display comprised only four targets and the motor response was restricted to simple pronation and supination of the forearm. To address this issue, Jordan and colleagues (2005) constructed an apparatus to mimic the task requirements in the Smyrnis and colleagues experiments. Eight targets formed a circular display with the start position located in the center. Each target was formed by an LED-illuminated spring-loaded microswitch. The start position was also a switch that was illuminated (by an LED) when depressed by the participant's right index finger. The go signal was the center LED being extinguished. These results indicated once again that RT is significantly shorter in the nonmemorized delay condition. The results could not be explained by a speed–accuracy trade-off, as MT was also significantly faster in the nonmemorized delay condition. It is possible that these results represent a species difference. Perhaps in monkeys the memorized delay task increases arousal and attention, which in turn has a positive effect on preparation and facilitates faster response initiation.

Theleritis, Smyrnis, Mantas, and Evdokimidis (2004) adopted a different approach to precuing, memory, and performance of reaching movements. They examined the effect of memory load on directional accuracy by serially presenting 2, 3, or 4 targets (from a set of 16 possible targets) followed by a cue (one of the targets in the presented set) signaling the subject to move to the target that would have appeared next in the set. Directional accuracy diminished as the size of the set of possible targets increased. Not surprisingly, RT also increased as the set size increased. Thus memory load as well as memorization altered both movement planning time and accuracy of performance. In a related experiment Pellizzer, Hedges, and Villaneuva (2006) investigated the effects that the amount of information and the time available to use the information have on RT as an index of the speed of planning directed movements. Generally RT increased when the number of distractors (possible target locations other than the one that was cued) presented in the cue period increased, especially when the cue period was short (100-800 ms). The effect of distractor cues was not different for cue durations varying between 800 and 1,600 ms. Thus both the amount of information to be processed (or filtered) and the duration available for preparation affected movement planning as measured by RT.

Summary and Future Directions

The interaction among vision (and visual feedback), memory, precuing, and time available for movement planning produces a range of possible effects on the speed and accuracy of performance and motor preparation. The sometimes obvious and other times very subtle differences in the specific task demands and multitude of experimental designs are one source of difficulty in coming to grips with this diverse literature. In general, movement planning appears to be more effective in the presence of real-time visual feedback, especially if the performance measure is associated with accuracy and outcome variability. In many studies focusing on speed of preparation, trials that result in performance errors are discarded as though the error was in some way intentional. Perhaps it would be valuable for experimenters, especially those focusing on movement planning and speeded response initiation, to view data from error trials as a separate analysis that could inform the literature on movement planning.

When considering future directions in the area of vision and movement planning in the context of goal-directed action, one advantage we have is that we can speculate without constraint! If, in a cricket match, a top-class batsman faces a first-rate bowler, it appears that both performers engage vision in the process of planning their movements. Yet even with 20/20 vision, the batsman in particular is limited not by the quality and quantity of visual information but by the speed and efficiency of his own biology, whether it be in reacting and moving or in processing the remembered and instantaneous online visual information. In our laboratory a significant research focus is on trying to describe the underlying mechanisms that might explain how goal-directed action is planned. Naturally, these mechanisms are underpinned by the biology of the organism—we are especially interested in the work of the brain and muscles in this regard. From a measurement perspective, real-time electromyography (EMG), electroencephalography (EEG), and TMS offer a powerful suite of tools with which to address questions of how the brain controls movement. Until now the application of these tools has been limited to laboratory-type tasks and as such has been met with valid criticism in terms of authenticity and relevance to real-world visuomotor tasks.

In the future such criticism may well be muted. Virtual reality through Xbox and PlayStation has enabled us to bring goal-directed action into the laboratory (and living room or den). If they can be appropriately interfaced to EEG, EMG, and TMS, these simulation devices offer opportunities to investigate in depth the junction between the biology of the performer and the performance environment. Furthermore, coupling virtual reality simulators to high-resolution instruments could allow goal-directed action to be examined in ways similar to those used to assess airline pilot training. This raises the intriguing question of whether the top-class batsman would be able to improve visuomotor performance by practicing on a cricket test simulator.

At a more fundamental level, research on vision and movement planning could be advanced by giving consideration to the entire visual system, including saccadic eye movement along with the two visual systems. Given existing evidence indicating that the eyes lead the hands, the role of saccadic eye movement must be incorporated into any new model of vision and action.

In sum, the future for research in vision and movement planning is both challenging and exciting. Closer coupling of biology and behavior to address system and performance questions and employment of virtual reality and movement-specific simulators to address questions of visuomotor skill development and enhancement will be at the forefront.

CHAPTER 5

Memory-Guided Reaching: What the Visuomotor System Knows and How Long It Knows It

MATTHEW HEATH, KRISTINA A. NEELY, OLAV KRIGOLSON, AND GORDON BINSTED

Reaching to or grasping a target is not limited by the ability to see that target. Indeed, you are likely able to grasp your morning cup of coffee with remarkable precision and without fear of scalding your hand all while keeping your eyes on this text (i.e., perform a memory-guided action). Of course, the ability to grasp the unseen cup must be supported by obligatory (previous) knowledge of its location, and, as such, is likely to draw upon visual inputs that are distinct from grasping a visible cup (i.e., visually guided or closed-loop action). This chapter contrasts visually guided and memory-guided responses and provides a basis for understanding how performers interact with targets that are not seen. Our goals for this chapter are threefold. First, we outline behavioral work on the temporal persistence of the visual information supporting memory-guided actions. Second, we draw upon clinical neuropsychology, neuroimaging, and behavioral work to provide a functional distinction between the visual information supporting visually guided actions and the visual information supporting memory-guided actions. Third, we examine whether the novelty or the visuomotor uncertainty attached to a movement environment affects the timeline by which stored target information is used to support the

This work was supported by a Natural Sciences and Engineering Research Council of Canada Discovery Grant and a Petro-Canada Young Innovator Award to MH.

sensorimotor transformation underlying motor output. At the end of the chapter we introduce work employing the Bereitschaftspotential and the reafferente potentiale as a means to correlate active electrophysiological processes in premotor and primary motor cortical areas to the behavioral antecedents of memory-guided actions.

The Temporal Durability of Stored Target Information

In his classic 1899 work, R.S. Woodworth made a notable observation on our ability to interact with an object without directly looking at it. He aptly developed this notion in his commentary on dyads of highly skilled workmen who, using hammers to drive hand drills, rarely (if ever) missed the target (i.e., the hand drill) and frequently completed a discrete response without directly viewing the target. Woodworth speculated that response accuracy in the absence of vision is driven by a kinesthetic sense of the serial action; however, he also commented that accuracy is in part driven by a visual memory of target location. Thus, a logical question derived from Woodworth's latter point is how long a stored sensory-based (specifically, visually based) target representation can persist in memory and be used to support motor output.

The first systematic examination of the temporal durability of the stored target information supporting reaching movements was undertaken by Elliott and coworkers (e.g., Elliott, 1988; Elliott & Calvert, 1990; Elliott, Calvert, Jaeger, & Jones, 1990; Elliott and Madalena, 1987; for review see Elliott, 1990).[1] In particular, Elliott and Madalena examined the accuracy of reaches performed in three visual conditions: (1) a visible limb and target throughout a movement (visually guided or closed-loop reaching), (2) occlusion of limb and target vision at movement onset (open-loop reaching), and (3) occlusion of limb and target vision 2,000, 5,000, and 10,000 ms before response cuing (memory-guided reaching). As expected, closed-loop reaches were more accurate than their open-loop counterparts (Adamovich, Berkinblit, Fookson, & Poizner, 1994; Elliott & Allard, 1985; Keele & Posner, 1968), and total end-point error was greater for the memory-guided reaches than it was for open-loop reaches. Given these data, Elliott and Madalena proposed that highly accurate stored target information is available to the motor system for up to 2,000 ms for "online error reduction during the movement" (p. 36). Indeed, Elliott and Madalena's results are cited frequently in the current visuomotor control literature and have been interpreted as indicating that, for delays less than 2,000 ms, stored target information provides an equivalent substitute for direct target vision (e.g., Glover, 2004; Hu, Eagleson, & Goodale, 1999; Hu and Goodale, 2000; Milner, Paulignan, Dijkerman, Michel, & Jeannerod, 1999).

The literature's interpretation of Elliott and Madalena's (1987) results is intriguing; however, strong support for this assertion requires a demonstration that memory-guided actions are as accurate as open-loop responses are for a sufficiently brief delay (see also Elliott & Calvert, 1990). Recall that in the Elliott and Madalena study, the shortest memory delay was 2,000 ms and the error in that condition was greater than it was in the open-loop condition (the condition in which direct target vision was available during movement planning). In an attempt to examine more directly the time frame by which stored target information is available to the motor system, our group provided the first systematic examinations of the end-point bias (i.e., constant error) and stability (i.e., variable error) characterizing closed-loop and open-loop reaches relative to memory-guided responses following brief and longer delays. In one study (Westwood, Heath, & Roy, 2001), we observed that radial end-point error was significantly greater for open-loop reaches than it was for closed-loop reaches and that error was even greater for delay conditions of 500, 1,000, 1,500, and 2,000 ms (which did not differ from one another). Moreover, a follow-up study contrasting open-loop reaches and memory-guided reaches of 0, 500, and 2,000 ms of delay (Westwood, Heath, & Roy, 2003) showed enhanced target under-shooting and amplified end-point variability across memory conditions versus open-loop conditions (for examples of undershooting bias see also Heath, 2005; Heath & Binsted, 2007). Thus, results from our group show a significant accumulation in end-point error following even the briefest memory delay (i.e., 0 ms), a result countering the claim that veridical stored target information is available to the motor system for any appreciable length of time following visual occlusion.

One direct interpretation from Elliott and Madalena's (1987) study that has proved to be particularly robust relates to the ability of stored target information to persist in memory for considerable delay durations (up to 10,000 ms; Lemay & Proteau, 2001), though this information provides a less accurate referent relative to continuous target vision. In fact, most of the work completed by our group has shown that the accuracy of memory-guided responses does not diminish over increasing visual delays (i.e., <5,000 ms; Westwood et al., 2001; Heath, 2005; Heath & Binsted, 2007; Heath & Westwood, 2003; Heath, Westwood, & Binsted, 2004). What has been found to change, however, is the spatial variability of movement end points, an observation that demonstrates amplification over delays. Thus, results for end-point accuracy and variability support the contention that stored target information provides the motor system with a reasonably accurate and temporally durable—albeit unstable—substitute for direct target vision. As discussed in the following section, we believe that the ability of stored target information to be maintained across considerable delays, as well as the performance features characterizing this ability (i.e., increased error and end-point variability), reflects the use of a visual processing stream that is functional and anatomically distinct from closed-loop actions (Goodale & Milner, 1992).

Visual Awareness and the Evocation of Visually Guided and Memory-Guided Reaches

What is the nature of the visual information used to support goal-directed actions? Do visually derived (visually guided and open-loop) and memory-guided responses rely on dissociable visual resources? Considering the nature of the visual information supporting visually derived actions, it is often thought that obligatory introspection of a target is required to complete a successful response. After all, the percept of a target (e.g., the impression of its size, shape, and texture) permeates the successful completion of visually defined actions. Interestingly, however, ample evidence indicates that awareness is not a prerequisite of visually derived actions. Indeed, a striking dissociation between awareness and action is demonstrated in individuals with action blindsight (for review see Danckert & Rossetti, 2005; Weiskrantz, 2008). Action blindsight is a neurological disorder in which individuals with damage to the primary visual cortex (V1) lack the ability to consciously perceive or identify objects in their contralesional visual field. In spite of the inability to access or develop conscious target information, individuals with action blindsight are able to track and point to visually defined targets in their scotoma (for the classic report of patient D.B. see Weiskrantz, Warrington, Sanders, & Marshall, 1974). A more subtle demonstration of action without awareness is associated with damage to the inferotemporal cortex (James, Culham, Humphrey, Milner, & Goodale, 2003). A particular example is provided by patient D.F., who exhibits a striking deficit in perceiving the orientation of a target as well as identifying line forms (i.e., visual form agnosia). Interestingly, however, D.F. is able to interact appropriately with a visible target (for review see Goodale & Milner, 1992) and can automatically adjust her limb trajectory to accommodate obstacles to her movement path (Rice, McIntosh, Schindler, Mon-Williams, Démonet, & Milner, 2006). Further supporting the notion of dissociable conscious awareness and visuomotor control are studies involving individuals with optic ataxia, a visual deficit arising from lesions to the posterior parietal cortex (PPC; for review see Milner, Dijkerman, McIntosh, Rossetti, & Pisella, 2003). Individuals in this group are able to identify targets within their visual fields but demonstrate early and late movement planning errors in visually guided actions directed to those same objects. Thus, evidence from the clinical neuropsychology literature indicates that visually derived responses operate without explicit perceptual awareness of extrinsic and intrinsic target features.

A basis for understanding the separation between visual awareness and motor output is rooted in Goodale and Milner's influential perception–action model (PAM; Goodale & Milner, 1992). Specifically, the PAM asserts that projections from V1 to the inferotemporal cortex comprise a conscious visuoperceptual network termed the *ventral visual pathway*. The ventral visual pathway plays the major role in building a stable perceptual representation of our visual world and thus allows for the recognition of objects. In contrast, V1 projections, or extrangeniculate projections, from the pulvinar to the PPC comprise dedicated visuomotor networks termed the *dorsal visual pathway* (Felleman & Van Essen, 1991). According to the PAM, the dorsal visual pathway relies on euclidean object features and does not require a conscious visual percept for movement planning or control. Thus, in the face of impaired visuoperceptual abilities, the PAM predicts that individuals with action blindsight or visual agnosia can retain specific visuomotor abilities because the structural deficits characterizing the aforementioned do not affect the integrity of visual inputs to the dorsal visual pathway.

Action without awareness, and thus support for the theoretical tenets of the PAM, is also observed in nonclinical populations and has been demonstrated frequently via the double-step paradigm (Bridgeman, Lewis, Heit, & Nagle, 1979; Goodale, Pelisson, Prablanc, 1986). In the double-step paradigm, participants orient their visual gaze to a home position before receiving an imperative to initiate a goal-directed response to a visible target. On a limited and unexpected number of trials, the position of the target is switched to a new location before or at peak ocular velocity. Because the target's location is altered during peak ocular velocity, saccadic suppression renders participants unable to consciously detect the change in target location. In spite of being unaware of the change in target location, participants modify their reach trajectories to account for the new target position. Moreover, the automatic corrections characterizing the double-step paradigm are disrupted by naturally occurring (optic ataxia) or artificially induced (via TMS) lesions to the PPC (Pisella et al., 2000). Such a pattern of results provides accumulating evidence for the role of the dorsal visual pathway in implicit visuomotor control.

More recent work has shown that unconscious visuomotor processing includes the integration of features more wide ranging than the exogenous change in target location characterizing the double-step paradigm. Indeed, Cressman and coworkers (Cressman, Franks, Enns, & Chua, 2007) reported that unconsciously presented endogenous cues can be integrated and used to evoke online corrections to a masked target location. Moreover, we have shown that an intrinsic object property (i.e., size) can be processed unconsciously and used to support the planning and control of a visually derived reaching task (Binsted, Brownell, Vorontsova, Heath, & Saucier, 2007; see also Heath, Neely, Yakimishyn, & Binsted, 2008). In our work, we used a variant of Di Lollo and colleagues' four-dot object-substitution masking paradigm (Di Lollo, Enns, & Rensink, 2000; for review see Enns & Di Lollo, 2000) and asked participants to complete perceptual reports and reaching responses. In this paradigm, an array of differently sized circles (1.5, 2.5, 3.5, 4.5, and 5.5 cm) are presented rapidly (13 ms) to participants. Within the array a target circle is identified by four small dots (the four-dot mask) that surround but do not touch the target. When the array and four-dot mask disappeared concurrently (i.e., nonmasked trials), participants were able to provide an accurate verbal report of the size of the target circle. When the four-dot mask persisted (for 320 ms) following offset of the array (i.e., masked trials), participants were unable to accurately report target size (i.e., masked trials). According to Di Lollo and colleagues' (2000) computational model of object substitution masking, concurrent blanking of the circles array allows participants to process target information based on a visible persistence maintained at high-level (and conscious) visual processing areas (i.e., the ventral visual pathway). In contrast, when the four-dot mask remains visible following offset of the circles array, reentrant processing of the mask at a low-level visual processing area (V1) conflicts with the visible persistence maintained at high-level visual processing areas. Put another way, persistence of the four-dot mask renders the original stimulus information (i.e., the circles array including the target object) unavailable for conscious verbal report. During the reaching trials, however, participants' trajectories scaled to the veridical size of the target object (see figure 2 of Binsted et al., 2007). MT and peak velocity values increased and decreased, respectively, as a function of increasing target size, a finding directly in line with Fitts' (1954) classic speed–accuracy trade-off. Our results argue, once again, that a conscious visual percept is not required to support the metrical parameterization of a visually derived response.

The PAM holds that dorsal stream information is evanescent and so is used to support motor output only when direct visual input from the movement environment is available at the time of response planning (Westwood & Goodale, 2003). It has been proposed that in the absence of direct visual input, memory-guided responses are mediated by a cognitive representation laid down and maintained by the visuoperceptual networks of the ventral visual pathway. At least three lines of evidence support this view. First, the retained visuomotor abilities characterizing action blindsight and visual agnosia are impaired significantly in the context of memory-guided action. Recall that D.F. elicits metrical scaling of grasp and trajectory parameters when she grasps or reaches to a visible target; however, when vision of a target object is removed before the initiation of a response (e.g., 5,000 ms beforehand), D.F. is no longer able to scale her grasp or trajectory to the size or orientation of the target (Goodale, Jakobson, & Keillor, 1994). Demonstrating a functionally distinct deficit, individuals with optic ataxia exhibit improved trajectory scaling when they use memory-based information to execute their actions (e.g., Milner et al., 2003). For example, Milner and coworkers (Milner et al., 1999) reported that the accuracy of target pointing actually improves for participants with optic ataxia when they reach to a target that has been removed from vision in advance of response cuing (e.g., 5,000 ms in advance; see also Schindler, Rice, McIntosh, Rossetti, Vighetto, & Milner, 2004 for obstacle avoidance behaviors of subjects with optic ataxia). In the former case, memory-guided action is impaired due to ventral stream lesions and the inability to develop or access a memory-based representation for action output. In the latter case, performance during memory-guided action improves because memory-guided responses can bypass, in part, the impaired visuomotor networks of the dorsal visual pathway and access a memory-based target representation laid down and maintained by intact visuoperceptual networks of the ventral visual pathway (see also Himmelbach & Karnath, 2005).

A second line of evidence supporting the putative role of the ventral visual pathway in memory-guided reaching and grasping is provided by neuroimaging and TMS work. Extensive neuroimaging and neurophysiology work reports that dorsal visuomotor networks exhibit reliable activation across visually guided and memory-guided responses (Bueno, Jarvis, Batista, & Andersen, 2002). Such evidence suggests that parietal network activation is not restricted to visually guided responses but instead reflects aggregation of global movement parameters for goal-directed actions in general. However, in a study specifically designed to examine a ventral visual area, Singhal, Kaufman, Valyear, and Culham (2006) found that memory-guided, but not visually guided, actions elicit reactivation of a ventral visual area (i.e., the lateral occipital cortex) at the time of movement cuing. Additionally, Rice and colleagues (Rice, Cross, Tunik, Grafton, & Culham, 2008) applied selective TMS to a dorsal (i.e., the anterior intraparietal sulcus) and ventral (i.e., Lateral occipital complex [LO]) area at, and 100 ms following, the onset of visually guided and memory-guided grasps. In line with the neuroimaging literature, it was found that disrupting the dorsal visuomotor area produced kinematic anomalies (affected maximal grip aperture and velocity of maximal grip aperture) in both conditions. Applying TMS to the ventral visual region, however, selectively disrupted the kinematic specification of memory-guided grasps. A parsimonious explanation for the aforementioned findings is that memory-based information developed and maintained by the ventral visual pathway is used at the time of response cuing as a substitute for direct vision of a target and that such information is combined with additional movement parameters specified by dorsal visuomotor networks. Indeed, the fact that ventral and dorsal visual networks are active during memory-guided actions suggests that the two visual pathways interact via their extensive interconnections (Merigan & Maunsell, 1993) or via independent influences through recurrent projections with the prefrontal cortex (Ungerleider, Courtney, & Haxby, 1998).

The third line of evidence stems from work examining how visually guided and memory-guided responses are influenced by context-dependent illusory or nonillusory geometric structure surrounding a target. Briefly, and as discussed in more detail by Westwood (see chapter 13), evidence suggests that visually guided reaching and grasping responses are refractory to the cognitive properties of pictorial illusions (Aglioti, DeSouza, &

Goodale, 1995; Bridgeman, Peery, & Anand, 1997 ; Haffenden & Goodale, 1998; Heath, Rival, Westwood, & Neely, 2005; Westwood, Heath, & Roy, 2000). This idea, however, is tempered by a growing body of work indicating that pictorial illusions and nonillusory geometric features produce a small but reliable effect on the planning and control of action (Ehresman, Saucier, Heath, & Binsted, 2008; Elliott & Lee, 1995; Heath, Neely, & Binsted, 2007; Neely, Binsted, & Heath, 2008; Neely, Tessmer, Binsted, & Heath, 2008). In spite of the equivocal findings on visually guided actions, the memory-guided reaching and grasping literature provides a clear indication that illusory and nonillusory cues affect the early and late kinematic specification of a response. In demonstration of this issue, our group has shown that memory-guided responses directed to a target surrounded by nonillusory contextual cues produce reach or grasp trajectories with greater online corrections and enhanced end-point accuracy and stability relative to memory-guided reaches performed in a neutral or otherwise empty visual background (Krigolson & Heath, 2004). Furthermore, the proximity of the visual cues to the target provides a more salient benefit to the accuracy of the memory-guided responses than to the accuracy of their visually guided counterparts (Krigolson, Clark, Heath, & Binsted, 2007). Presumably, the fact that contextual visual cues exhibit a more salient effect on memory-guided—as opposed to visually guided—responses indicates that the former draws upon a conscious percept based on spatial relationships between target and nontarget items.

As previously indicated, there is ample evidence that a conscious representation is necessary to support memory-guided actions. Interestingly, however, we have discovered that under certain response sets, memory-guided responses can be evoked without participant awareness of physical target properties. Recall that an earlier study by our group (Binsted et al., 2007) showed that visually derived reaches scale to physical target size in the absence of conscious awareness of that extrinsic target property. In an extension of that work, we recently employed an adapted version of the four-dot object-substitution masking paradigm to examine the scaling of memory-guided reach trajectories to unconsciously derived visual information (Heath, Neely, Yakimishyn, & Binsted, 2008). Participants were presented briefly with masked or nonmasked targets and were cued to initiate a reaching response immediately at presentation of the target or following a visual delay of 1,000 or 2,000 ms. Given the proposed real-time nature of dorsal visual networks, we hypothesized that unconscious target information would be unavailable to support visuomotor performance for any appreciable time of delay. Contrary to our predictions, our results showed that the reaches cued across the three conditions yielded equivalent scaling to target size. In other words, in spite of a lack of awareness of target size, the participants' MT and peak velocities were scaled to the differently sized target for up to 2,000 ms of delay. Although such a finding flies in the face of traditional views concerning the cognitive nature of information supporting memory-guided responses, it is possible that the exogenous nature of the stimulus presentation used in our investigation (i.e., a 13 ms presentation) mediated reach trajectories via extrangeniculate connections to dorsal visuomotor networks and permitted such networks to maintain unconscious target information to support the control of memory-guided actions. Future work by our group is aimed at determining whether static and dynamic visual stimuli differentially engage conscious versus unconscious visuomotor processes for memory-guided actions. In particular, we will use a visual masking technique in combination with single-pulse TMS applied to putative ventral and dorsal visual networks during different visual delay intervals to examine selective differences in the visual inputs serving visually guided and memory-guided responses.

Visual Coordinates or a Fully Specified Movement Plan

Goal-directed actions require the transfer of sensory information (i.e., target size and location) into appropriate motor coordinates at some point before movement onset (Flanders, Helms Tillery, & Soechting, 1992; Henriques, Klier, Smith, Lowy, & Crawford 1998). Concerning visually guided responses, it has been proposed that dorsal stream visuomotor mechanisms transform visual target coordinates from a retinal to some body-centered frame (e.g., head-, shoulder-, or arm-centered frame; Berkinblit, Fookson, Smetanin, Adamovich, & Poizner, 1995; McIntyre, Stratta, & Lacquaniti, 1997), or a frame, of visual reference, at the time of response cuing. In other words, a movement plan is developed in real time, and not before, to account for possible changes in visual coordinates arising from moment-to-moment alterations in head and body position or target location (Westwood & Goodale, 2003). Furthermore, the classic work of Henry and Rogers (1960) demonstrating that movement planning times increase with movement complexity and the spatial demands of a task provides robust evidence that the internal structure of a motor plan is instantiated at the time of response cuing and not before (see chapters 4 and 6).

Although real-time planning generally predominates visually derived and guided actions, disrupting preparatory set leads to the development of a movement plan before movement initiation; that is, the visual coordinates of a target are used to precompute the kinematic parameters of a movement (i.e., off-line mode of control). In support of this view, work from our group has shown that real-time movement planning can be nullified when a performer faces a novel movement environment or amplified visuomotor uncertainty. For example, in one study (Heath, Rival, & Binsted, 2004) we asked participants to complete grasps (both closed loop and open loop) under a condition in which grip aperture was shaped, in advance of movement onset, to the perceived size of an object embedded within arrows-in and arrows-out Müller-Lyer figures (see also Heath & Rival, 2005; Heath, Rival, Neely, & Krigolson, 2006). As shown in figure 5.1, the premovement shaping of grip aperture, as well as grip aperture throughout the unfolding grasp trajectory, was reliably influenced by the illusions of the Müller-Lyer figures. This finding counters an earlier study (Heath et al., 2005; see also Westwood et al., 2000) in which visually guided grasps initiated with a typical starting posture (i.e., the thumb and forefinger pinched lightly together) were refractory to the same Müller-Lyer figures. We reasoned that the between-experiment difference in the sensitivity of grasp trajectories to the Müller-Lyer figures was related to the time frame of sensorimotor transformation supporting action output. In the latter case (Heath et al., 2005), the neutral or typical premovement posture resulted in real-time sensorimotor transformations and thus advantaged the metrical processing properties of the dorsal visual pathway. In the former case (Heath, Rival, et al., 2004), the preshaping of the grip aperture disrupted preparatory set and the normally real-time transfer of visual to motor coordinates (i.e., off-line mode of control). Indeed, the fact that grip apertures were reliably influenced by the Müller-Lyer figures in this response context suggests

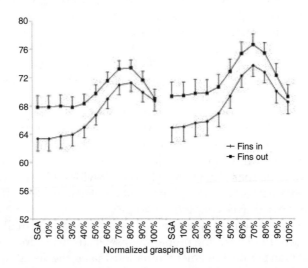

▶ **Figure 5.1**   Grip aperture (mm) as a function of *(left)* closed-loop conditions and *(right)* open-loop conditions and arrows-in and arrows-out Müller-Lyer figures during the shaping of a stable grip aperture (SGA) before movement onset and grip aperture at discrete stages during the movement trajectory. Using the perceived size of the object embedded in the Müller-Lyer figure to formulate grip aperture resulted in a grasp trajectory that was reliably influenced by the context-dependent features of the visual array.

Experimental Brain Research, 158, 2004a, pgs. 378-384, "Can the motor system resolve a premovement bias in grip aperture? Online analysis of grasping the Müller-Lyer illusion," M. Heath, C. Rival, and G. Binsted, ©Springer. With kind permission of Springer Science+Business Media.

that perception-based networks of the ventral pathway mediate off-line sensorimotor transformations.

Another framework our group has used to understand the time frame of sensorimotor transformations involves visuomotor uncertainty and altering the predictability of visual feedback. As mentioned previously, evidence indicates that visually guided reaches performed in a predictable environment (i.e., visual feedback is always available) are structured in real time and supported by online, feedback-based modifications to the unfolding movement trajectory (online control; for review see Elliott, Helsen, & Chua, 2001). When the availability of visual feedback cannot be predicted in advance of movement onset, however, actions elicit few, if any, corrections to the unfolding trajectory (Elliott & Allard, 1985; Jakobson & Goodale, 1991; Khan, Elliott, Coull, Chua, & Lyons, 2002; Zelaznik, Hawkins, & Kisselburgh, 1983). Our group sought to extend earlier work manipulating the predicted availability of visual feedback to determine whether visuomotor uncertainty affects online feedback use as well as the nature of the visual information supporting motor output. To accomplish that objective, we (Heath, Rival, & Neely, 2006) required participants to grasp an object embedded in the same Müller-Lyer figures mentioned previously (see Heath, Rival, et al., 2004; Heath & Rival, 2005; Heath et al., 2005) in visually guided (closed-loop) and visually derived (open-loop) grasping environments. Grasps were performed under feedback schedules in which closed-loop and open-loop responses were performed in separate trial blocks (a blocked feedback schedule) and under schedules in which closed-loop and open-loop trials were randomly interleaved on a trial-by-trial basis (a random feedback schedule). We found that closed-loop responses performed in the blocked feedback schedule were refractory, whereas open-loop grasps (performed in both the blocked and random feedback schedules) as well as closed-loop grasps performed in the random feedback schedule were reliably tricked by the Müller-Lyer illusion. We reasoned that closed-loop grasps performed in a blocked feedback schedule are immune to the Müller-Lyer figures because advance knowledge of the availability of visual feedback leads to real-time sensorimotor transformations and evokes an online grasp trajectory supported by the dorsal visual pathway. In contrast, knowledge that visual feedback would be unavailable (open-loop blocked feedback schedule) or unpredictable (closed-loop and open-loop random feedback schedule) resulted in off-line movement planning and the precomputing of movement parameters via visual inputs from the perceptual networks of the ventral visual pathway.

Building on the work just described, we conducted a more recent study (e.g., Neely, Tessmer, et al., 2008) in which we manipulated visuomotor uncertainty during a pointing response directed to the induced Roelofs effect (IRE; Bridgeman et al., 1997). In brief, the IRE is a pictorial illusion in which a luminous target is presented within a centered, off-proximal (or offset-left) or off-distal (or offset-right) frame. In previous work, we demonstrated that the IRE gives rise to perceptual and motor responses that are biased in a direction opposite the frame shift (Neely, Heath, & Binsted, 2008; see also Coello, Richaud, Magne, & Rossetti, 2003; Bridgeman et al., 1997). Thus, for our latter study we employed the IRE in the context of goal-directed reaching, as opposed to grasping, to examine the control properties of unfolding reach trajectories. In other words, we sought to determine whether response modes influence the nature of the visual information supporting motor output. The end-point accuracy and the spatial correlations (R^2 values) relating limb position at different kinematic markers (i.e., 25%, 50%, and 75% of MT) and ultimate movement end-points were computed to examine whether actions planned online versus off-line are influenced differentially by the IRE. Spatial correlations for closed-loop reaches in the blocked feedback schedule were modest, and end points were largely refractory to the IRE. In contrast, open-loop reaches (in both blocked and random feedback schedules) as well as closed-loop reaches in the random feedback schedule demonstrated robust R^2 values with end points influenced by the IRE (see figure 5.2 for R^2 analysis). In line with previous work (e.g., Elliott, Binsted, & Heath, 1999; Heath, Rival, et al., 2004; Heath, 2005; Heath et al., 2007; Messier & Kalaska, 1997), we interpreted the different patterns of R^2 values to reflect two modes of reaching control. Specifically, the low R^2 values observed during closed-loop trials in the blocked feedback schedule evidenced real-time movement control and the attenuation of movement planning errors via online, feedback-based movement corrections. In turn, the more robust R^2 values of open-loop trials (in both blocked and random feedback schedules) as well as closed-loop trials in the random feedback schedule reflected an off-line mode of control in which responses are structured in advance of movement onset via central planning mechanisms; that is, movement parameters are computed in advance of response cuing. Certainly, the finding that distinct R^2 values gave rise to end points that are differentially sensitive to the IRE evidences the separate nature and timeline of sensory-to-motor transformations supporting online and off-line modes of movement control.

Concerning the time frame of the sensorimotor transformations subserving memory-guided reaches, a logical assumption stemming from the work just described is that such actions are supported by a movement plan computed before response cuing and, in particular, before occlusion of the target. This assertion was supported by an early study by our group, in which we examined the trajectory parameters and end-point characteristics of closed-loop, open-loop, and memory-guided reaches of 0, 200, 400, and 600 ms of delay (Heath, Westwood, & Binsted, 2004). In line with previous work (e.g., Westwood et al., 2001, 2003), visually guided reaches were more accurate and less variable than were their open-loop and memory-guided counterparts. Furthermore, visually guided

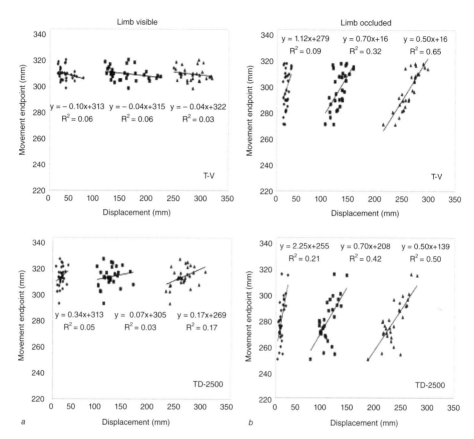

▶ **Figure 5.2** The proportion of variance (R^2) in movement end points explained by the position of the limb at peak acceleration, peak velocity, and peak deceleration. These values were taken from (a) limb-visible and (b) limb-occluded trials performed by an exemplar participant to a target that was visible (T-V) or was occluded 2,500 ms (TD-2500) in advance of response cuing. T-V and TD-2500 limb-visible trials elicited weak R^2 values throughout the time course of reach trajectories. In contrast, T-V and TD-2500 limb-occluded trials yielded robust R^2 values during the latter stage of reach trajectories.

Adapted, by permission, from M. Heath, 2005, "Role of limb and target vision in the online control of memory-guided reaches," *Motor Control* 9: 281-311.

reaches showed that the spatial position of the limb at peak acceleration, peak velocity, and peak deceleration did not robustly predict ultimate movement end points (i.e., weak R^2 values). In contrast, open-loop and memory-guided responses elicited robust spatial correlations during the middle and late stages of reach trajectories. Our initial interpretation of this finding was that sensory information related to a remembered target is not available to support the real-time sensorimotor transformation associated with an online mode of reaching, thereby resulting in the precomputing of movement parameters.

One methodological consideration arising from the Heath, Westwood, and Binsted (2004) study is that the effects of removing target and limb information were not disentangled—target information and limb information were manipulated concurrently via liquid-crystal shutter goggles. As such, both limb vision and target vision were available to performers during closed-loop reaches, and both were occluded during open-loop and memory-guided reaches. This is a notable limitation because ego-motion cues have been shown to influence the nature of the visual information supporting motor output as well as the timing of online limb adjustments (Chua & Elliott, 1993). In yet another study (Heath & Westwood, 2003), our group demonstrated the importance of this issue by using a video-based memory-guided aiming task during which we manipulated feedback about virtual limb position. Specifically, we created a situation in which participants could not precompute an upcoming memory-guided response due to trial-to-trial variation of the spatial relationships associated with the movement of a mouse and the movement of a cursor on a screen. Thus our participants were required to use real-time sensorimotor transformations to move their visible limb (i.e., the cursor) into the remembered target location. We found that participants were able to complete reasonably accurate memory-based reaching movements for up to 5,000 ms of delay in spite of the varied spatial environment. In other words, participants accessed a stored sensory-based representation of target location and used that information in combination with vision of their moving limb to achieve the real-time sensorimotor transformations necessary to support an online mode of reaching control. In a second demonstration (Heath, 2005), we manipulated limb and target vision in a virtual aiming environment in order to examine three-dimensional limb trajectories across a range of memory delays (see Neely, Heath, & Binsted, 2008 for a full description of the aiming environment). Figure 5.2 shows the R^2 values associated with limb-visible and limb-occluded trials across a range of conditions in which the target was visible, was occluded at movement onset, or was occluded for some length (0, 500, 1,500, or 2,500 ms) of memory delay preceding response cuing. As demonstrated by figure 5.2, the presence of target vision during reaching trials did not influence the structuring of responses; rather, the robust R^2 values across reaches performed without limb vision suggest that actions were structured in advance of movement onset via central planning mechanisms. In contrast, the weak R^2 values characterizing reaches performed with online limb vision evidence primarily online, feedback-based limb control. Thus, it appears that the presence or absence of ego-motion cues affects the time frame of the sensorimotor transformations serving motor output. Moreover, convergent evidence suggests that stored sensory information related to a memory-based target location does not simply provide a static representation to support off-line movement planning; rather, stored target information, when paired with ego-motion cues, provides a dynamic visual referent with which participants effect real-time sensorimotor transformations necessary to make online adjustments to an unfolding movement trajectory.

Memory-Guided Reaches and the Relationship Between End-Point Error and Corticomotor Potentials

The Bereitschaftspotential (BP) and the reafferente potentiale (RP) are event-related corticomotor potentials that reflect activity in the supplementary motor area (SMA) and primary motor cortex (M1) related to movement planning and execution. Research examining the BP suggests that it can be divided into two principal subcomponents, the earlier of which reflects motor-planning processes within the SMA (e.g., Cui & Deecke, 1999) and the latter of which reflects premovement activity within the lateral premotor area (LPA; Yazawa et al., 2000) and M1 (Gerloff, Uenishi, & Hallett, 1998; Shibasaki & Hallett, 2006). Following movement onset, the RP can also be subdivided into smaller components. Although less is known about the RP subcomponents, they are thought to reflect movement-related activity within the SMA, LPA, and M1 (Cui & Deecke, 1999; Shibasaki & Hallett, 2006). Moreover, RP subcomponents are thought to reflect the processing of sensory feedback (Shibasaki, Barrett, Halliday, & Halliday, 1980) or reafferent activity from motor areas (Cui & Deecke, 1999). Most studies examining the BP and RP have focused on simple finger movements and grasp formation, although recent research has demonstrated the existence of parietal corticomotor potentials associated with preparatory hand movements toward tools and other complex objects (Wheaton, Yakota, & Hallett, 2005). In our current research we are using the event-related potential (ERP) technique to examine the BP and RP as a means to correlate the electrophysiological and behavioral antecedents of memory-guided reaching. For instance, we (Krigolson, Heath, & Holroyd, 2008) had participants make manual aiming movements to targets in closed-loop and memory-guided conditions and examined the corticomotor potentials just preceding and just following movement onset. Specifically, participants made video-based aiming movements under three visual conditions. In the first condition (closed loop), participants viewed a target for 2 s and then were cued by an auditory tone to make a rapid aiming movement to the presented target. In the other conditions, participants again previewed the target for 2 s, and then the target was occluded for 1,000 (D1000) or 2,000 (D2000) ms before response cuing. We found that memory-guided reaches undershot target location and were more variable than were their visually guided counterparts, and during the visually guided reaching participants spent more time moving after peak velocity (c.f., Heath, Westwood, & Binsted, 2004; Heath, 2005;

Westwood et al., 2001, 2003). This finding presumably reflects enhanced feedback-based processing (Elliott et al., 1999). Interestingly, the ERP waveforms locked to movement onset revealed key differences between the corticomotor potentials associated with movement execution (the RP) and the corticomotor potentials associated with movement planning (the BP). Specifically, BP amplitudes preceding movement onset did not vary as a function of the different visual conditions; however, immediately following movement onset the RP waveforms began to differ, with the RP for closed-loop reaches being associated with greater mean negative amplitude when compared with the RP for memory-guided reaches across the reaching trajectory. Furthermore, as demonstrated in figure 5.3, the

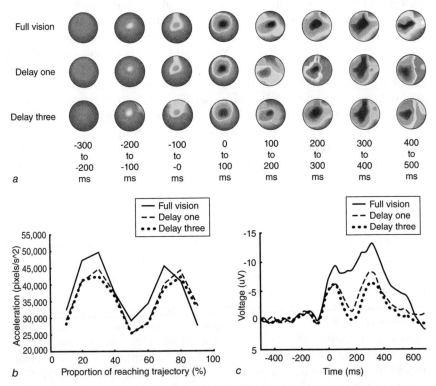

▶ **Figure 5.3** (a) Scalp topographies highlighting corticomotor potentials (in light gray) for closed-loop conditions and delay conditions of 1,000 and 3,000 ms. As demonstrated in (b), closed-loop trials elicited corticomotor potentials that were larger than those elicited by 1,000 and 3,000 ms delay trials (which did not differ). In turn, (c) acceleration profiles for each visual condition, when compared with part b, demonstrate a relationship between peak acceleration and peak corticomotor potential.

Reprinted, by permission, from S. Hansen, D. Elliott, and M.A. Khan, 2008, "Quantifying the variability of three-dimensional aiming movements using ellipsoids," *Motor Control* 12: 241-251.

profiles of corticomotor potentials paralleled the profiles of reach accelera-tion, and the amplitudes of the corticomotor potentials scaled to the reach end points (i.e., the magnitude of the undershooting bias).

The differences in the RP reported in this study provide a basis for explaining the behavioral differences characterizing visually guided and memory-guided reaches. Specifically, we propose that the target undershooting of memory-guided reaches relates to a reduction in the amplitude of within-movement corticomotor potentials. This reduc-tion can be thought of as a reduction in force, which in turn results in reduced acceleration. What remains unclear is why these differences occur. A compelling explanation relates to a compression of visual space as a function of memory. Indeed, a recent hypothesis derived from our group (Heath & Binsted, 2007) asserts that remembered visual space is contracted toward the body. As such, a target location held in memory is represented as being closer to the body than it actually is. Thus, when a memory-guided reaching movement is planned and executed, it is made based on a compressed visual representation of peripersonal space. Importantly, our electrophysiological evidence supports the notion of a compressed representation of remembered target location, as memory-guided responses elicited reduced corticomotor potentials across the time frame of unfolding reach trajectories. In further exploration of this hypothesis, our group is currently applying the ERP technique to reaches performed to memory-based targets located distally (i.e., causing reach-ing away from the body) or proximally (i.e., causing reaching toward the body) to a common home position. Our goal is to determine whether the undershooting and overshooting bias characterizing respective reaches to remembered targets in distal and proximal space is reflected by the magnitude of corticomotor potentials.

Conclusions and Future Directions

The goal of this review has been to argue that a temporally durable target representation is available to the motor system to support memory-guided actions. We showed that even for the briefest of delays (0 ms), stored target information does not provide an equivalent substitute for direct target viewing. Moreover, evidence reviewed here suggests that the nature of the visual information supporting memory-guided actions and the ability to access such information for movement planning and control depend on a myriad of factors such as the presence or absence of ego-motion cues, visuomotor uncertainty, and the novelty of a movement environment. Future studies need to determine how these factors interact to support memory-guided action.

Endnotes

1. A number of studies by Thomson (e.g., 1983) report on the accuracy of a locomotor task in conditions in which responses are initiated following an immediate delay or some duration of visual occlusion. We do not review Thomson's work here because it does not include the requisite control condition (i.e., visually guided movement) to examine the temporal decay of stored target information. Moreover, a detailed discussion of Thomson's work has been outlined previously (Elliott, 1990).

2. There is some controversy as to whether persons with action blindsight are able to initiate a metrical response after a visual delay. On the one hand some report that persons with action blindsight are not able to evoke metrical delayed reaching responses (see Danckert & Rossetti, 2005). On the other hand, the cuing paradigm used in Weiskrantz and colleagues' (1977) classic study of patient D.B. afforded a delay of approximately 1,000 ms between offset of the visual target object and reach trajectory onset. For further discussion of this issue, see Heath, Maraj, Godbolt, & Binsted (2008).

CHAPTER 6

The Preparation and Control of Multiple-Target Aiming Movements

MICHAEL A. KHAN, WERNER F. HELSEN, AND IAN M. FRANKS

It is well known that the processes associated with specifying and organizing a response increase as a function of the number of response elements (Henry & Rogers, 1960; Klapp, 1995). These additional preparatory processes have been observed through increases in latencies preceding response initiation (i.e., RT). However, the influence of response complexity has not been limited to RT. Increasing the complexity of a response affects processes not only before response initiation but also during movement execution (Smiley-Oyen & Worringham, 1996; Van Donkelaar & Franks, 1991). While some researchers have focused on the influence of response complexity on RT, others have highlighted the effect of response elements on the time it takes to execute movements, known as *movement time* (MT) (Adam et al., 2000). Like RT, MT does not vary with response complexity in a straightforward manner, and understanding the factors that influence this relationship has remained a challenge for researchers interested in the processes associated with movement preparation and execution.

Interestingly, researchers investigating the effects of response complexity have tended to focus on RT and MT separately. The goal of this chapter is to bring the evidence surrounding these two foci together. We first review how RT is influenced by the number of elements in a response. We then extend our discussion to the preparation and control of multiple-target aiming movements. In doing so, we distinguish between preparatory processes before movement initiation and control processes during movement execution. While distinctions are made between movement preparation and movement control, we also offer proposals on the interdependency between these processes.

The Influence of Response Complexity on Reaction Time

In their classic study, Henry and Rogers (1960) demonstrated that RT is directly related to the number of elements in a response. They showed that RT for lifting a finger off a key is faster when performed alone than when followed by subsequent actions (e.g., grasping a ball). This lengthening of RT as response complexity increases was attributed to the greater time needed to program more complex movements. According to Henry and Rogers, the programming of complex responses involves "a larger amount of stored information . . . and thus the neural impulses will require more time for coordination and direction into the eventual motor neurons and muscles" (p. 450).

While generally it has been accepted that the time required to program a response increases as a function of response complexity, the question of what aspect of response complexity is responsible for increasing programming time has been a matter of much debate. In this regard, researchers have investigated the effects of the number of response elements (Fischman, 1984; Sternberg, Monsell, Knoll, & Wright, 1978), the response duration (Klapp & Erwin, 1976), and the movement accuracy (Lajoie & Franks, 1997; Sidaway, 1991) on RT (for a review see Klapp, 1996). A second issue that has received much attention concerns the varying effects of response complexity on simple versus choice RT tasks (Henry, 1980; Klapp, Abbott, Coffman, Snider, & Young, 1979; Klapp, Wyatt, & Lingo, 1974). Participants performing simple RT tasks know what response to produce before the stimulus is presented. In contrast, participants performing choice RT tasks do not know the required response until stimulus presentation. Hence, choice RT is longer than simple RT since response selection processes must occur during the RT interval in choice RT tasks. Also, it is possible that response programming can occur before the RT interval in simple RT tasks since the required response is known in advance of the stimulus. On this basis, it might be expected that simple RT does not increase as a function of response complexity since programming can be performed in advance of the RT interval. In choice RT tasks, the response is specified by the stimulus, and programming must occur after stimulus presentation. Hence, the effect of response complexity should be greater in choice RT tasks than it is in simple RT tasks. However, while choice RT has been shown to be greater than simple RT, the influence of response complexity on RT has not been straightforward.

In a series of experiments using Morse code responses, Klapp (1995) showed that the duration of single-element responses (e.g., dit versus dah) influenced choice RT but not simple RT. Alternatively, while simple RT increased as the number of response elements increased (e.g., dit versus dit, dah, dah, dit), the number of elements had no effect on choice RT. Klapp accounted for these results by proposing a two-process model of response programming in which he referred to *INT* as the programming of internal features of individual elements (e.g., duration) and *SEQ* as the ordering of elements. In simple RT, INT is performed before the stimulus presentation, whereas SEQ occurs during the RT interval. Therefore, simple RT is influenced by the number of elements in a response since it takes longer to perform SEQ as the number of elements increases. In choice RT, preprogramming is not possible, and both INT and SEQ must occur during RT. Assuming that both processes occur in parallel and that INT takes longer than SEQ, the duration of individual elements but not the number of elements influences choice RT.

In a subsequent study, Klapp (2003) extended the results he obtained for Morse code responses to speech articulation. He showed that for situations in which the syllables of a word can be integrated into a chunk, simple RT is not influenced by the number of syllables given in a task, while choice RT increases as the number of syllables increases. In contrast, under conditions preventing the integration of syllables, simple RT but not choice RT increases as a function of the number of syllables in the task. Hence, like choice RT and simple RT from the Morse code experiments, choice RT in these speech experiments was influenced by the internal features or complexity of a chunk whereas simple RT increased as a function of the number of elements in a response.

Interestingly, Klapp (2003) also showed that when the number of syllables but not the actual syllables themselves are precued before stimulus presentation, RT increases as a function of the number of elements. Hence, in contrast to RT in Klapp's other experiments, RT in this experiment was influenced by the number of response elements when the entire response was not known in advance of the stimulus (i.e., choice RT task). Klapp reasoned that since the content of the syllables was not known in advance of the stimulus, both INT and SEQ must be occurring during the RT interval. Hence, the finding that RT depends on the number of syllables was inconsistent with his original idea that INT and SEQ occur in parallel and that INT determines RT because it takes longer than SEQ takes. Klapp therefore modified his theory by proposing that SEQ involves the scanning of an abstract time frame rather than the sequencing of the actual elements or chunks. This time frame specifies the time of initiation of each chunk without specific reference to the content of the chunks. In simple RT, the time frame is loaded into a buffer before the presentation of the stimulus. During the RT interval, the time frame is activated and scanned to locate the starting point. This scanning process takes longer as the number of elements increases and hence simple RT increases for responses involving more elements. Similarly, the abstract time frame can be loaded into a buffer before the stimulus presentation when the number of elements but not the nature of the elements is precued. Hence, RT increases as the number of elements and the time to perform the scanning process increase. In choice RT situations in which the number of elements is not precued, the time frame is retrieved immediately before the response and therefore does not have to be scanned. Hence, choice RT does not increase as a function of the number of elements in a sequence.

The pattern of RT results obtained by Klapp (1995, 2003) has also been reported in studies employing rapid aiming movements. For example, Khan, Lawrence, Buckolz, and Franks (2006) performed a series of experiments in which participants performed single- or two-target aiming responses. The movements consisted of sliding a pen along a track that was attached to a digitizing tablet. Participants performed either a single movement to a target or a reversal movement in which they moved to one target and then reversed direction to stop at a second target. Similarly to Klapp (1995, 2003), Khan and colleagues found that simple RT was greater for the two-target response compared with the single-target response, whereas choice RT was not influenced by the number of elements in the response.

In a subsequent study, Khan, Mourton, Buckolz, and Franks (2007) extended the results of Klapp (2003) to show that RT increases as a function of the number of response elements when the number of elements but not other features of the response is precued in advance. Before the stimulus presentation, participants were informed about (1) both the required number of elements and the required movement amplitude, (2) the number of elements but not the movement amplitude, (3) the movement amplitude but not the number of elements, or (4) nothing regarding the required response. The results indicated that RT increases as a function of the number of response elements when the entire response is precued and when the number of elements but not the movement amplitude is specified before the stimulus presentation. RT was not influenced by the number of response elements when only the amplitude was precued or when no information was given about the required response. Therefore, it appears that a necessary condition for RT to increase as a function of response elements is that the number of elements is known in advance of the RT interval. RT is directly related to the number of response elements when the entire response or just the number of elements is known in advance of the stimulus presentation. Response elements do not influence RT when the number of response elements is not known until stimulus presentation.

In summary, RT increases as a function of the number of response elements when the number of elements is known before stimulus presentation. However, RT remains unaffected when the number of elements is not specified until stimulus presentation. Although Klapp (1995, 2003) has offered elegant explanations of this pattern of results, these findings are counterintuitive if we assume that programming takes place before the

RT interval in simple RT tasks. As mentioned earlier, when the number of elements is known in advance of stimulus presentation, programming can potentially occur during the foreperiod. Hence, RT should not be influenced by response programming since these processes occur outside of the RT interval. On the other hand, when the number of elements is not known until stimulus presentation, programming processes take place during the RT interval. Therefore, the number of elements in a response should have a greater influence on choice RT than it has on simple RT—not the opposite. In the following sections, we consider alternatives to Klapp's model of response programming by taking into account the processes occurring during movement execution and how they relate to events preceding response initiation.

Online Programming Hypothesis

One possible interpretation of the finding that the number of response elements influences simple RT more than choice RT is that participants distribute the programming of elements differently under simple RT and choice RT situations. Although RT has been used as an index of response programming time, RT may not fully capture the processes involved in response preparation, and programming might be continued during movement execution (i.e., continued online; Glencross, 1980; Smiley-Oyen & Worringham, 1996). There are several lines of evidence supporting online programming. For example, the effect that the number of response elements has on RT is not linear but instead decreases as the number of elements increases (Canic & Franks, 1989; Henry & Rogers, 1960; Klapp et al., 1979). MT for initial elements has been shown to be longer for multiple-element responses than it is for single-element responses (Chamberlin & Magill, 1989). Also, response complexity has a larger effect on RT when movements are performed as fast as possible compared with slower speeds (van Donkelaar & Franks, 1991). It seems that when responses are relatively complex, participants program the initial elements of the response during RT but then delay the programming of later elements until after the RT interval, providing they have sufficient time to do so during movement execution. If movements are programmed online, response complexity may have a reduced effect on RT since fewer elements are programmed during the RT interval.

If response preparation involves the storage of elements in a short-term buffer (Henry & Rogers, 1960), it may be that only a limited number of elements can be programmed at any point in time. Since in simple RT tasks it is possible to prepare responses during the foreperiod, there is the potential to hold more elements in short-term memory before movement initiation. Hence, more complex responses should result in longer RTs if the translation of movement commands to the neuromotor centers cannot take place until stimulus presentation (Henry, 1980). However, since in choice RT tasks the responses cannot be prepared during the foreperiod, participants may minimize RT by programming fewer elements in advance of movement initiation (Chamberlin & Magill, 1989; Klapp et al., 1979). Hence, when compared with simple RT, choice RT is influenced less by the number of elements in a sequence because the extent to which responses are programmed online is greater.

In order to test this hypothesis, Khan and coworkers (2006) analyzed movement durations of single- and two-target reversal movements performed under simple RT and choice RT conditions. They hypothesized that if online programming occurs in choice RT tasks but not in simple RT tasks, MT to the first target should be longer in choice RT conditions than in simple RT conditions because of the additional processing demand during movement execution. However, MT was actually longer in the simple RT tasks than it was in the choice RT tasks, with this difference being greater for the two-target responses. This evidence suggests that the extent to which aiming movements are controlled online is greater in simple RT tasks than it is in choice RT tasks.

In order to further assess processing demands both before and during movement execution in simple RT tasks and choice RT tasks, Khan and coworkers (2006) required participants to perform a secondary (probe) task (a key press in response to a tone) in conjunction with an aiming task. RT for the secondary tasks was greater in the two-target condition compared with the one-target condition regardless of whether the probe occurred before or after movement initiation. This was the case in both simple RT and choice RT conditions. This result suggests that online processes were present in both RT tasks. More importantly, however, introducing a secondary task during movement execution caused a greater deterioration in aiming accuracy in the simple RT task. This large decrement suggests that there are additional processes occurring during movement execution for the simple RT task but not during movement execution for the choice RT task. Khan and coworkers (2006) hypothesized that these additional processes are associated with enhancing the integration of response elements through the utilization of visual feedback. In two-target aiming movements, the implementation of the second element depends on the spatial and temporal characteristics of the movement toward the first target (Vindras & Viviani, 2005). In the simple RT condition, participants knew in advance when a two-element response would be required. Hence, they may have programmed movements with longer durations so that they could visually monitor the execution of the first element to facilitate the implementation of the second element. We now turn our attention to the concept of movement integration and the interdependencies of control processes underlying individual elements.

Movement Integration

For sequential aiming movements in which participants are required to move to a target and then continue—in the same direction—to a second target, MT to the first target is typically slower than it is when participants are required to stop at the first target (Chamberlin & Magill, 1989; Helsen, Adam, Elliott, & Buekers, 2001; Lavrysen et al., 2003). This one-target advantage (OTA) is a very stable phenomenon that perseveres regardless of manipulations of vision, hand preference, and hand use (Adam, Helsen, Elliott, & Buekers, 2001; Lavrysen, Helsen, Elliott, & Adam, 2002; Lavrysen et al., 2003).

Different interpretations have been put forward to explain the OTA. These vary in the extent to which the lengthening of MT can be attributed to planning versus online control. On the one hand, the increased MT observed during the first part of a two-target movement could indeed be attributed to planning processes implemented while the first part is still in progress (Fischman & Reeve, 1992). On the other hand, the first movement might be performed in a more controlled or constrained manner in order to provide an ideal starting position for the second movement (Chamberlin & Magill, 1989). A third hypothesis combines the advance planning and online control explanations. The movement integration hypothesis (Adam et al., 2000; Helsen et al., 2001) states that the second movement is prepared in advance but that there is also a certain cost associated with implementing the program for the second movement just before its start. According to Adam and colleagues (2000), the OTA arises from an overlap of the control processes underlying the movements to the first and second targets. In order to facilitate a smooth and efficient transition between response elements, the performer implements the processes associated with the second element while executing the first element. Hence, the movements to the two targets are not controlled separately and strictly serially. Instead, executive control processes are increased during the production of the first element in two-target responses, and this increase leads to interference and hence the OTA. In this regard, Adam and colleagues (2000) distinguished between the online programming hypothesis and the movement integration hypothesis (also see Lavrysen et al., 2002). Online programming involves both the construction of a motor program and the implementation of the program during movement execution. By contrast, according to the movement integration hypothesis, program construction is performed before response initiation, but the implementation of the second element is performed online as the first element is executed. This implementation process causes interference and hence the OTA.

The one notable exception to the OTA is when the second element involves a reversal in direction. In this case, a two-target advantage arises in which MT to the first target is shorter for dual-element responses compared with single-element responses (Adam, van der Bruggen, & Bekkering, 1993; Khan et al., 2006). Researchers have accounted for the two-target advantage by looking at the patterns of muscle activity underlying rapid aiming movements. Single-target movements are characterized by a triphasic pattern of muscle activity. First there is initial agonist activity that accelerates the limb toward the target. Next is a burst of antagonist activity that decelerates the limb upon approaching the target. Third is a second burst of agonist activity that dampens mechanical oscillations at the end of the movement. The second agonist burst counteracts any tendency of the limb to reverse direction due to the storage of elastic energy from a rapidly lengthening antagonist muscle. In two-target reversal movements, there is no need for this second burst of agonist activity since the elastic properties of the muscle can be exploited to save energy in moving the limb in the reverse direction (i.e., reciprocal conversion between kinetic and potential energy; Guiard, 1993). Moreover, the antagonist muscle forces used to decelerate the first element also act as the agonist on the second element. This dual purpose of antagonist activity allows for optimal integration between elements, giving rise to the two-target MT advantage.

To evaluate the trade-off between planning and control processes in multiple-target responses, Lavrysen and coworkers (2003) manipulated visual feedback during either the first part or the second part of a two-part movement. They hypothesized that a reduced opportunity for online control would shift the timing of the preparatory processes and that these temporal costs would provide insight into how movement reversals and movement extensions are prepared and executed. Their results indicated that although online visual processing is important for accurate limb control, humans can adopt a more preplanned mode of control when visual information is less available. Moreover, performers demonstrated differences in the way single-element movements, movement reversals, and movement extensions were prepared. Consistent with the position of Adam and colleagues (2000) and Helsen and colleagues (2001) with respect to the movement integration hypothesis, the finding that OTA was absent for a movement reversal indicates that the two elements of a reversal movement may be prepared as a single unit. In this context, it is not surprising that the availability of visual feedback affected the execution of reversal movements and single movements similarly. Evidence for an advance planning contribution to the OTA also came from the kinematics, which suggested that participants perform a more constrained first movement when that movement is followed by a second extension movement. Specifically, participants achieved lower peak velocities and took longer to achieve peak velocity when they were making a movement extension than when they were making a movement reversal or a single movement. Presumably, by producing a weaker initial impulse in the extension situation, participants reduce end-point variability (Schmidt, Zelaznik, Hawkins, Frank, & Quinn, 1979) and place themselves in a better position to hit the first target and begin the second movement. Therefore, it appears that under normal afferent circumstances both advance planning and online control processes contribute to the OTA for MT. When the availability of online visual information is reduced, the performer simply adopts a different control strategy in which advance planning plays a greater role.

Apart from the role of vision in planning and updating a movement, there are probably other mechanisms leading to the OTA. The transition from one movement to another is made possible by a delicate balance between the muscular forces needed to brake the limb and the muscular forces needed to accelerate the limb (Helsen et al., 2001). In the case of the two-target movement extension, these antagonist and agonist forces do not act in the same direction and thus interfere with one another. However, in the case of the two-target movement reversal, there is a smaller loss in efficiency, since the same muscular forces used to slow down the first movement can be used to propel the second. Thus, in this light, an evaluation of EMG signals could be most interesting in the study of the mechanisms behind the OTA. Savelberg, Adam, Verhaegh, and Helsen (2002) evaluated the EMG signals of flexor and extensor muscles during two-target aiming and indeed found that in the two-movement conditions, implementation of the second movement began during execution of the first movement.

The implementation of the second movement during the final part of the first movement is based on both preplanned and online information. In addition to being affected by the cost of the implementation processes, the first movement is performed in a more constrained manner to provide a good starting position for the next movement and to maximize the efficiency of the agonist and antagonist muscular work. More generally, fast goal-directed movements are preplanned according to the specific task demands and are subject to corrections according to information that becomes available as the movement unfolds.

Since the requirement to hit a second target influences the movement made to the first target, the presence of both the OTA and the two-target advantage implies that the elements in a response are not controlled separately; rather, the control processes underlying the movements to the two targets are interdependent. Furthermore, changing the properties of the second target influences control of the movement to the first target. For example, when the size of the second target is reduced, MT to the first target increases while the dispersion of movement end points decreases (Rand, Alberts, Stelmach, & Bloedel, 1997; Sidaway, Sekiya, & Fairweather, 1995). Cameron, Franks, Enns, and Chua (2007) have also shown that adjustment to a perturbation in target location is less in two-target responses than it is in single-target responses and that perturbing the location of the second target biases accuracy at the first target in the direction of the perturbation.

This interdependency between the two response elements is influenced by certain task variables that affect the transition between target movements. When the size of the first target is relatively large, manipulating the size of the second target influences the control of the movement to the first target. When the size of the first target is small, the second target size does not influence the execution of the first movement (Adam et al., 1995; Rand & Stelmach, 2000). Also, Adam and colleagues (1993) have shown that the two-target advantage emerges when targets are large but not when targets are small. When the accuracy demands at the first target are very high, the pause between the target movements increases, thereby disrupting the transition between antagonist muscle forces and agonist muscle forces (see also Adam & Paas, 1996). It seems that when the first target is small, the two movements to the two targets are organized as separate units rather than as an integrated chunk.

In addition to the size of the targets, the physical characteristics of the movements influence the integration between the two elements. The two-target advantage typically emerges for sliding movements that involve a low degree of friction and no physical contact with the targets (Adam et al., 1993; Khan et al., 2006). Since these movements take place in a single plane of motion, there is a tight coupling between antagonist muscle forces on the first element and agonist activity on the second element. The degree of integration between muscle forces is less in three-dimensional aiming movements that involve contact with targets. In these cases, integration between muscular forces acting on both elements is disrupted, and hence the two-target advantage does not emerge (Adam et al., 2000). Also, in single-target responses that involve relatively frictionless sliding movements, it is perhaps necessary to produce slower movements in order to reduce mechanical oscillations at the end of the movement so that the limb comes to rest at the target. In reversal movements, there is no need to dampen oscillations by reducing the velocity of the limb since the elastic properties of the muscle can be exploited on the reversal component.

At this point, it is important to distinguish the mechanisms underlying integration between elements in two-target extensions and integration between elements in two-target reversals. In extension movements, the OTA is said to result from the implementation of executive control processes associated with the second element during execution of the first element. This explanation of the OTA implies that the programming of the second element is not completed before movement initiation and that interference arises from cognitive processes operating online. While the OTA is due to interference at a cognitive level, the two-target advantage in reversal movements emerges from the muscular forces associated with the mechanical characteristics of changing direction. As mentioned earlier, since in reversal movements the antagonist in the first movement acts as the agonist in the second movement, it may be that control processes associated with the reversal are linked with control processes of the first element in a single program and executed before response initiation. Hence, in contrast to extension movements, reversal movements may not involve the implementation of the second element during the production of the first element.

In order to test the degree to which reversal movements are prepared before response initiation or during movement execution, Khan, Tremblay, Cheung, Luis, and Mourton (2008) employed a perturbation paradigm in which the task requirements changed from a one-target response to a two-target response and vice versa. A second aim of the study was to test whether reversal movements are organized as a single unit or as two discrete units of action. Of interest was the participants' ability to change with changing task requirements and under which conditions the two-target advantage would emerge. In the first experiment, participants were instructed to prepare movements to a single target. On some of the trials, a second target was presented at the same time the first target was presented, at movement onset, or at peak velocity to the first target. Khan and colleagues reasoned that if the two-target advantage is a result of preparatory processes preceding movement initiation, the two-target advantage would be observed only when the second target was presented simultaneously with the first. In the second experiment, participants were instructed to prepare two-target reversal movements. On some of the trials, the second target was not presented at target presentation or was removed at movement onset or peak velocity to the first target. In these cases, participants were required to move to the first target but prevent movement to the second target. The researchers hypothesized that if reversal movements are prepared as a single unit of action before response initiation rather than as two discrete movements, the ability to inhibit movement to the second target would be difficult once the movement was initiated.

The results of both experiments revealed that MT to the first target was determined by the information available at stimulus presentation. MT was shorter when two targets as opposed to one target appeared at stimulus presentation (i.e., there was a two-target advantage). Changing the task requirements at movement onset or later did not influence MT. It also was difficult for participants to switch task demands once the movement was initiated. There was a smooth transition between elements when the two targets were presented simultaneously but not when the second target appeared at movement onset or peak velocity. Furthermore, when two targets were presented and the second target disappeared as early as movement onset, a significant movement to the second target was observed and the production of the first movement was relatively unaffected. Previous research has shown that adjustments in limb trajectories to a perturbation in target position occur as quickly as 100 ms after the change in target position (Paulignan, Mackenzie, Marteniuk, & Jeannerod, 1990). Also, evidence from research employing the go–stop paradigm has shown that stopping latencies are approximately 140 ms (McGarry, Chua, & Franks, 2003; McGarry & Franks 1997). In the study of Khan and colleagues (2008), MT to the first target was greater than 250 ms. This result suggests that participants had enough time to implement and integrate response elements during movement execution or inhibit the second movement when the task requirements changed at movement onset. The inability to add and integrate additional elements as well as inhibit the reversal component provides support for the hypothesis that reversal responses are organized as a single unit of action.

Planning and Movement Integration

Increases in RT as a function of response complexity have been taken as evidence that movements are programmed in advance of response initiation. However, there is also evidence that movement programming processes are not fully captured in the RT interval and that programming occurs during movement execution. These two lines of evidence can be viewed as contradictory since the presence of online programming implies that movements are not planned entirely in advance. Hence, the influence of response complexity on RT should be reduced if movements are programmed online rather than before response initiation. On the contrary, recent findings have revealed that increasing the number of response elements leads to increased RT as well as additional processes during movement execution, especially when the number of elements is specified in advance. In the remainder of this chapter, we offer an account for the preparation and control of multiple-target movements that distinguishes between the processes that occur before response initiation and those that unfold during movement execution.

Supporting the idea that more complex movements take longer to program during the RT interval is the finding that RT increases as a function of the number of response elements when the number of elements is known in advance of the stimulus (Khan et al., 2006, 2007; Klapp, 1995, 2003). This relationship holds when either the characteristics of the entire response or just the required number of elements is known before the stimulus presentation (Khan et al., 2007; Klapp, 2003). Also, it is extremely difficult to alter the number of response elements once the movement is initiated (Khan et al., 2008). Taken together, these lines of evidence suggest that motor programming specific to the number of response elements takes place before the initiation of the response.

As discussed earlier, the influence of advance information about the number of response elements is not limited to the RT interval. Additional control processes occur during movement execution when the number of elements is known in advance. MT to the first target of a two-target response is greater when the required number of elements is known before the stimulus (Khan et al., 2006, 2007). Also, movement to the first target in two-target responses is susceptible to dual-task interference when the number of elements is known in advance of the stimulus. Ketelaars, Khan, and Franks (1999) demonstrated grouping between the muscle activity underlying the reversal in an elbow extension and flexion response and the muscle activity associated with a probe task (a bite response to a tone). In addition, Khan and coworkers (2006) showed that RT to a probe task was greater for two-element movements than it was for single-element movements, regardless of whether the probe occurred during RT or movement execution. Moreover, the interference between tasks was greater when advance information on the number of elements was available before the stimulus. When the probe was presented during movement execution, accuracy at the first target deteriorated only when the number of elements was specified in advance.

Therefore, while we have proposed that two-target movements are organized before response initiation, it is possible that the implementation of control processes occurs during movement execution. In distinguishing between the movement integration hypothesis and the online programming hypothesis for two-target extension movements, Adam and colleagues (2000) have proposed that movements to both targets are specified and organized before response initiation but that the implementation of the second element does not occur until execution of the first element. Along these lines, we propose that the organization of multiple-target movements involves specifying the general pattern of muscle activity before response initiation but that the implementation and fine-tuning of the second element occurs during movement execution. Similar proposals have been made by Vindras and Viviani (2005), who claim that while the major features of two-element movements may be planned during RT, fine-tuning is necessary for movement toward the second target because of variability in movement toward the first target. We propose that it is the organization of the pattern of muscle activity during RT that takes longer for multiple-element movements than for single-element movements. Once the features of the response that pertain to the number of elements are established, it is difficult to modify the number of elements after the response is initiated. While the organization of response elements occurs before response initiation, participants plan their movements to optimize the integration between elements when they know in advance that a multiple-target response is required. According to Khan and coworkers (2006), movements are planned with longer durations so that the execution of the first element is visually monitored to time the implementation of the second element (also see Ketelaars et al., 1999).

The importance of vision has been demonstrated for sequential aiming movements in which the second element is in the same direction as the first. Ricker and colleagues (1999) have shown that RT is shorter when visual feedback is available during movement execution than it is when vision is occluded to the first target. Perhaps organization of the overall movement plan is more complete when vision is occluded. Also, when vision to the first target was occluded, pause times at the first target and MT to the second target were lengthened. It seems that when vision is available, the control processes underlying movement to the second target are implemented during the first element. When vision is occluded, participants are forced to delay the preparation of the second element until the first element is completed.

In summary, it seems that visual feedback plays a dual role toward the completion of the first element in two-target movements. As discussed in earlier chapters, during single-target movements vision is used to correct errors in the limb trajectory so that the limb stops accurately on the target. In two-target aiming movements, vision is used not only to adjust the limb trajectory to the first target but also to modify the movement parameters for the second element. In two-target extension movements, a longer distance traveled on the first element has to be compensated for by a shorter distance traveled on the second element and vice versa. For reversal movements, visual feedback processing during execution of the first element is perhaps even more critical since the transition from antagonist to agonist activity means that accuracy at the first target is determined by when the reversal component is implemented (Ketelaars et al., 1999).

Future Directions

The evidence presented in this chapter clearly demonstrates that the influence of response complexity on RT and MT should not be considered in isolation. An effect of response complexity on RT does not preclude an effect on MT and vice versa. In two-target movements, there is an overlap of control processes occurring during RT and movement toward the first and second targets. While events occurring during RT and movement execution are interdependent, there is a functional distinction between processes. Future work should attempt to identify and understand these functional differences. Toward this goal, researchers have employed movement precuing and target perturbation in multiple-target aiming. It has already been shown that RT increases when the number of response elements is known in advance, even when other features of the response are not known (Khan et al., 2007; Klapp, 2003). Also, when the number of elements is specified in advance of the stimulus, participants adopt strategies that enhance the integration between response elements. Further work is needed to investigate response preparation and movement execution under invalid precue conditions. This work would allow researchers to examine the cost of reprogramming movement parameters during RT and its corresponding effects on movement execution. For example, if the general pattern of muscle activation is determined by the number of elements in the response, reprogramming this feature of the response may be more costly than modifying other features during movement execution (e.g., amplitude or target size). Similarly, Khan and coworkers (2008) have shown that for reversal movements, participants have difficulty changing the number of elements in a response when the number of targets is perturbed at movement onset or later. To determine the case for extension movements, further work is needed in which target perturbation techniques are applied to extension movements. The cognitive and neuromuscular mechanisms underlying movement integration in two-target reversal movements are different from those underlying two-target extension movements. This also applies to sliding movements in a single plane that rely more on muscular forces to terminate movements when compared with three-dimensional aiming movements. In this regard, it would be interesting to examine online adjustments to movements and the interactive effects of when either the number of targets or another movement feature is perturbed in multiple-target aiming. This would allow us to further develop a comprehensive framework underlying the interdependency in movement planning and the integration between response elements at both cognitive and neuromuscular levels.

CHAPTER 7

Rapid Regulation of Limb Trajectories: Response to Perturbation

STEVE HANSEN, LAWRENCE E.M. GRIERSON,
MICHAEL A. KHAN, AND DIGBY ELLIOTT

One of the classic controversies in motor control is the extent to which discrete goal-directed movements unfold as planned or are modified based on response-produced feedback or changing environmental demands. An approach for examining the flexibility of movement planning and online control is to introduce an unexpected perturbation either during or some time after movement initiation. Of interest is how the perceptual–motor system is able to adapt to change in the task or environmental circumstance. In this chapter, we review research examining the effect of perturbations on the movement execution, movement goal, perceived goal, and visual context in which the action unfolds. Overall this research indicates that the visuomotor system is extremely flexible in adapting movement trajectories to rapidly changing task demands.

In general, the visual control of movement is studied through measurements of goal-directed behavior that describe the timing and spatial characteristics of a movement as it unfolds (e.g., Khan et al., 2006). Performance measures such as RT, MT, and end-point error describe overall performance or outcome. However, measuring and comparing the characteristics of the trajectory to the terminal outcome of the movement provide valuable additional information for researchers about the underlying visuomotor control processes responsible for the behavior observed after a perturbation (Elliott, Helsen, & Chua, 2001).

In the two-component model of goal-directed aiming (Woodworth, 1899), the kinematic events during the initial portions of the movement reflect movement planning toward the target, while later kinematic events reflect the processing of sensory feedback during the corrective process. The location of peak velocity has been associated with the separation point between the initial, planned portion of the movement and the latter, feedback-based portion of the movement (e.g., Elliott, Binsted, & Heath, 1999). Subsequently, decreased trial-to-trial spatial variability in the location of peak acceleration and peak velocity indicates increased planning efficiency (Khan & Franks, 2003), and decreased spatial variability at peak deceleration and movement end point indicates more efficient use of sensory feedback (Khan, Elliott, Coull, Chua, & Lyons, 2002).

Various other measures have been identified during the quest to discover the processes underlying visuomotor control. For example, Crossman and Goodeve (1963/1983) counted the number of discontinuities in the acceleration profile to quantify corrections to the initially executed movement (see also Elliott, Hansen, Mendoza, & Tremblay, 2004). Elliott and colleagues (1999) interpreted the average time elapsed between peak velocity and movement termination as an indication of the processes associated with vision gathered during movement execution. Khan, Franks, and Goodman (1998) employed an index of error correction effectiveness that quantified the ability of participants to correct for errors in the executed movement by normalizing the movement error before and after a correction. The variability in the locations of various kinematic markers throughout the movement trajectory over a series of trials has been used to infer the presence of corrective processes associated with vision (Darling & Cooke, 1987; Khan et al., 2002; Messier & Kalaska, 1999). More recently, several researchers have correlated the distance traveled at movement termination with the distance traveled at earlier kinematic markers such as peak velocity, or the primary submovement end point, to quantify the effectiveness of the corrective processes (Desmurget et al., 2005; Elliott et al., 1999; Heath, Westwood, & Binsted, 2004; Messier & Kalaska, 1999). However, the principal evidence for visuomotor processes occurring during a movement comes from trajectory corrections (Crossman & Goodeve, 1963/1983; see chapter 2 for a more detailed description of these various kinematic indexes). Perturbations induce changes in the kinematic measures, and theoretical inferences are made based on the direction and magnitude of these changes.

Although most models of the visual control of rapid action associate the initial portions of a movement with preplanning and the latter portions with online control, not all models concur with this view. Models explaining the control of rapid movements range from those positing complete preprogramming and execution without subsequent adjustment (e.g., Plamondon, 1995) to two-component models positing an initial movement to acquire the target area and subsequent adjustments to the trajectory near the target (Meyer, Abrams, Kornblum, Wright, & Smith, 1988; Woodworth, 1899). Finally, there are other models suggesting that sensory information gathering and concurrent adjustments to the movement trajectory occur continuously throughout the movement (Crossman & Goodeve, 1963/1983; Elliott, Carson, Goodman, & Chua, 1991; Elliot et al., 2001, 2004). In other words, models of the visual control of rapid movement range from completely open loop to entirely closed loop.

Discrete aiming movements are typically used to investigate visual control processes because they have an identifiable point of initiation and termination. Aiming movements are also relatively easy to observe and quantify with modern techniques. Researchers have employed multiple paradigms to investigate the processes underlying rapid and efficient action. These have included manipulations of practice (Elliott, Chua, Pollock, & Lyons, 1995; Proteau, 1995), vision of the limb (Elliott, Lyons, & Dyson, 1997; Pélisson, Prablanc, Goodale, & Jeannerod, 1986; Prablanc, Echallier, Komilis, & Jeannerod, 1979), vision of the target (Carlton, 1981b), and vision of both the limb and the target (Keele & Posner, 1968; Woodworth, 1899). In addition, researchers have changed the target location or size upon movement initiation (Elliott, Lyons, Chua, Goodman, & Carson, 1995; Heath, Hodges, Chua, & Elliott, 1998), manipulated the environmental context (Proteau & Masson, 1997), or altered the temporal and spatial association between the effector and the movement environment (Hansen, Elliott, & Tremblay, 2007; Redding & Wallace, 2001, 2002; Smith & Bowen, 1980). The important methodological questions have included how, when, and where to introduce manipulations within perturbation protocols investigating visual control processes.

Visual Occlusion

The traditional method of studying the visual regulation of manual aiming is to eliminate visual information and then examine the resulting behavior. Many researchers employ visual occlusion to investigate visual regulation because of the mechanical and theoretical simplicity of the manipulation. The ambient environment, target, and effector each contribute vital information toward the creation of an efficient visual representation of the environment for planning and control of goal-directed action. Vision can significantly increase the accuracy of aiming movements even in samples of the environment revealed as little as 40 ms (Hansen, Cullen, & Elliott, 2005). Visual occlusion eliminates the opportunity to use visual feedback to make corrections during the movement. Participants are then forced to complete their movement under visual open-loop control.

Investigators typically employ either a temporal or a spatial criterion for occluding vision. Temporal studies typically compare full-vision trials with trials that remove vision at movement initiation or for a fixed duration before movement initiation (Elliott et al., 1991; Keele & Posner, 1968;

Meyer et al., 1988; Pratt & Abrams, 1996). Contributions of premovement visual information can also be examined when the occlusion occurs before the movement (Elliott & Madalena, 1987; see chapter 5). In comparison to temporally based occlusion methods, spatial studies compare full-vision trials with trials that visually occlude portions of the movement (Carlton, 1981a; Chua & Elliott, 1993; Khan & Franks, 2003; Whiting & Sharp, 1974). The reasoning behind spatial occlusion is that it can be used to examine the importance of vision at the start and end of the movement and thus can be used to contrast the predictions made by the various models of manual control.

Researchers using temporal occlusion have assumed that the minimal time required for visually based feedback is determined by the time at which there are no differences in the observed errors between full-vision and no-vision conditions (Keele & Posner, 1968). The first researcher to establish a time for visual processing was Woodworth (1899). In an experiment using a rotating drum, Woodworth occluded vision at movement initiation by asking participants to close their eyes and then had participants perform reciprocal aiming movements across the drum to the beat of a metronome. From this work, Woodworth (1899) estimated the visual processing time to be 450 ms.

Decades later, Keele and Posner (1968) pointed out that Woodworth (1899) overestimated the visual processing time because he calculated this latency from a reciprocal aiming movement and did not take into account the time spent reversing the movement. In their experiment, Keele and Posner (1968) had participants perform discrete aiming movements within four different time ranges. The results revealed a significant difference between full-vision trials and no-vision trials in the 250 ms condition. In addition, during the 150 ms condition, the number of missed targets in the full-vision trials was equal to that of the no-vision trials. In the no-vision trials, though participants attempted to perform their movements in less than 150 ms, they required 190 ms on average. From these results, Keele and Posner (1968) concluded that the visual processing time is between 190 and 260 ms.

In another series of studies on discrete aiming experiments, Zelaznik, Hawkins, and Kisselburgh (1983) estimated the time to be less than 200 ms. The results from each of four experiments completed by Zelaznik and colleagues indicated an accuracy advantage for the full-vision condition compared with the no-vision condition. The advantage held even for movements 120 ms in duration. Thus Zelaznik and colleagues found it reasonable to assume that visual regulation processes could occur within 70 to 100 ms. Reasons for the discrepancies between the results of Keele and Posner (1968) and Zelaznik and colleagues (1983) may involve the predictability of the visual condition in the subsequent trial or differences in the measurement of movement accuracy (see Zelaznik et al. for a review).

In response to Keele and Posner (1968), Carlton (1981a) conducted a spatial occlusion study to investigate the time needed to process visual information. Carlton had participants aim to targets while a shield covered none of the movement or the initial 25%, 50%, 75%, or 93% of the movement. Carlton found a significant increase in MT between the 50% no-vision condition and the 75% no-vision condition. In addition, the rate of errors also increased significantly between the 50% and 75% conditions. Film analysis of the movements indicated that the time between the visual acquisition of the stylus and the movement end point was approximately 135 ms. From these results, Carlton estimated the visual processing time to be 135 ms.

Provided with a reasonably accurate visual processing time, Carlton (1981b) then independently occluded the visual elements associated with an aiming movement in order to determine the importance of each individual component for movement accuracy. In this study, Carlton had participants complete their manual aiming movements under full vision, no-vision, target-only, stylus-only, and target- and stylus-only conditions. He found that vision of the stylus was more important than vision of the target to maintain accuracy and suggested that a short-term visual representation of the environment might exist. A sustainable representation of the environment could provide the performer with information about the position of the target once vision was occluded (see chapters 4 and 5).

During experiments examining the contributions of the stylus and target information associated with the hypothesized visual representation, Elliott (1988) observed that participants could maintain a high degree of accuracy when they were presented continuously with the position of the stylus. In a second experiment, Elliott (1988) used phosphorescent paint to add target information and observed that doing so increased movement accuracy (when compared with when the target was absent during aiming). The results of Elliott demonstrated that vision of the stylus is important for reducing terminal error when the potential for the target information remained in either a physical or a representational form. The latter results were consistent with previous work by Elliott and Madalena (1987), who demonstrated that providing information of the target location in the absence of stylus information only partially eliminated the decay of accuracy observed during the complete no-vision condition. Perhaps as Carlton (1981b) suggested, visual information from the stylus is also required for optimal terminal accuracy. However, in the context of the results from Elliott (1988), the results of Carlton (1981b) may indicate that the vision of the stylus was only important when the potential for a visual representation of the target persisted (see chapter 5).

The overall importance of visual information regarding the effector is the topic of some debate. For example, in a subsequent study to the no-vision delay experiments of Elliott and Madalena (1987), Elliott and coworkers (1991) eliminated vision of a handheld stylus when performers initiated their aiming movements. Vision of the effector before and during the movements was found to be important in determining movement accuracy (Elliott et al., 1991). However, other researchers have found that vision of the limb is not as important for movement outcome. For example, Prablanc, Pélisson, and Goodale (1986) demonstrated that in a simple manual aiming task participants can modify their movements as efficiently with or without vision of the limb.

Instead of occluding the entire trajectory or various elements of the aiming task, several researchers have occluded portions of the movement trajectory to investigate the relative importance of vision gathered early and late in the action. For example, in order to examine the optimized submovement model of control (Meyer et al., 1988), Chua and Elliott (1993) occluded vision of the cursor during the initial half or the last half of a movement. In addition to performing the partial-vision trials, the participants also performed trials under conditions of full vision and no vision at movement initiation. Participants made more accurate movements when vision was available, but vision was most useful for movement regulation and making efficient modifications when it was available in the last half of the movement. In order to maintain a smooth trajectory, participants picked up and processed the relevant information before the end of the primary submovement (Chua & Elliott, 1993).

Like Chua and Elliott (1993), Khan and Franks (2003) investigated the two-component model of visually guided action (Woodworth, 1899) by examining the contribution of vision to the corrective portion of a movement by limiting vision to the initial portion of the action. Khan and Franks (2003) had participants aim to a target under no-vision, 50% first-portion vision, 75% first-portion vision, and full-vision conditions. The researchers posited that increasing the amount of vision available in the latter portions of the movement would decrease end-point error by providing the participants with the opportunity to use vision to execute discrete corrections following the initial ballistic phase of the movement. In addition, they posited that vision available for the initial portions of the movement might contribute to the off-line planning and online adjustment of the initial portion of the trajectory in a more continuous manner (Elliott et al., 1995). The added contribution of the study was the manner in which the off-line and online adjustments in the primary component were quantified (see chapter 2). First, more efficient preplanning of the ballistic phase of the movement was observed in the reduction of trial-to-trial spatial variability in the location of early kinematic markers. Second, trajectory modulation during the initial phase of the movement was quantified by an average increase in the distance traveled and a reduction in end-point variability of the initial impulse because continuous adjustments do not appear in the kinematic data as discrete events. The results indicated that both the primary and secondary components of the aiming movements were improved in the 75%

and full-vision conditions. When compared with the no-vision condition, vision of the initial 50% of the movement produced no benefits on accuracy during acquisition of the aiming task. Therefore, providing vision in latter portions of the trajectory improved the correction phase of the movement (e.g., Carlton, 1981a; Chua & Elliott, 1993), the planning of the initial phase (e.g., Khan et al., 2002; Khan & Franks, 2000; Lhuisset & Proteau, 2002), and continuous adjustment of the initial portion of the trajectory (e.g., Proteau & Masson, 1997). These results again demonstrate the robust effect that vision has on the terminal accuracy of manual aiming and the control of the limb throughout the trajectory (see figure 7.1).

A limitation of visual occlusion is that it places constraints on the task that differ from those of the typical aiming task (also see chapter 15). Control of the movement may differ if the participant knows that the occlusion will occur halfway in the movement (Chua & Elliott, 1993; Elliott & Allard, 1985). Specifically, guiding or correcting the trajectory of the limb from a sudden visual appearance of the stylus is not similar to visually guiding the limb continuously throughout the movement regardless of the movement duration. If the occlusion occurs early or late, the participant may choose to plan a longer or shorter initial movement and then spend a longer or shorter time using online control. In either case, the behavior differs from normal in order to optimize the use of the limited vision.

Visual occlusion forces the sensory system to adjust to the unexpected requirements of the task. Thus, the no-vision versus full-vision paradigm eliminates the regular interaction of the sensory system, thereby inducing a substitution of processes, or a dependence on open-loop processes. In order to address this problem, researchers have manipulated multiple environmental elements, including the ambient environment, the target, and the effector, without occluding any of the elements (Heath et al., 1998; Prablanc et al., 1986; Proteau & Masson, 1997).

Physically Changing the Target

Visual control research from the 1950s and early 1960s had a major influence on the theoretical approach to movement behavior research and ergonomic design (e.g., Crossman & Goodeve, 1963/1983; Fitts, 1954; Fitts & Peterson, 1964; Keele & Posner, 1968). Much of that research was based on the idea that visual information presented to the system drives or dictates the interaction with the environment. In accordance with this theory, the relationship between the target width and the movement amplitude provides specific information to the organism. Specifically, movement amplitude dictates the muscular forces required to propel the limb into the vicinity of the target. In addition, target width dictates the necessity for time-consuming visual–motor or proprioceptive–motor adjustments for final target acquisition. In

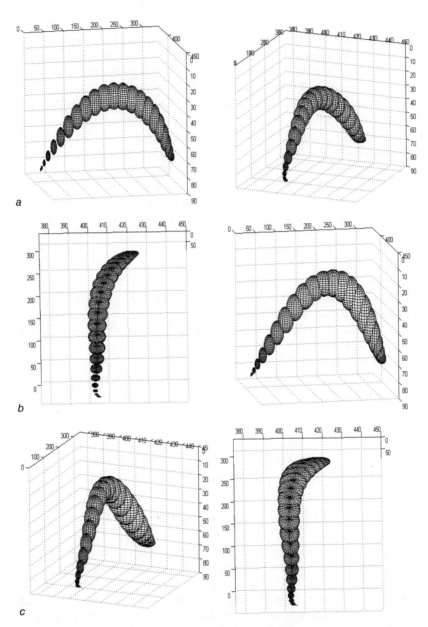

▶ **Figure 7.1** Three-dimensional representations of variability created from the ellipsoid method described in chapter 2. Depicted in the figure is the spatial variability associated with movements made by two participants under full-vision and no-vision conditions. There are *(a)* lateral, *(b)* dorsolateral, and *(c)* superior views of the ellipsoids for each condition. In all three perspectives, differences in three-dimensional variability between the two conditions emerge very early in the movement trajectory (at approximately 100 ms).

Reprinted, by permission, from S. Hansen, D. Elliott, and M.A. Khan, 2008, "Quantifying the variability of three-dimensional aiming movements using ellipsoids," *Motor Control* 12: 241-251.

other terms, when a person is given strict accuracy constraints, a specific target affords an action of a set duration (Gibson, 1977). The relationship between the temporal duration and the amount of information is directly proportional. The slope of the increase in MT with an increase in information has been shown to depend on the effector used to complete the movement (Langolf, Chaffin, & Foulke, 1976). The relationship remains evident under different gravitational constraints (Jüngling, Bock, & Girgenrath, 2002), underwater (Kerr, 1978), and with imaginary targets (Maruff et al., 1999).

Researchers can investigate visual motor processes by manipulating the relationship of the target width and amplitude to acquire the same predicted MT based on the information that the performer has to process (e.g., MacKenzie, Marteniuk, Dugas, Liske, & Eickmeier, 1987). Similar accuracy and MT performances can be acquired when the target displays the same amount of information even though the target width and movement amplitude are half of the previous dimensions (Fitts, 1954). In the absence of environmental perturbation, the manipulation of either the time requirements or the accuracy constraints allows for the examination of the speed–accuracy trade-off and to a lesser extent the strategic control of action (e.g., Elliott et al., 2004; Rabbit, 1981; Schmidt, Zelaznik, Hawkins, Frank, & Quinn, 1979).

Researchers can burden the system by requiring participants to maintain accuracy while completing their movements in shorter amounts of time. In this manner, it is possible to examine how participants cope with the added demand of acquiring the target in a normally insufficient duration. As mentioned earlier, when this manipulation is combined with the occlusion of vision, it has added utility for determining temporal limitations of visual regulation (Keele & Posner, 1968).

Perturbations of the target location and size are employed to investigate the temporal and spatial limitations of visual regulation. Experiments in this context are based on the premise that the initial movement behavior is associated with the previous planning of the movement and adjustments in the limb trajectory or deviations from the unperturbed condition are associated with sensorimotor feedback. Research has shown that the latter portions of goal-directed movements are influenced by vision gathered early in the movement (Heath et al., 1998) and that the initial portions of action can be corrected if movement error can be detected rapidly (Paulignan, MacKenzie, Marteniuk, & Jeannerod, 1991; Pélisson et al., 1986).

In the context of the two-component model, shorter amounts of time before and longer amounts of time after the acquisition of peak velocity can indicate time-consuming movement corrections in the latter portion of the movement. For example, Heath and colleagues (1998) demonstrated that presenting a target during the movement planning stage influences the time before peak velocity. The time after peak velocity is determined by the size of the target introduced after movement initiation (see also Fernandez,

Warren, & Bootsma, 2006; Hansen & Elliott, 2009). Heath and colleagues (1998) posited that the change in the target characteristics altered the timing of the movement because the change introduced or removed the necessity for corrective modifications in the trajectory. A similar explanation is that the change in timing resulted from modifications in the information processing constraints associated with the new task characteristics. Specifically, increasing target width reduced the amount of information that required processing during the movement, resulting in a simultaneous reduction in the amount of time required to complete the movement. In comparison, increases in MT are associated with increases in the complexity of the information processed during the movement, which are brought on by decreasing target width. The time course of the adjustments to the change in target characteristics is relevant for researchers interested in visual regulation in the absence of complete occlusion.

The initial portions of movement trajectories are also amenable to changes in target position. For example, participants in the study of Pélisson and coworkers (1986) were capable of acquiring a target that changed position during a saccadic eye movement toward the target. The target was acquired without vision of the effector, without conscious awareness that the target had moved, and, more importantly, without evidence of discrete corrections in the trajectory. The latter finding indicates that the initial portions of the movement trajectory typically associated with advance planning of the movement can be adjusted rapidly without incurring temporal costs associated with target overshoots and undershoots (see Elliott et al., 2004). Similarly, Paulignan and colleagues (1991) discovered that participants could adjust the trajectory of a prehension movement within 100 ms of initiation if the target was moved at the start of the action. By using TMS in conjunction with this type of target-stepping paradigm, Desmurget and coworkers (1999) were able to stimulate the PPC in order to disrupt the trajectory corrections of pointing movements of an unseen limb to targets that changed position. In comparison to models predicting that initial behavior is completed as planned and that the latter portion of movement trajectories is adjusted based on sensorimotor feedback (e.g., Heath et al., 1998), the latter studies indicate that even the early portions of action can be adjusted rapidly when task constraints change.

Visual Illusions

An alternative to observing movement planning and execution in an unperturbed context is to deceive the visual system with visual illusions. In a reaching task or an aiming task, visual illusions can change the perceived target size or required amplitude of the movement (Coren, 1986). Similarly to the physical perturbation of task characteristics, the presentation of size-contrast illusions before and during movement execution can be used to investigate visual–motor control processes (Haffenden & Goodale, 1998; Handlovsky, Hansen, Lee, & Elliott, 2004). Influences of visual illusions on movement control parallel those of physical changes to the environment. However, rather than the rapid adjustment of the trajectory elicited by studies employing new task constraints, the behavior of interest in illusion studies is temporal duration and limits of the detection and response to the erroneous information. Illusions often require major trajectory adjustments because movement planning or initial execution is influenced by the illusion.

Recent neurophysiological models of visual control posit that specific movement outcomes result from the different neural systems needed to perceive and respond to the relevant environmental information (Milner & Goodale, 1995; Ungerleider & Mishkin, 1982). Specifically, Milner and Goodale (1995) proposed a functional dissociation between the dorsal and ventral visual streams. The function of the brain areas associated with the termination of the dorsal and ventral visual streams is the core of the hypothesis. The ventral stream physically terminates in the inferior temporal areas of the brain and is associated with object identification, perception, and allocentric spatial coding. In comparison, the dorsal stream terminates in the superior parietal areas of the brain and is associated with movement execution in an egocentric frame of reference. While the debate over visual control continues to focus on the relative contribution or function of these anatomical subsystems for goal-directed movement, the deceptiveness of visual illusions provides an excellent medium to explore hypotheses related to a functional separation of sensorimotor systems.

Debate over the influence of diverging visual information on movement executions has added a level of complexity to the investigation of visual–motor control. In this context, visual illusions are employed to investigate the contributions of the ventral and dorsal streams to the perception of the environment and goal-directed actions (e.g., Mendoza, Elliott, Meegan, Lyons, & Welsh, 2006). Illusions influence movement behavior because they affect the relevant spatial information in the environment. Differences in perceptual and motor performance should exist depending on the visual information gathered and the structures receiving that information (see Mendoza, Hansen, Glazebrook, Keetch, & Elliott, 2005; chapter 13).

Theoretically, a functional dissociation in movement execution can be observed because memory-dependent aiming is executed with reference to a representation that is decayed in the dorsal stream but maintained in the ventral stream (Westwood & Goodale, 2003). As such, the relative contributions of the two visual streams are investigated by introducing memory constraints (Binsted & Elliott, 1999; Elliott & Lee, 1995; Haffenden & Goodale, 1998; Westwood, Chapman, & Roy, 2000; Westwood & Goodale, 2003; Westwood, Heath, & Roy, 2000) in combination with size-contrast illusions because it is posited that the ventral visual stream is affected by the illusion while the dorsal stream is not (Haffenden & Goodale, 1998).

Although the idea of a functional dissociation between perceptual decision making and action is appealing, both rapid aiming and grasping paradigms have produced contradictory results (Aglioti, DeSouza, & Goodale, 1995; Binsted & Elliott, 1999; Handlovsky et al., 2004; Westwood & Goodale, 2003). Some researchers reported that the illusion influenced target perception but did not influence movement execution unless execution was dependent on memory representations of the environment (Westwood et al., 2000). Other researchers observed that the illusion affected both target perception and action toward the target (Franz, Gegenfurtner, Bülthoff, & Fahle, 2000). Consequently, Glover and Dixon (2002) suggested that illusory contexts affect movement preparation but not movement execution. However, recent evidence indicates that illusion influences movement preparation and execution in an additive manner (Handlovsky et al., 2004; Mendoza et al., 2006).

Overall, individual variation in response to visual illusions makes the employment of illusions difficult (Coren, 1986). Inferences from such studies should be interpreted cautiously. These issues are covered more fully in chapter 13.

Changing the Visual Context

An additional means of investigating visual regulation is to manipulate the associations between the effector and the environment by inducing temporal delays (Smith & Bowen, 1980), moving the visual background (Proteau & Masson, 1997), or using prisms to displace visual information relative to proprioceptive information (Hansen et al., 2007; Redding & Wallace, 2001, 2002, 2003). Participants expect the relationship between sensory input and motor output to be in concordance based on their experience. However, evidence indicates that individuals can adjust their movements rapidly once execution errors are detected (Pélisson et al., 1986).

In deceptive contexts, adjustments can be advantageous or detrimental because they can occur even if the error is detected when limb velocity is misperceived due to a moving background. For example, Proteau and Masson (1997) manipulated the background of a computer screen so that it moved in the opposite direction (experiment 1) or in the same direction (experiment 2) as a cursor controlled by a force transducer. The perturbation induced the impression that the cursor was moving more slowly or faster than it really was. Although participants undershot the target in both conditions, they terminated their movements earlier when the background moved in the opposite direction, indicating that they perceived the cursor to be moving faster than it actually was. More importantly, Proteau and

Masson (1997) parsed the movements during data analyses in such a way that there was no opportunity for discrete visual corrections to be included in the trajectory analyses. Therefore, the results indicated that the initial portion of the movement response typically associated with advance planning was modified continuously, without an abrupt change in force production that would be associated with discrete error correction.

Similar to the work of Paulignan and colleagues (1991), studies by Proteau and Masson (1997) provided evidence that vision could be employed rapidly to adjust the initial impulse of a movement. The latter work is in contrast with the notion that the initial component of a rapid movement occurs without influence of sensory feedback and simply unfolds as planned while the performer gathers information for movement corrections within later portions of the trajectory.

In addition to Proteau and Masson (1997), Smith and Bowen (1980) presented data consistent with the idea that movements can be modified rapidly. Smith and Bowen (1980) used high-speed video to examine the influence of delaying and displacing visual information of the entire work space during rapid goal-directed action. They observed that discrete changes in the movement trajectories occurred more often than every 200 ms. Delayed visual information deteriorated movement accuracy for movements less than 160 ms in duration. Evidently, interfering with the relationship between the acquired visual information and the effector is an effective method of inducing rapid adjustments of the limb during goal-directed action.

An interesting means of creating discordance between the visual environment and the movement completed in the environment is to employ prisms (e.g., Redding & Wallace, 2003). Prisms displace vision of the effector and environment relative to the motor representation of the movement. Thus, prisms can be used to disrupt the expected interaction between the participant and the outcomes within the work space. Researchers have used Fresnel prisms to examine sensorimotor adaptive processes (Redding & Wallace, 2003) and motor development (Hay, 1979) and to prevent ceiling performance effects during goal-directed action (Elliott & Allard, 1985; Elliott & Jaeger, 1988). Typical prism experiments involve three testing phases. First, a pre-exposure phase provides baseline measurements of performance. Second, an exposure phase allows participants to calibrate and align to the displacement. Third, a post-exposure phase investigates adaptation to the prism by measuring the magnitude of the negative after-effect (compensation of the perceptual–motor system in the opposite direction of the displacement).

Although the triphase methodology is effective for exploring the calibration and alignment to visual displacement (for reviews on prism adaptation, see Redding & Wallace, 2002; Welch, 1978), researchers have recently employed prisms to investigate rapid adjustments to visual displacement (Hansen et al., 2007; Redding & Wallace, 2003). For example, Redding and Wallace (2003) studied a phenomenon termed *first-trial adaptation to prism exposure.* In this phenomenon, participants terminate their initial movement only 5° from the target location even though the prism displaces their vision by 10° in total. In other words, participants rapidly engage in visual–motor processing and then cease their movements closer to the actual target location than is expected given the total magnitude of the perturbation. This adaptation indicates rapid online calibration of the sensorimotor system to the incompatibility.

The relative importance of these types of visual regulation processes can be emphasized when the direction of the displacement is unpredictable (Elliott, Calvert, Jaeger, & Jones, 1990; Hansen et al., 2007). Rapid adjustments to the displacement benefit the participant in these situations. However, alignment of the sensorimotor system to a specific displacement of the environment is detrimental. For example, Elliott and colleagues (1990) revealed the benefits of the decay of displaced visual information before movement onset. Participants were exposed to an orientation of the prism for 2 s and then made aiming movements under conditions of full vision, no vision, no vision with a 2 s delay, or no vision with a 10 s delay. Participants were much more accurate in the delay conditions and more accurate with a longer delay before movement initiation. In addition, in a series of rapid aiming experiments, Hansen and coworkers (2007) introduced (experiment 2) and removed (experiment 3) left and right orientations of a Fresnel prism. Early presentation and removal of the displacement influenced movement outcome in both experiment 2 and experiment 3. Interestingly, male and female participants reacted differently to the stimulus. Female participants were partial to the visual context presented during movement execution, while male behavior depended on the visual information presented before the movement regardless of when the manipulation occurred. Speculations remain surrounding the locus of the latter results. Specifically, the behaviors could result from cognitive strategies, processes associated with visual regulation, or physical differences in neural and anatomical structures. However, it is evident that human behavior is flexible to changes in the environmental context irrespective of the locus of the gender differences in behavior.

Deceiving the Control Processes

Occlusion experiments designed to determine the relative importance of early and late visual information from the movement trajectory have yielded mixed results. Grierson and Elliott (2008, 2009) recently suggested that discrepancies in the perturbation literature might be explained by two distinctly different forms of online control. Building on the work of Woodworth (1899), they have proposed that feedback-based control late in the trajectory relies on a comparison of the relative position of the limb with the position of the target as the limb approaches the target. For this type of control, aiming error is reduced by a discrete modification to the movement path. If the final limb position will fall short of the target, a second acceleration is introduced to propel the limb the extra distance. If the final limb position will overshoot the target, a discrete reversal is necessary. These adjustments, made late in the movement, occur only after the limb has entered foveal vision and is in the vicinity of the target.

In contrast to Woodworth's notion that the initial part of a movement is ballistic and not amenable to online control (see also Meyer et al., 1988), Grierson and Elliott (2008) suggested that there is a very early type of visual regulation based on a comparison of early dynamic information from the limb (e.g., limb velocity and direction) with an internal model or representation of the expected sensory consequences of the movement (see Wolpert & Miall, 1996). This type of vision regulation results from a graded adjustment to primary impulses used to accelerate and decelerate the limb and can occur quite early because the error reduction process is based on a comparator established before movement initiation.

To test their ideas about early and late control, Grierson and Elliott (2008, 2009) introduced separate perturbations designed to affect each of these forms of regulation. For example, they used a moving background to influence the perceived velocity of the limb movement (a manipulation designed to affect early control), as well as a Müller-Lyer illusion to perturb the perceived position of the target (a manipulation designed to affect late control). Consistent with their hypothesis, Grierson and Elliott (2009) found that the Müller-Lyer illusion had a late effect on the corrective process, whereas the moving background affected early limb control.

In another study, Grierson and Elliott (2009) abandoned an illusion-based approach and actually altered the target position at movement initiation. In addition, they used an air compressor to physically perturb the velocity of the limb at about the time of peak acceleration. They again found evidence for early and late online regulation of limb trajectories.

Online Perturbations

Advances in optoelectronics have provided the opportunity to perturb the environmental context based on the participant's concurrent actions. Arguably, introducing perturbations at specific predetermined spatial and temporal locations in a movement can change a participant's approach to the task. Subsequently, the kinematics of the movement trajectories would vary artificially from those associated with movement in an unperturbed situation, defeating the purpose of disrupting the system. A further caveat is that spatial and temporal perturbation studies can introduce the manipulation before or after the initiation of corrective processes associated with vision obtained during the trial. Participants who are proficient at the action under investigation might even finish their movements when a temporal manipulation is employed. Introducing perturbations based on the kinematics of the concurrent action provides an alternative to spatial and temporal perturbations. It also offers the opportunity to perturb the movements at specific kinematic markers in order to investigate visual control models that highlight the importance of those markers (Elliott et al., 1999). Recently, Hansen, Tremblay, and Elliott (2008) introduced a Fresnel prism that displaced vision of the environment by 14.25° when participants reached peak acceleration, peak velocity, and an estimated time of peak deceleration. Movements were significantly influenced when the perturbation was introduced at peak acceleration. Actions terminated farther in the direction of the perturbation when the manipulation was introduced early. Participants were capable of completing their movements as without disruption when the perturbation was introduced at peak velocity or later in the trajectory. Presumably, actions were completed based on the vision gathered before movement initiation and during early portions of the trajectory. The latter experiment provided support for the notion that individuals can adjust their trajectories rapidly by using visual information provided early during discrete action.

Other researchers have employed concurrent perturbations to examine the attentional processes associated with movement planning and control. For example, Ketelaars, Khan, and Franks (1999) presented probe stimuli to participants when they reached peak acceleration and peak velocity of single-target extension and two-target extension and flexion movements. Participants were required to execute a bite response on a bite bar when the probe stimulus was presented while they attempted to perform the arm movements. Bite responses to the probe stimulus were coupled with the subsequent movement responses of the limb. Increases in probe RT were associated with the planning of the subsequent movement and the execution of the corrective modifications to the concurrent movement. In other words, the time spent in executing the later portion of the first movement and the time spent in transition between the first and second movements increased when a bite response was required during the first movement.

In general, online perturbations provide a method of introducing manipulations without incurring the potential caveats of spatial and temporal perturbation. Tying perturbations to the kinematics of movement provides an interesting venue of investigation for researchers. Theoretically, these techniques can be used to examine visual regulation in the absence of conscious anticipation (Hansen et al., 2008).

Manipulating Certainty of the Visual Environment

Uncertainty and predictability of the environment can contribute to visual motor behaviors (Hansen, Glazebrook, Anson, Weeks, & Elliott, 2006; Zelaznik et al., 1983). Previous knowledge about the goal of simple aiming movements and the availability of sensory feedback during movement execution can influence the strategic approach taken by the performer (Hansen et al., 2006). For example, in a study by Hansen and colleagues (2006), participants who were certain of the target location and the visual environment in advance of the response imperative adopted a closed-loop strategy of limb control that depended on visual feedback. Specifically, performers displayed a shorter RT and a longer MT when they were aware of the target location and the availability of vision. Hansen and colleagues proposed that these temporal effects indicated that participants initiated their action quickly with the knowledge that they could employ visual information to correct trajectory errors during the ensuing action. However, RT was longer and MT was shorter when individuals were uncertain of the ensuing visual context and target location or knew that they would not be able to see the environment during the aiming response. Thus participants were selecting a response based on a worst-case assumption about the information that would be available during movement execution (Zelaznik et al., 1983). In this situation, visual occlusion is the worst-case scenario, and participants adopted a more feed-forward approach to the task (Hansen et al., 2006).

Conditions of certainty and uncertainty are dichotomized along a spectrum of familiarity. Performers draw from a knowledge base of previous performances and their capacity to perform with certainty of the visual conditions involved in a task. Arguably, performers can also misperceive their capacity to perform a task relative to the expected outcome of themselves and observers. Performers can select a default setting when presented with the worst-case scenario. In other words, they can rely on a course of action that has proved to be effective in similar situations. The course of action might not produce the maximal outcome when conditions are optimal (i.e., full-vision conditions), but it should produce the maximum gain in the current situation, in which the potential for optimal conditions is low. Individuals should be able to employ vision when available and kinesthesis when vision is not available following movement initiation. When the visual situation is unknown, the gains associated with having vision to correct movement errors are not worth the outcome that will result should a movement executed in expectation of vision have to be completed with vision occluded (Hansen et al., 2006).

Although Hansen and colleagues (2006) provided evidence that individuals require complete task-relevant information to modify their behavior, Trommershäuser, Matis, Maloney, and Landy (2006) provided evidence that individuals can plan and execute aiming movements despite a delayed (0, 200, and 400 ms) and unpredictable appearance of a penalty zone in the vicinity of the target. Terminal movement efficiency decreased only when the penalty zone was presented during latter portions of the movement (i.e., 400 ms from the stimulus onset). This finding indicates that the participants incorporated the presented knowledge of the area to avoid and then modify their trajectories during the movement. In an earlier study, Trommershäuser, Gepshtein, Maloney, Landy, and Banks (2005) reported evidence of the capacity to engage in this type of incorporating process without conscious knowledge. Trommershaüser and colleagues (2005) induced trajectory variability into the cursor representation of the effector during rapid upper-limb movements. Participants did not compensate for the systematic variability on individual trials. However, they adjusted their movement trajectories to the imposed variability following moderate practice ($n < 120$ trials). Participants reported that they were unaware that there was systematic variability added to the cursor movement when quizzed by the experimenter.

The latter experiments occluded vision of the environment or limb. However, knowledge of the target location is also of utmost importance. In an experiment designed to examine the influence of target uncertainty on movement planning and execution, Elliott and Calvert (1990) had participants aim in a simple RT or choice RT situation under conditions of full vision or under one of three conditions of no vision. Vision was occluded at or before movement initiation (stimulus onset or 2 s before stimulus onset, respectively) in order to investigate the influence of the decay of the visual environment on movement performance when participants had to recall one spatial location or a choice between two locations. Although RT and MT were significantly lower in the target-known condition, target uncertainty had little influence when combined with the visual conditions. Movement accuracy decreased with an increase in the availability of visual information at a cost of increased MT. The latter result indicates that the individuals employed the visual information about the target and environment when they knew that it would be available.

A dependence on vision can be detrimental in many situations (e.g., Proteau, 1992). Familiarity with the sensory consequences of actions following practice reinforces the gross behavior and the control of the fine adjustments that occur during the movement. Visual cues about the target, effector, and environment provide information for future control in that specific context. Specifically, some researchers advocate that manipulating the conditions of the afferent information provided to participants leads to decrements in performance, especially with extended practice (Proteau, 1992; Proteau & Cournoyer, 1990; Proteau, Marteniuk, & Levesque, 1992). However, other researchers have demonstrated that individuals are flexible when it comes to the afferent information gathered and attended to during movement (Tremblay, Welsh, & Elliott, 2001; Tremblay & Proteau, 1998). Perturbing the expected environmental context is a robust means of examining the processes and behaviors participants have developed following practice under specific visual contexts. For example, Tremblay and colleagues (2001) had participants complete computer mouse movements with and without vision of the cursor in an experiment designed to investigate the importance of vision of the limb during practice. Participants in the variable-practice groups executed movements to five different targets. Constant-practice participants completed movements to the same target throughout the protocol. Half the participants in each group practiced their movements with full vision or no vision of the cursor. Interestingly, participants in the target-only condition managed to reduce their end-point error even after practice. This finding is in contrast to the expectations of models predicting that practice causes participants to become dependent on the visual information gathered from the effector (e.g., Proteau, 1992). This result potentially was caused by an augmented dependence on kinesthesis for increases in accuracy during movements to the various targets (Tremblay et al., 2001). Tremblay and Proteau (1998) suggested that individuals dominantly attend to a single source of afferent information with practice of a task. Evidently, individuals are flexible in deciding which source of afferent information is most beneficial.

Future Directions

In addition to using the visual perturbations mentioned throughout this chapter, researchers have recently employed TMS (Desmurget et al., 1999), other neural disruptions such as galvanic vestibular stimulation, and physical disruptions such as tendon vibration in their studies of goal-directed movement. In all cases, researchers follow similar logic when ascertaining when and where to introduce the perturbation. In other words, the model under investigation still drives the manipulations employed to observe adaptations in behavior irrespective of the afferent or efferent system under investigation. Research on the function of other afferent and efferent systems such as the vestibular and proprioceptive systems in isolation will also be of interest for motor control researchers in the near future. Observing interactions of multiple afferent and efferent processes provides more ecologically valid information on the function of the human systems that can surpass the knowledge acquired by examining the systems in isolation.

In the future, perturbations to examine the sensorimotor system will be combined with neuroimaging techniques to determine the neural correlates of control. Discovering the locus of neural control of movements is becoming possible as medical imaging techniques grow increasingly available to researchers. The gauntlet thrown down is to ensure that the pattern of neural activation can be associated directly with the perturbation introduced to the participant. Doing so involves ensuring the viability of the manipulation and testing numerous individuals spanning various population characteristics to assure that the results can be generalized to the general population.

Unfortunately for researchers who prefer to control for as many variables as possible, the behavior of mature participants does not occur in isolation.

Mature observers have an inherent knowledge of the capacity of their motor system to interact with the environment due to practice over their life span, recent practice, and concurrent actions. Experience with various situations helps the performer to formulate possibilities for interaction with the environment that can result in beneficial or detrimental effects. In essence, individuals have the capacity to engage in the process of learned causality, relating stimuli from the environment and the capacity of their bodies to a causal outcome.

The human sensorimotor system functions normally when perturbed, but the flexibility of the active processes allows for adaptation to the imposed obstruction from the environment. This adaptation to the stimulus based on visual and proprioceptive information for movement adjustment is of relevance to sensorimotor researchers. Both feedback processes during action and changes to the planning of impending actions based on integrated information contribute to observed behavior. Selecting and deselecting the active visual and proprioceptive processes before and during the action might be as simple as choosing a scalpel for surgery and a chef's knife for chopping onions. Previous sections of this chapter presented evidence for adaptive processes in multiple contexts that suggests that a variety of processes are available and can be accessed depending on the environmental context and the previous experience.

Overall, the complex mixture of theories, influential variables, observations, and subsequent hypotheses creates a challenging field for visual control researchers. Uncovering the sensorimotor processes controlling goal-directed movements is an arduous task. The process is complicated further by the necessity to consider independent variables such as the effectors involved in the task and the perturbation paradigm employed. As such, evidence for individual differences in human motor development, psychological capabilities, and motor performance indicate the need to employ individual characteristics as independent variables during the examination of goal-directed movements of adult humans. Actions involving multiple effectors provide additional complexity to the investigation of the underlying visual control processes. In general, human movement control is flexible but is subject to the performer's experience with the task conditions. The observed behavior therefore results from the characteristics of the performer and the performer's experience with the experimental context.

CHAPTER 8

Visual Field Asymmetries in the Control of Target-Directed Movements

MICHAEL A. KHAN AND GORDON BINSTED

When reaching to a location in space, people typically fixate on the target either before initiating limb movement or very early in the limb trajectory (Abrams, Meyer, & Kornblum, 1990; see chapter 11 for a review of eye–hand coordination). This coordinated eye–hand action places the hand within the peripheral vision early in the movement and within the central vision when nearing the target. In addition, because in many reaching and pointing movements the hand starts at a position close to the body and then moves out toward a point in space, the hand is typically in the lower visual field throughout its trajectory to the target. Thus researchers have postulated that different parts of the visual field have distinct functional roles in the control of target-directed aiming movements.

In this chapter, we examine how changes in the location where the limb (or target) appears on the retina influence a person's ability to prepare and control aiming movements. We consider the issue of whether differences in visuomotor processing between central vision and peripheral vision are due to the position of the limb in the visual field (and any processing benefits this provides) or the time that is available to process visual information as the limb traverses peripheral and central vision. Then we consider whether visual feedback from peripheral and central vision is used differentially to correct errors during limb movement or to modify movement commands on subsequent trials. Finally, we direct our attention to comparing the upper and lower visual fields, looking at differences in perceptual processing, attention (resolution and shifting), and visuomotor control associated with target-directed movements (for a review see Danckert & Goodale, 2004).

The focus of this chapter is on visual field asymmetries in visuomotor performance. Specifically, we investigate the proposition that the lower visual field provides an advantage in the control of target-directed movements.

Peripheral Vision Versus Central Vision

Taking into consideration observed anisotropies in retinal ganglion distributions (see Rovamo, 1978; Popovic & Sjöstrand, 2001; Wässle, Grünert, Röhrenbeck, & Boycott, 1989), Paillard and Amblard (1985) forwarded a model of visuomotor control that postulates distinct functional roles for peripheral vision and central vision. Specifically, Paillard and Amblard proposed that information from peripheral and central vision is processed via two semi-independent visual systems. The kinetic channel processes high-speed visual information from peripheral vision and plays an important role in the control of movement direction. The static channel operates in central vision and plays a major role in controlling movement amplitude during the homing-in phase of the limb trajectory when limb velocities are relatively low.

As previously mentioned, the limb crosses the peripheral visual field during the early stages of an aiming movement and crosses through the central vision during the later stages. Based on Woodworth's (1899) seminal idea that aiming movements consist of a ballistic initial impulse followed by feedback-based error correction, an extensive body of research has investigated the importance of visual feedback from early and late in the movement trajectory. On the one hand, studies have found that visual feedback from early in the movement is not critical for aiming accuracy and that vision over the last half of the movement is necessary for optimal accuracy (Beaubaton & Hay, 1986; Carlton, 1981). On the other hand, other studies have revealed that vision over the first half of the movement is important for aiming accuracy. Notably, Spijkers and colleagues (Spijkers & Lochner, 1994; Spijkers & Spellerberg, 1995) have shown that visually occluding the initial part of the limb trajectory reduces the percentage of target hits. Unlike manipulations of early vision, visual occlusion extended to the second half of the movement results in significant increases in MT and error rates (e.g., Carlton, 1981).

While the efficacy of visual feedback during the early and late stages of movement is somewhat contentious, these manipulations also have implications for understanding the roles of peripheral vision and central vision. Since many of the studies manipulating early and late vision are not performed with the intent of comparing peripheral vision with central vision, they vary considerably in terms of task (e.g., single-dimensional versus multidimensional movements), error measurements (e.g., separate versus combined amplitude and directional error measurements), visual angle between start and target position, and MT. We now take a more systematic look at the roles of central vision and peripheral vision in the control of movement direction, variability, and amplitude.

Directional Control

In order to isolate the control of movement direction, researchers traditionally have employed aiming tasks in which there is no amplitude constraint. In such directional aiming tasks, participants move through the target in a sweeping manner similar to striking a ball. Hence, in directional aiming tasks and in contrast to more conventional aiming tasks, the limb does not stop at the target (velocity > 0). More importantly, when participants fixate on the target, vision during the early part of the movement is in effect peripheral vision, while vision during the last part of movement corresponds to central vision. As would be expected, accuracy is highest when vision of the entire movement is available compared with when no vision is available. More importantly, Bard, Hay, & Fleury (1985) have shown that information provided early in the movement trajectory (i.e., when movement is in the peripheral visual field) is sufficient to achieve optimal levels of directional accuracy. Interestingly, there is also an advantage gained from having vision available in the late part of the movement (i.e., when movement is in the central visual field). Subsequently, Bard, Paillard, Fleury, Hay, and Larue (1990) showed that both peripheral vision (70°-20° eccentricity) and central vision (10°-0° eccentricity) improve directional accuracy when compared with no vision. While the benefit of peripheral vision was consistent with the two-channel model proposed by Paillard and Amblard (1985), the contribution of central vision to feedback control was not expected.

One possible account of the role of central vision in improving performance is that feedback is not used to correct errors in the limb trajectory during movement execution (online); rather, movement parameters are adjusted on subsequent trials (off-line; see also chapter 2). Furthermore, feedback from central vision is available only late in the movement and hence there may not be enough time for feedback loops to operate during movement execution, especially when MT is relatively short. Participants may be using information about where the limb passes the target on trial n as a form of knowledge of results (KR) to improve programming on trial $n + 1$.

In order to further understand the roles of peripheral and central vision in the control of movement direction, Proteau and colleagues undertook a series of studies in which they systematically investigated the capabilities and limitations of the two visual fields. In the first of these studies, Abahnini, Proteau, and Temprado (1997) required participants to perform aiming movements with vision occluded centrally or peripherally (c.f., Bard et al., 1990). Regardless of the overall viewing condition (monocular or binocular), accuracy levels in the peripheral-vision (44°-12° eccentricity) and central-vision (12°-0° eccentricity) conditions were as high as they were in the full-vision condition. Abahnini and colleagues noted that in the central-vision condition, vision was available for only 79 ms; hence, they proposed that participants did not have enough time to process this information and make corrections before the limb reached the target.

In order to test whether information from central vision is used as a form of KR to program subsequent movements, the researchers performed a second experiment that included a condition in which the hand was visible only as it crossed the target. In this experiment, MT was also increased to investigate whether peripheral vision would be useful at slower movement speeds ($55°/s$ versus speeds greater than $100°/s$). As in their first experiment, accuracy levels in both the peripheral-vision and the central-vision conditions were as high as they were in the full-vision condition. Thus the authors concluded that the kinetic channel (Paillard & Amblard, 1985) is operational for relatively slow stimuli moving across the peripheral visual field. Furthermore, being able to see the hand as it passes the target results in higher accuracy when compared with the no-vision condition. Although accuracy levels were not as high as they were under the central-vision condition, these results show that information about where the hand passes the target can be used to program subsequent movements.

In the peripheral-vision condition employed by Abahnini and colleagues (1997), the opaque shield occluded vision in central vision but allowed the hand to be visible as it crossed the targets. Hence, terminal feedback was similar across viewing conditions, potentially explaining why performance was comparable in the full-vision, peripheral-vision, and central-vision conditions. Addressing this concern, Abahnini and Proteau (1999) employed a video-based aiming task during which they manipulated visual feedback by varying the visibility of the cursor. The target was always present, and results were again similar to those obtained with the more conventional aiming task. When the peripheral visual field was defined as $10°$ eccentricity and beyond, accuracy levels were similar for the full-vision, peripheral-vision, and central-vision conditions. Interestingly, when peripheral vision was constrained to $14°$ eccentricity, accuracy was better than it was in the no-vision condition but not as good as it was in the full-vision and central-vision conditions. Therefore, it seems that information obtained within $14°$ and $10°$ of visual angle is critical for optimal control of movement direction. This speculation was supported in a follow-up examination (Proteau, Boivin, Linossier, & Abahnini, 2000) that closely controlled the range of viewing (i.e., $40°-0°$, $40°-10°$, $40°-20°$, $40°-30°$, $20°-10°$, or not visible throughout the trajectory). The study demonstrated that the most critical information from peripheral vision for the directional control of aiming movements was $20°$ to $10°$ of visual angle. Information beyond $20°$ did not appear to be useful for the control of movement direction. In order to investigate whether the benefit of visual feedback from $20°$ to $10°$ of visual angle is due to online or off-line processing, Proteau and colleagues analyzed the first trial in each visual condition; since these trials are not preceded by any feedback, they should not be influenced by off-line processing. Data in these initial trials again demonstrated the importance of information gathered between 10° and 20° eccentricity. Hence, it seems that the benefit of visual feedback is indeed due to online processing.

The question of how information arising from central and peripheral inputs underlies visual feedback (online or off-line processing) has also been addressed by analyzing variability in limb trajectory (see chapter 2). In contrast to the directional aiming tasks described for the previously discussed studies, Bédard and Proteau (2003) required participants to end their movement on the target, thus enabling the use of kinematic landmarks (e.g., peak acceleration, peak velocity, peak deceleration) for determination of online processes. Overall, variability in the position of the limb orthogonal to the primary direction of movement increased at each successive kinematic marker. The rate at which directional variability increased was lower when participants could see the cursor over the entire movement trajectory when compared with when the cursor was visible in peripheral vision between visual angles of 40° to 25° and 40° to 15°. Furthermore, variability rose at a lower rate in these two peripheral-vision conditions when compared with when the cursor was not seen throughout the movement. Since variability in all vision conditions increased linearly as the movement progressed, Bédard and Proteau concluded that the benefit of peripheral vision was due to off-line processing and not online control.

In the study of Bédard and Proteau (2003), MT ranged between 240 and 310 ms. These MT values may have been too short too enable online corrections to occur in the video-based aiming task employed (also see Khan et al., 2003). Hence, in a subsequent study Bédard and Proteau (2004) increased MT up to 900 ms. Furthermore, they computed coefficients of variability at each kinematic marker (i.e., variability divided by the distance traveled to the target). The reasoning behind this analysis was that online corrections could be inferred only if coefficients of variability decreased as MT decreased. Consistent with their previous study (Bédard & Proteau, 2003), and in agreement with an off-line use of central visual cues, coefficients of variability did not vary throughout the trajectory when MT was relatively short (300 ms). However, when MT was 400 ms or greater, coefficients of variability decreased as the movement progressed in all conditions providing vision. Thus, when sufficient time was available, vision from either peripheral or central vision could be utilized to implement corrections during movement execution. Hence, Bédard and Proteau suggested that peripheral vision and central vision may not have specialized functions for the online control of movement—instead, utilization occurs simply by way of opportunity.

In the task employed by Bédard and Proteau (2004), participants were required to stop on the target. Since limb velocities were low at the end of the movement, the limb spent more time in central vision than it would for a purely directional aiming task in which there is no need to reduce limb velocity upon approaching the target. Therefore, Khan, Lawrence, Franks, and Buckolz (2004) were interested in whether the contributions of peripheral and central vision in the control of movement direction were indeed determined by the time available to process visual information and whether the actual location of visual information in the visual field had any effect. Similar to Proteau and colleagues, Khan and colleagues employed a video-based aiming task in which participants performed aiming movements away from the body on a horizontal digitizing tablet. In experiment 1, participants fixated on the target, and the task was performed with vision of the cursor throughout the movement, with vision of the cursor through 40° to 10° (peripheral or early vision), with vision of the cursor through 10° to 0° (central or late vision), or without vision of the cursor. Importantly for this investigation, participants were instructed to move through the targets in 450 ms. Since the task did not have an amplitude requirement, variability of limb trajectories at 25%, 50%, 75%, and 100% of the distance from the start position to the target was analyzed. This analysis revealed that variability was lowest in the full-vision and peripheral-vision (early) conditions compared with the central-vision (late) condition, which in turn was less variable than the no-vision condition (see figure 8.1a). More importantly, trend analyses indicated that variability increased linearly for the no-vision and central-vision (late) conditions, while variability leveled off toward the end of the movement in the peripheral-vision (early) and full-vision conditions (i.e., there was a significant quadratic component). From calculating the ratios in variability between each visual condition (full, peripheral, central) and the no-vision condition, it was confirmed that the forms of the variability profiles were different in the full-vision and peripheral-vision conditions compared with the no-vision condition, whereas there was no difference between the central-vision and the no-vision conditions. Khan and colleagues consequently proposed that peripheral vision is used to modify the limb trajectory during movement execution while central vision is used off-line to improve the programming of subsequent trials. Note that in the study of Bédard and Proteau (2004) the cursor was visible centrally for approximately 169 ms, leading to evidence of online control. Conversely, in the investigation by Khan and colleagues (2004), the cursor was visible in central vision for only 83 ms, yielding data more consistent with off-line processing.

In order to further assess whether the ability to process peripheral vision online is due to its early availability in the limb trajectory or the actual location of this information in the visual field, Khan and colleagues (2004, experiment 2) required participants to fixate on the home position rather than the target. Doing so placed visual information from early in the movement in central vision rather than peripheral vision. Similarly to when participants fixated on the target, variability was lowest when visual feedback was available over the entire trajectory and when vision was available early in the movement (see figure 8.1*b*). Variability was also lower when vision was available late in the movement when compared with when the cursor was not visible. The analysis of the ratios in variability revealed that the forms of the variability profile were different in the full-vision and early vision conditions compared with the no-vision and late-vision conditions. Hence, as when fixated on the target, participants were able to process early visual feedback online and benefited from late visual feedback through off-line processing. This finding suggests that the time available to process visual feedback rather than the actual location of vision in the visual field is the major determinant of the functional differences between peripheral vision and central vision.

Despite this reasonable conclusion, there remains considerable evidence suggesting that when early visual information is available in peripheral vision, the visuomotor system is more adept at processing visual feedback. When comparing the variability profiles for the early vision conditions, it can be seen that a quadratic profile emerged when early vision was in the peripheral visual field (figure 8.1*a*), whereas variability increased linearly when early visual information was in central vision (figure 8.1*b*). Hence, variability increased at a lower rate when early visual information was in the peripheral compared to central visual field. This finding does suggest that a functional difference exists between central vision and peripheral vision in the utilization of visual feedback to modify limb trajectories during movement execution.

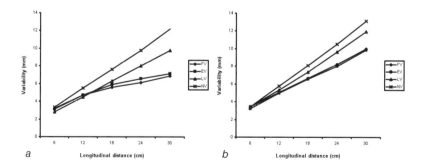

▶ **Figure 8.1** Variability in direction at longitudinal distances to the target of 6, 12, 18, 24, and 30 cm for full-vision (FV), early vision (EV), late-vision (LV), and no-vision (NV) conditions when participants (*a*) fixated on the target and (*b*) fixated on the start position. In (*a*), early vision was in the peripheral visual field while late vision was in the central visual field. In (*b*), early vision was in the central visual field while late vision was in the peripheral visual field.

Experimental Brain Research, 158, 2004, pgs. 241-251, "The utilization of peripheral and central vision in the control of movement direction," M.A. Khan et al., ©Springer. With kind permission of Springer Science+Business Media.

Amplitude Control

As discussed in the previous section, researchers typically investigate the control of movement direction by using tasks for which participants move through the target, which means that the velocity of the limb is greater than 0 at the location of the target. In contrast, when a task specifies the amplitude of the movement, the limb must come to a complete stop on the target. The requisite acceleration and braking result in a bell-shaped velocity profile in which the velocity of the limb is 0 at the beginning and end of the movement. In some cases, studies employ aiming tasks that constrain limb movements in a single dimension and hence there is no direction requirement. Other studies use three-dimensional aiming tasks that have both direction and amplitude components. Regardless of whether single-dimension or multiple-dimension tasks are employed, the requirement to stop on the target means that the velocity will be low when the limb is in the central visual field. Providing that the movement amplitude is large enough, limb velocities will be high as the limb crosses the peripheral visual field.

In order to investigate the contributions of peripheral vision and central vision in the control of movement amplitude, Bard and colleagues (1990) locked their handheld lever in one dimension. Hence, movement direction was constrained in one direction and participants were required to control only the amplitude of the movement. Consistent with Paillard and Amblard's (1985) two–visual channels model, the findings of Bard and colleagues showed that peripheral vision did not improve the accuracy of movement amplitude when compared with when no vision was available. However, when central vision was available, there was a significant improvement in accuracy.

Following from the work of Bard and colleagues (1990), a number of studies have used three-dimensional aiming tasks to reveal similar findings. For example, Temprado, Vieilledent, and Proteau (1996) showed that when early visual feedback is available between visual angles of 59° and 40°, accuracy in movement amplitude is no better than it is without vision. When visual feedback is available in the last part of the trajectory from 40° to 0° of visual angle, amplitude accuracy is as high as when vision is available over the entire trajectory of the limb. Similarly, Bédard and Proteau (2001, 2003) showed that the availability of peripheral vision (from 40°-15° eccentricity) did not benefit the control of movement amplitude.

As when examining the direction component of aiming movements, it is important to determine whether the benefit of visual feedback in the control of movement amplitude is due to online or off-line processing. In order to address this issue, Bédard and Proteau (2004) computed coefficients of variation in distance traveled at peak acceleration, peak velocity, peak deceleration, and movement end. Recall that a reduction in coefficient of variation indicates that limb trajectories are modified during movement execution. Like the direction component of an aiming movement, the co-efficients of amplitude variability did not differ between kinematic land-marks when MT was 300 ms. However, when MT ranged between 500 and 900 ms, there were significant reductions in coefficients of variability between peak velocity and movement end point for the full-vision, periph-eral-vision (40°-15°), and central-vision (15°-0°) conditions. This indicates that when MT is sufficiently long, both peripheral vision and central vision can be used to control movement amplitude.

While the studies of Bédard and Proteau (2003, 2004) employed video-based aiming tasks in which movement of the limb is represented by a cursor on a monitor, Lawrence, Khan, Buckolz, and Oldham (2006) extended the investigation of peripheral and central vision to a conventional aiming task. The analysis of variability at various kinematic markers revealed that the variability in distance traveled was greater for the no-vision and peripheral-vision (40°-10° eccentricity) conditions than it was for the full-vision and central-vision (10°-0° eccentricity) conditions at peak deceleration and movement end point. The peripheral-vision and no-vision conditions did not differ from each other, while the central-vision and full-vision conditions shared similar variability. Comparisons of the variability profiles revealed that the ratio in variability between the full-vision and no-vision conditions and between the peripheral-vision and no-vision conditions decreased from peak acceleration to peak velocity. There were also significant decreases in the variability ratios between the full-vision and no-vision conditions and the central-vision and no-vision conditions from peak deceleration to movement end. Hence, consistent with the findings of Bédard and Proteau (2004), it appears that information from both peripheral vision and central vision is processed during movement execution. However, when informa-tion is available in the peripheral visual field, limb trajectory modifica-tions early in the movement are not sufficient to influence final end-point accuracy. In contrast, modifications to the limb trajectory made late in the movement have a significant effect on end-point accuracy when central vision is available.

In the study of Lawrence and colleagues (2006), the distance traveled at peak velocity, peak deceleration, and movement end was greater in the peripheral-vision condition than it was in the full-vision, central-vision, and no-vision conditions. This finding is consistent with evidence reveal-ing a magnification effect of the perifoveal retinal areas that results in an overestimation of eccentricity (Bock, 1986). It may be that in the peripheral-vision condition, the eccentricity of the early part of the trajectory was overestimated and so participants moved farther than they did when vision of the early part of the trajectory was unavailable (during the no-vision and central-vision conditions). When vision was available throughout the trajectory, participants were able to compensate for the early effects of peri-foveal magnification toward the later stages of the movement. Again, these findings suggest that information from the visual periphery is processed but not to the extent of having a positive effect on end-point accuracy.

In summary, although the amount of literature examining the relative roles of peripheral and central vision is quite limited, combining it with comparable investigations from the more ubiquitous literature on visual feedback generates a reasonable picture. Contrary to the dichotomous predictions of Paillard and Amblard (1985), the utilization of peripheral and central vision is not easily separated into kinetic and static processing streams. Although there does appear to be a moderate preference for garnering online control cues from the periphery, a considerable portion of this kinetic property may be attributable to sufficiency of processing time (and not extrafoveal retinal properties). Similarly, the superficially static properties are largely associated with diminished access to information; when sufficient processing time is provided, central sources are able to modulate ongoing action. Additionally, central vision appears to provide cues for the modification of upcoming actions, thus permitting errors in the current trial to positively influence performance on subsequent trials.

Upper Visual Field Versus Lower Visual Field

In his 1990 review, Previc made a number of sweeping statements regarding behavioral asymmetries across the horizontal margin of the retina. In particular, he summarized a number of studies indicating the facilitation of perceptual and attentional performance in the upper visual field. In a complementary fashion, anatomical evidence suggests that the capacity for the production and rapid adjustment of movements may not be distributed equally across the retina. Notably, the lower visual field demonstrates preferential connections with the subregions of the PPC that are implicated in the online control of movement (e.g., area V6a, Maunsell & van Essen, 1987; area MT, Galletti, Fattori, Gamberini, & Kutz, 1999). Moreover, it has been hypothesized that the disproportionate number of projections from the lower visual field to the dorsal regions of the visual cortex (see chapter 13) induce a processing benefit for online visual feedback control in the lower visual field (Danckert & Goodale, 2001; for a review, see Previc, 1990, 1996), a feature consistent with the improved ability of humans to manipulate tools in near-peripersonal space.

In order to compare visuomotor processing between the upper and lower visual fields, Danckert and Goodale (2001) required participants to perform horizontal repetitive aiming movements from left to right to targets of varying sizes. Participants performed the aiming task while fixating either above or below the targets and the trajectory of the hand. When participants fixated above the work space, the task was performed in the lower visual field. Conversely, when participants fixated below the targets and hand, movements were performed in the upper visual field. Danckert and Goodale reported that MT increased linearly as a function of index of difficulty (ID) when movements were performed in the lower but not the upper visual field—one of the few instances of a failure to replicate Fitts' law (Fitts, 1954). On this basis, Danckert and Goodale claimed that the lower visual field was superior in the control of visually guided movements. However, there was no difference in accuracy between the lower and upper visual fields for the smallest target size (i.e., the condition in which visual control should be most critical). Furthermore, while movements toward larger targets were more accurate in the lower visual field, this accuracy was obtained at the cost of greater MT. Hence, the greater slope of the relationship between MT and ID for movements performed in the lower visual field could be interpreted as a trade-off between speed and accuracy and not necessarily as more efficient use of visual feedback in the lower visual field.

The study of Danckert and Goodale (2001) motivated several other investigations comparing visual control between the upper and lower visual fields. Binsted and Heath (2005) questioned whether the advantage of the lower visual field was due to utilization of visual feedback during movement execution or better planning in advance of response initiation. Their study employed a discrete aiming task instead of a reciprocal aiming task so that planning and online control processes could be assessed independently. Also, they used a wider range of ID that would test visual control processes at higher IDs than those used by Danckert and Goodale. In contrast to Danckert and Goodale, Binsted and Heath did not find any difference in the slope of the relationship between MT and ID between visual fields. Despite a lack of difference in speed–accuracy trade-off, end-point variability was generally lower for movements performed in the lower visual field. However, several lines of evidence suggested that this difference in variable error was not due to online control processes. First, the availability of target vision during movement execution had relatively little effect in the lower visual field. Second, time after peak velocity did not differ between visual fields. Third and finally, the correlation between limb position at peak velocity and movement end did not differ between the upper and lower visual fields. These findings led Binsted and Heath to conclude that any advantage of the lower visual field was due to better planning or more precise execution of the movement plan.

While Binsted and Heath (2005) showed similar speed–accuracy trade-offs in the upper and lower visual fields, a subsequent study by Khan and Lawrence (2005) provided contradictory evidence suggesting that the lower field has an advantage for the online control of aiming movements. The major difference characterizing the Khan and Lawrence study was that it employed a time-constrained task instead of a time-minimization task. In the studies of Danckert and Goodale (2001) and Binsted and Heath (2005), participants were instructed to move as quickly and as accurately as possible. Under such instructions, participants had a certain degree of flexibility in trading speed for accuracy. Indeed, in both of these studies, MT versus ID functions were derived when there were differences in error measurements between the upper and lower visual fields. In order to minimize any contamination from speed–accuracy trade-offs, Khan and Lawrence instructed participants to perform aiming movements in 400 ms. Since MT was controlled between the upper and lower visual fields, error measurements became the primary variable of interest. The subsequent analysis revealed that limb trajectories were less variable in the lower visual field late in the movement; there were no differences in variability at peak acceleration or peak velocity. Also, correlations between limb position at peak velocity and movement end discovered that the extent to which end position was determined by the position at peak velocity was less in the lower visual field than it was in the upper visual field. These findings demonstrate that modifications to limb trajectories were more effective in reducing error when movements were performed in the lower visual field.

In an attempt to isolate the relative efficacy of online adjustments across visual fields, Krigolson and Heath (2006) employed a target perturbation paradigm in which the target was displaced 3 cm closer to or farther from the start position at the time of movement onset. The magnitude of this perturbation meant that participants were consciously aware of the change in target position (see chapter 7). Similar to previous results (Binsted & Heath, 2005; Khan & Lawrence, 2005), the spatial distribution of spatial end points was less in the upper visual field compared with the lower visual field. However, there was no evidence that adjustments to the perturbation were more efficient in the lower field, as MT to targets and the associated kinematic measures did not vary between visual fields.

From the relatively few studies comparing the upper and lower visual fields in terms of visual control in aiming movements, one consistent finding is that the variability of movement end points is less when movements are performed in the lower visual field (Binsted & Heath, 2005; Khan & Lawrence, 2005; Krigolson & Heath, 2006). Examinations of variability profiles and correlations between kinematic markers have revealed that this advantage is due to online control, at least for temporally constrained movements (Khan & Lawrence, 2005). However, an advantage of the lower visual field for speed–accuracy relationships has not been consistent (c.f., Binsted & Heath, 2005; Danckert & Goodale, 2001), and adjustments to perturbations are not more efficient in the lower visual field (Krigolson & Heath, 2006). As noted by Krigolson and Heath (2006), one reason for the discrepant findings may be the instructions given to participants. Khan and Lawrence (2005) employed a temporally constrained task in which MT was not required to be shorter than 400 ms and found that online control was superior in the lower visual field. Binsted and Heath (2005) emphasized movement speed and did not find an advantage for the lower visual field. Danckert and Goodale (2001) reported more reliable speed–accuracy relationships in the lower visual field compared with the upper visual field when both movement speed and accuracy were emphasized. However, when providing the same task instructions, Krigolson and Heath (2006) did not find any difference between visual fields for adjustments to target perturbations.

These findings suggest that the advantage for visuomotor control in the lower visual field may be due to very specific visuomotor processes associated with fine-tuning at the end of the movement. For tasks emphasizing the importance of movement planning, perhaps driven to some extent by the instruction to move as fast as possible, a visual field asymmetry does not materialize. Similarly, specialized mechanisms of the lower visual field may not mediate gross adjustments in perturbation tasks that can be implemented through changes to the motor plan (see chapter 7). As suggested by Danckert and Goodale (2004), the advantage of the lower visual field may be associated with visual control processes that involve assessing the velocity and position of the moving hand as it approaches the target. It may be that these fine adjustments that are based on the movement of the hand enable movement end points to be more consistent in the lower visual field compared with the upper visual field.

Conclusions and Future Directions

Throughout this chapter we have explored asymmetries in the use of visual information presented to the human retina. Although the early anatomical findings predict a specialization for peripheral vision and the lower visual field for the online regulation of movement and, somewhat more controversially, the use of upper and central inputs for the preparation of future action, the behavioral findings are more diverse. While it does appear that actions are accurate when made in the lower visual field, it is equivocal whether this advantage is due to improved movement preparation or planning (or perhaps other factors such as visual acuity or unconscious processing; see Binsted, Brownell, Vorontsova, Heath, & Saucier 2007). Similarly, despite a relatively consistent finding of the preferential use of peripheral cues for online control, central vision appears capable of diverse motor functions, from online control (when sufficient time is provided) to trial-to-trial plasticity.

In order to garner a clearer picture of the behavioral consequences of retinal asymmetries, we need more direct examinations of the anatomical substrates. Notably, the disruption of pathways via magnetic stimulations (TMS) or the active monitoring of cortical activity (with EEG) will enable use to answer more pointed questions regarding the efficacy of the previously reported pathways and the degree to which they are active during goal-directed pointing.

Part II

Sensory and Neural Systems for Vision and Action

Part II extends the research associated with this volume to neurophysiological and biological systems. Although goal-directed behavior is still the primary concern, the authors contributing to this part make a systematic attempt to reveal the sensory and physiological processes and systems responsible for fast, accurate, and efficient performance. Because the overall concern is visuomotor behavior, it is appropriate to start this part with the role of eye movements in limb control.

In chapter 9, Bennett and Barnes direct their attention toward pursuit eye and head movements designed to track moving objects through the environment. These movements provide us not only with visual information about the location and movement of objects in the environment but also with nonvisual information from extraretinal signals associated with motor commands sent to the eyes. Building on evidence from studies examining eye movements when the target object is occluded, the authors present a model of ocular pursuit that accounts for reflexive and predictive control of the eyes.

Chapters 10 and 11 continue along these lines but deal more specifically with the interaction between ocular systems and manual systems. In chapter 10, Binsted, Brownell, Rolheiser, and Heath explore the ocular system responsible for discrete visuomotor behaviors. Using both behavioral and neurophysiological evidence, they discuss various viewpoints on the mechanisms underlying eye–hand coordination. In chapter 11, Helsen, Feys, Heremans, and Lavrysen take the review of vision and limb control one step further. The first part of the chapter discusses eye–head–hand coordination in healthy subjects, while the second part shows how important insights into normal functioning can be gained by examining neural pathology. To set the stage for the next chapter, which is on lateralization of goal-directed behavior, Helsen and colleagues also review how eye–hand coordination varies depending on which hand is used to achieve the movement goal.

Chapters 12, 13, and 14 move beyond the visual sensory systems to explore how cortical and subcortical neural systems use the information provided by the eyes to achieve different movement goals. In chapter 12, Sainburg explores how sensorimotor processing differs between the two cerebral hemispheres of the brain and how that affects precise limb control and lateral advantages or disadvantages for the left and right hand. The chapter reviews not only the neural systems that provide the foundation for limb asymmetries in performance and human handedness but also the genetic and environmental influences that affect how performance asymmetries are expressed in different task contexts.

Central to chapters 13 and 14 is Milner and Goodale's (1995) extremely influential model of visual processing, which was first introduced in part I (chapters 4 and 5; see also chapter 8). According to the perception–action model, the ventral visual stream, which terminates in the inferior parietal areas of the brain, is responsible for perceptual judgments that are mediated by conscious awareness and language. On the other hand, the dorsal stream, which terminates in the superior parietal areas of the brain, is specialized for the visual control of action. In chapter 13, Westwood explores this dissociation while providing a critical review of the literature on the influence of visual illusions on perceptual judgments, movement planning, and control. Like several chapters in part I, chapter 13 deals with issues such as visual frame of reference and memory in limb control, but this time these issues are addressed within the context of the Milner and Goodale model. Although Westwood deals exclusively with work involving healthy young adults, Carey, in chapter 14, explores the neuropsychological evidence for the ventral and dorsal perception–action dichotomy by reviewing behavioral and neuroimaging research conducted with patients with brain injury to one or the other of these visual systems. Together chapters 13 and 14 provide the most comprehensive evaluation of the perception–action model currently available.

The six chapters in part II of this volume provide a solid foundation for further examination of the sensory and neural systems responsible for precision goal-directed behavior. Work reviewed in this part demonstrates to researchers who have taken a primarily behavioral approach to their work how advances in both behavioral and neurophysiological methods have made the biological systems associated with skilled performance more accessible.

CHAPTER 9

Prediction in Ocular Pursuit

SIMON J. BENNETT AND GRAHAM R. BARNES

As the previous chapters highlighted so well, normal functioning in everyday life requires humans to interact with moving and static objects within a visually dynamic environment. Moving around inside and outside the home, such as when preparing food in the kitchen or climbing a stairway, requires us to pick up, intercept, or avoid surrounding objects. Failure to perceive the changing relationship between our body and an object of interest could lead to ineffective behavior that has the potential for serious consequences. For example, misperceiving the speed of an approaching car while waiting to cross a road could possibly result in collision. It is perhaps not surprising, therefore, that the human visual system has evolved highly specific mechanisms for processing motion that are capable of extracting very precise information about an object's position, direction, and speed as it moves across the retina (Anderson & Burr, 1985; McKee, 1981).

Although the human visual system can provide accurate object-related information from retinal input alone (i.e., when the eyes are fixated), when an object of interest moves relative to the retina, either because the self or the object is moving, our normal response is to move the eyes and head in an attempt to maintain the object image on the fovea. This can be achieved using image-stabilizing eye movements of the vestibulo-ocular reflex (VOR) and optokinetic reflex (OKR) or gaze-orienting eye movements such as saccades, smooth pursuit, and vergence. As well as keeping the object of interest in the region of high acuity to discriminate object characteristics such as size and shape, motor signals sent to move the eyes (i.e., efference copy) provide extraretinal information. This information is critical in interpreting retinal stimulation generated as the eyes pursue an object moving against a cluttered background (i.e., did the object move or did the observer move?).

Extraretinal information not only provides a stable perception of the world around us but also provides advanced information related to upcoming object motion. This information allows the observer to exhibit predictive eye movements that are not driven reflexively by online visual feedback. These predictive eye movements help the observer to overcome the delays involved in processing retinal feedback that would otherwise limit the ability to pursue a fast-moving object. In addition, predictive eye movements allow the observer to initiate and perpetuate the pursuit response when tracking an object in the absence of visual feedback. This ability is particularly important in situations where an object undergoes transient occlusion that does not permit integration of consecutive visual samples and the formation of a continuous percept of the object trajectory. Such situations are commonplace in everyday life (e.g., when the goalkeeper's view of the incoming free kick is occluded by the wall of defending players). Until recently, little was known about how the eyes move when visual feedback of a moving object is occluded and, therefore, about the underlying control mechanisms.

In this chapter, we describe the gaze-orienting eye movements that are used to keep the object image on the fovea. We then turn to the use of these eye movements in tracking smooth object motion as opposed to step changes in object position that elicit saccadic eye movements (for a discussion of saccadic eye movements in reaching and grasping, see chapters 10 and 11) or changes of object position in depth that require vergence eye movements. The main findings are from experiments that have examined the ocular response in situations where there is a temporary absence of visual feedback of the moving object. This should create problems for a control system that, according to traditional dictum, is under reflexive control driven by retinal input. Particular focus is given to work on ocular pursuit in which visual feedback from the moving object is temporarily unavailable, such as if the object undergoes transient occlusion or extinction. Using the findings in our laboratory as well as those of others, we present a model of ocular pursuit, including a novel arrangement of extraretinal input that accounts for both reflexive and predictive control of the eyes. Finally, we refer to work that has revealed the underlying neural substrate and then discuss potential directions for future research.

Gaze-Orienting Eye Movements

Movement of the eyes to maintain object foveation can be classified as saccades, smooth pursuit, or vergence. The first two categories involve conjugate eye movements in response to object motion in a single depth plane, whereas vergence involves disconjugate rotation of the eyes in opposite directions as the object moves in depth at distances of less than 2 m from the observer. Traditionally, these types of gaze-orienting eye movements were thought to have distinct but complementary roles supported by separate neural substrates. However, outside controlled laboratory settings, objects often move in a way that does not demand one type of eye movement in isolation from the others. It should not be surprising, therefore, that the gaze-orienting eye movements interact. For instance, it has been shown that vergence velocity increases when accompanied by a saccade, whereas saccade peak velocity decreases (Zee, FitzGibbon, & Optican, 1992). In the case of conjugate eye movements, it has been suggested that smooth pursuit velocity can be enhanced by previous saccadic activity in certain contexts (Lisberger, 1998).

It is also common for gaze-orienting eye movements to occur synchronously with head movement. This occurrence is particularly important in situations where the object is located far from the fovea and hence beyond the comfortable range of eye rotation within the orbit (approximately 50° in humans). Coordinating gaze-orienting movements of the eyes with movement of the head in order to foveate a moving object creates additional complications, most notably the need to suppress the VOR that would naturally cause the eyes to rotate in opposing direction to the head. However, when an object of interest is visible, the human oculomotor system overcomes these difficulties to produce gaze movements with gain comparable to the gain of eye movements in isolation (for a review, see Barnes, 1993). Despite the interaction between eye and head movements; this chapter focuses on conjugate eye movements performed with a fixed position of the head.

Saccades are fast eye movements (up to approximately 500°/s in humans) that can be made voluntarily without requiring special feedback conditions or experience. The drive to saccades can come from a variety of sources, including auditory and tactile inputs as well as remembered object locations. Saccades have stereotyped dynamics (Bahill, Clark, & Stark, 1975), which is evident in the consistent relationship among their amplitude, duration, and peak velocity (commonly known as *saccadic main sequence).* Average saccade latency is approximately 200 ms, but this is affected by many factors such as the amount of information to be processed, participant motivation and attention, object luminance, and saccadic refractory period (for a review, see Leigh & Zee, 2006).

Typically, saccades have been classified as a gaze-orienting eye movement that brings the static image of an object onto the fovea, such as when scanning a visual scene. However, when the object of interest is moving, saccades relocate the object image on the fovea if velocity control (i.e., smooth pursuit) is inadequate. Therefore, in the case of a moving object, smooth pursuit and saccades need to be well coordinated to maintain accurate pursuit (Erkelens, 2006). Recently, De Brouwer and colleagues (De Brouwer, Yuksel, Blohm, Missal, & Lefèvre, 2002) have shown that in addition to taking into account a sudden change in object position and velocity, the amplitude of catch-up saccades compensates for the eye displacement resulting from smooth pursuit during saccade programming. The implication is that the processing mechanism underlying saccades receives input from motion-sensing mechanisms that are probably also involved in controlling smooth pursuit.

Compared with saccades, smooth pursuit eye movements are relatively slow rotations (up to approximately 80°/s in humans) of the eye that attempt to match the velocity of the moving object and in doing so minimize retinal slip (i.e., the difference between eye velocity and object velocity) and object image blur. If retinal slip is less than 2 to 3°/s when making slower smooth pursuit eye movements (Barnes & Smith, 1981; Westheimer & McKee, 1975), vision is preserved and enables continuous monitoring of object characteristics. The latency of smooth pursuit onset is approximately 100 to 150 ms (Carl & Gellman, 1987; Robinson, Gordon, & Gordon, 1986), with the initial 40 ms of the smooth pursuit response to a step ramp being independent of the object motion (Krauzlis & Lisberger, 1994; Lisberger & Westbrook, 1985).

Traditionally, it was thought that smooth pursuit eye movements were driven reflexively by a negative feedback loop with retinal slip as input (Young & Stark, 1963). In other words, it was suggested that contrary to saccades, smooth pursuit eye movements are not under volitional control but are a reflexive response that occurs only in the presence of a moving object. However, there are observations indicating that different sensory inputs (e.g., tactile, limb motor commands) drive pursuit onset and continuation (for a review, see Berryhill, Chiu, & Hughes, 2006). Of most relevance to the current chapter is the finding that participants can use expectation about upcoming object motion to voluntarily initiate smooth pursuit in the absence of visual feedback. As we will discuss in more detail later, the implication is that smooth pursuit is not simply driven by reflexive mechanisms that receive delayed sensory input. Instead, smooth pursuit eye movements, like other gaze-orienting movements (saccades and vergence) and limb movements, are subject to volitional control.

Prediction in Ocular Pursuit

When an object moves relative to the retina with a frequency of direction change in excess of 0.5 Hz (Westheimer & McKee, 1975), the delay of the visual feedback loop does not permit accurate smooth ocular pursuit and maintenance of the object image on the fovea. One solution might be to make reflexive catch-up saccades to correct for the developing position error. However, due to the latency of saccades, which has been measured at approximately 150 ms during smooth pursuit (De Brouwer et al., 2002), the eye relying on saccades would continually lag behind the moving object. Observation of eye movement when tracking sinusoidal object motion of 1 Hz and 5° amplitude (Meyer, Lasker, & Robinson, 1985) shows that participants are quickly able to match both gain and phase of the stimulus.

Similar behavior can also be seen when participants pursue more complex mixed sinusoid trajectories (Barnes, Donnelly, & Eason, 1987) and can be accompanied by phase lead when the mixed sinusoid trajectories have low frequencies (Yasui & Young, 1984).

To account for the ability of smooth pursuit to match an object moving at constant velocity, it has been suggested that input from efference copy provides a basic prediction of future object motion (Krauzlis & Miles, 1996; Krauzlis & Lisberger, 1994; Robinson et al., 1986; Yasui & Young, 1975). Importantly, though, the low-level prediction in these accounts is still thought to be part of an underlying reflexive kernel that responds to visual feedback of object motion (see Churchland, Chou, & Lisberger, 2003). Specifically, the efference copy loop (referred to as *eye-velocity memory*) is modeled as an integral part of the reflexive mechanism and is believed to accumulate during the early stages of object pursuit as the eyes move in an attempt to nullify a velocity and acceleration error signal from visual feedback (Krauzlis & Lisberger, 1994; Lisberger, Morris, & Tychsen, 1981).

Although efference copy models can explain the smooth pursuit eye movements (e.g., onset and offset) in response to a step ramp in which the time of object motion onset and velocity is unknown, it is fair to say that they do not provide a satisfactory account of the more complex prediction that is required to pursue the type of object motion that is experienced in our normal surroundings. For instance, despite the efference copy loop quickly attaining a level close to that of an object moving to the left or right with constant velocity, which then enables it to perpetuate the ongoing response and overcome visual feedback delay, the loop is unable to produce the nonconstant eye velocity required to pursue accelerative object motion (e.g., sinusoidal trajectories or objects acted upon by gravity or friction). However, as discussed in the next section, even in conditions where an object moves with constant velocity, it can be difficult to explain smooth pursuit onset without invoking more complex predictive mechanisms.

Onset of Anticipatory Smooth Pursuit

Traditionally it was thought that people could not initiate smooth pursuit eye movements of more than 4 to 5°/s in the absence of a moving object to track (Heywood & Churcher, 1971). Some studies revealed low-velocity (<2°/s) eye movements occurring before object motion onset, but these were believed to be the consequence of habit formed over repeated presentations (Kowler & Steinman, 1979a, 1979b) that could, when appropriate, be overridden by cognitive control (Kowler, 1989). However, with regularly timed, repeated presentation of object motion stimuli (e.g., the step-ramp paradigm in which an object moves from a stationary location at a constant velocity between 200 and 1,000 ms), smooth pursuit eye movements of up to 30°/s precede the onset of object motion (Barnes & Asselman, 1991; Kao & Morrow, 1994).

Barnes and Asselman (1991) suggested that the repeated motion stimuli develop an internal representation of velocity-based information that can be released under volitional control to drive the ocular response in anticipation of object motion onset. This idea of internal representation is similar to the earlier suggestion that smooth pursuit in the absence of visual feedback is driven by a copy of the motor drive, but it assumes that the representation is held in a self-contained, short-term memory that is not reliant on the sustained integrity of the efference copy loop. In the more conventional models, the efference copy loop is arranged as a leaky integrator that decays when gain is less than unity and hence does not preserve its level; modeling the efference copy loop as a leaky integrator enabled Krauzlis and Miles (1996) to simulate the characteristic decay in smooth pursuit that occurs following the cessation of object motion. A consequence of such an arrangement is that it is difficult to account for the storage of information between presentations when the eye is no longer in motion. Indeed, to explain the anticipatory smooth pursuit eye movements that are observed across step-ramp presentations separated by a fixation of up to 14.4 s (Chakraborti, Barnes, & Collins, 2002), it would be necessary for the efference copy loop to be temporarily disengaged in order to remain uninfluenced by the lack of image or eye motion. Although potentially this could be achieved, several other findings regarding smooth pursuit onset are not so easily reconcilable.

Barnes, Grealy, and Collins (1997) examined smooth pursuit onset in conditions where participants either tracked the moving object with their eyes or kept their eyes fixated while the object image moved across the retina. The logic of this elegant manipulation is that a feedback loop receiving input from a copy of the ocular motor command would be unable to build up a representation of eye velocity during fixation. However, if the internal representation is held in a more persistent independent store that receives input from a source that is closer to the afferent source of velocity-based information, it could develop with sufficient exposure to the retinal slip generated as the object moves across the stationary retina. It was found that without fixation, smooth movement on the first presentation was initiated after object motion onset, but with repeated presentations, anticipatory smooth movements were observed. However, when the first attempt to move the eyes was preceded by three trials in the fixation condition, participants were immediately able to make anticipatory smooth eye movements that had a peak velocity equal to that of the third response without previous fixation.

Having shown that information related to object velocity could be stored and used to generate future anticipatory responses even in the absence of eye movement, Jarrett and Barnes (2002) next sought to determine if participants could volitionally scale the speed and direction of anticipatory smooth eye movements based on symbolic precues. This was an important manipulation because it would confirm the participants' volitional control over what many still thought of as a reflexive response (see also Jarrett & Barnes, 2001, 2005). The study found that participants were able to volitionally scale anticipatory smooth eye movements according to the direction (left versus right) and speed (10, 20, 30, and 40°/s) of information contained in the symbolic cues given before object motion. Moreover, there was no difference in smooth eye velocity between the randomized precued trials and the control trials in which direction and speed were received in blocked order.

Clearly, these examples indicate that the onset of anticipatory pursuit in the absence of visual feedback involves more than simple motor habit or a low-level prediction that perpetuates the ongoing response. The need to explain these predictive characteristics of smooth ocular pursuit while at the same time accounting for the reflexive response exhibited in conditions of uncertainty regarding the upcoming object motion was recognized by Barnes and Asselman (1991) and then later refined in Barnes and Wells (1999). In their novel model of ocular pursuit, Barnes and colleagues incorporated a direct loop that receives input from efference copy and an indirect (predictive) loop that accumulates and stores velocity-based information. Both loops receive retinal input derived from negative visual feedback. The storage of velocity-based information is achieved using a sample-and-hold mechanism with a sampling interval of 160 ms (coarser sampling intervals can be used). The model was able to simulate both anticipatory smooth pursuit onset and the predictive eye movements that are required to pursue more complex trajectories such as those of a waveform containing single and mixed sinusoidal frequencies.

More recent work from Barnes and Collins (2008) has shown that the formation of the more persistent internal representation within the indirect loop requires only brief exposure to object motion. For example, these researchers observed the increasing velocity of anticipatory smooth pursuit even when the object was initially exposed for only a brief time (50-100 ms) and then disappeared for 600 ms. The implication is that participants could sample the object motion, which was randomized in presentation, during the brief initial exposure and then use that information to control the magnitude of eye velocity produced in the absence of any visual input.

Anticipatory Smooth Pursuit During Transient Occlusion

Experiments on pursuit initiation and pursuit of sinusoidal trajectories have revealed much about the role of predictive and reflexive mechanisms. However, in our normal surroundings there are other instances in which it is advantageous to predict the upcoming object trajectory. For instance, it is common for objects to move behind opaque surfaces, which creates a trajectory involving transient occlusions. For a long occlusion (>200 ms), it is not possible to integrate consecutive visual samples into a spatio-temporally continuous percept. Still, in such situations the human perceptual system provides constancy of characteristics such as object shape, color, and trajectory. As a consequence, we understand that an occluded object has not simply vanished and hence there is a benefit to moving the eyes such that the object image will be on the fovea when it reappears.

One way to achieve prediction might be to use information from the occluder edges to plan and then execute a saccade that brings the eye to the reappearance position to coincide with reappearance time. Evidence from infants indicates that such a strategy develops by 21 wk and brings the eye to within 2° of the reappearance location with a lag of less than 200 ms (Rosander & von Hofsten, 2004). Although a potentially useful way to compensate for the loss of retinal input, failure to maintain smooth pursuit of a moving object during a transient occlusion will result in significant retinal velocity error at reappearance, which may cause difficulties for discriminating object characteristics. Therefore, a more advantageous strategy would be to maintain pursuit gain near unity during the transient occlusion, thereby eliminating the need to predict reappearance time and minimizing image blur.

Even though humans are able to maintain permanence of an object trajectory, we do not maintain smooth pursuit with gain near unity without contribution from visual feedback (Barnes, 1993). When participants pursue a moving object that disappears and is not expected to reappear, their eye velocity decays exponentially toward 0 (Mitrani & Dimitrov, 1978). When participants attempt to predict when the unseen moving object will reach a visually indicated location, they still do not maintain smooth pursuit and instead cover the occlusion distance with a saccade (Mrotek & Soechting, 2006). Expectation that the moving object will reappear later in its trajectory has been shown to modify smooth pursuit, with eye velocity decaying rapidly (within 190 ms) following object disappearance and then reaching a plateau (at approximately 450 ms) before being maintained (up to 4,000 ms) at a reduced gain (Becker & Fuchs, 1985). Similar smooth pursuit has been observed when attention is directed toward pushing the unseen object after disappearance (Pola & Wyatt, 1997).

These findings, particularly the relatively stereotypical decay in smooth pursuit, have been modeled as a decrease in the gain applied to the extra-retinal input that contributes to the visuomotor drive (Becker & Fuchs, 1985). More specifically, the decay in eye velocity results from a reduction in gain applied to the efference copy loop when visual feedback is removed, which by virtue of being arranged as a leaky integrator causes eye velocity to decrease toward 0 (Churchland et al., 2003; Krauzlis & Miles, 1996; Krauzlis & Lisberger, 1994).

Although this arrangement explains the gradual decay in smooth pursuit in the absence of visual feedback, as well as the enhancement (adaptation) of pursuit gain following learning with auditory stimuli (Madelain & Krauzlis, 2003), it has limited ability to account for an anticipatory increase in eye velocity back to existing levels that occurs during transient occlusion. This can be partly overcome by increasing the value of the gain signal acting within the efference copy loop to well above unity, but doing so could create undesirable instability in smooth pursuit following object reappearance (Dallos & Jones, 1963). The problems with this arrangement, therefore, are most evident when consecutive object motion is received in blocked order such that the time, location, and velocity of object reappearance are predictable. Under such conditions, Bennett and Barnes (2003) have found that although smooth pursuit decays from a level that matches the object velocity following object disappearance (e.g., at the onset of an occlusion), there is an anticipatory recovery in eye velocity preceding object reappearance (for qualitative evidence, see also Becker & Fuchs, 1985; Churchland et al., 2003). It was also reported that though the recovery in eye velocity during occlusion occurs in advance of object reappearance, it often occurs around a similar time for different durations (420, 660, and 900 ms) of transient occlusion. This results in eye velocity that reaches a peak and then decelerates beyond the moment of object reappearance until visual feedback became available.

The discovery of an early anticipatory recovery in smooth pursuit following object disappearance was confirmed by us (Bennett & Barnes, 2004) in a study using a longer and wider range (660, 1,140, and 1,620 ms) of occlusion intervals. Importantly, in this study we also manipulated the duration for which the moving object was initially visible before it disappeared (240, 480, and 720 ms). Under these conditions, the recovery in eye velocity occurred later when the moving object was initially visible for only 240 ms. Therefore, the recovery in eye velocity did not occur at the same time after object disappearance, such as if a fixed amount of time was required to register and respond to the loss of visual feedback (i.e., to elicit a decrease and then increase in gain acting on the extraretinal input). Rather, the recovery occurred when eye velocity approached a minimum threshold. This threshold took longer to reach when participants were pursuing the most briefly presented object (240 ms) because eye velocity had not reached its peak before object disappearance. Still, the recovery occurred well in advance of object reappearance, and thus although anticipatory in the sense that eye velocity did not simply decay to 0 or was maintained at a reduced gain, the timing of this recovery was once again not well suited to the duration of object occlusion (see figure 9.1).

Initially, we suggested that such a response was inappropriate because it resulted in retinal slip and blur as the object reappeared (Bennett & Barnes, 2003). However, we later realized that there are strategic benefits when the system responds early. First, because both position and velocity error

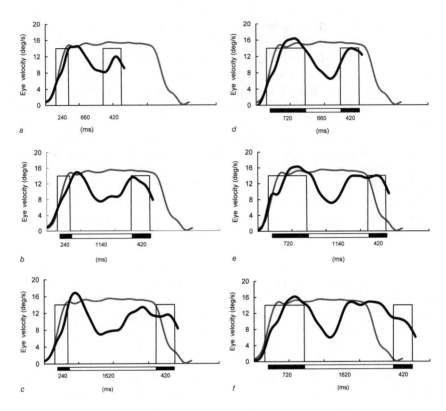

▶ **Figure 9.1**   Smooth eye velocity (thick black lines) and pursuit object (thin gray lines) versus time (ms) as a function of initial ramp duration (240 ms in panels *a, b, c;* 720 ms in panels *d, e, f*) and occlusion duration (660 ms in *a* and *d;* 1,140 ms in *b* and *e;* 1,620 ms in *c* and *f*). When time bars are black, pursuit object was visible (14°/s). Smooth eye velocity (gray lines) for control presentations is included for comparison.

accumulate following object disappearance with the decay in eye velocity, it may be advantageous to start reducing these errors as soon as possible rather than allowing them to reach unacceptable levels. For instance, exhibiting an early recovery followed by decay and then a further recovery in a long occlusion (see Bennett & Barnes, 2005a) will likely result in less position and velocity error at object reappearance when compared with allowing eye velocity to decay toward 0 before exhibiting a recovery just before reappearance. Second, by releasing a recovery when eye velocity approaches a threshold level, it becomes unnecessary to include a timing mechanism that represents the duration of the transient occlusion, hence freeing the limited capacity of working memory to represent information about object speed and direction (Pasternak & Zaksas, 2003). This could be particularly valuable when participants do not have sufficient experience to construct a reliable estimate of occlusion duration.

Predictive Smooth Pursuit During Transient Occlusion

As noted earlier, the finding of an anticipatory recovery in smooth pursuit during transient occlusion could be explained by increasing the value of the gain signal acting within the efference copy loop to a value greater than unity. Therefore, before reasonably rejecting this account, we (Bennett & Barnes, 2004) decided to examine the capacity of the mechanism controlling smooth pursuit during transient occlusion to exhibit predictive scaling up and down of eye velocity. To this end, we required participants to pursue a moving object that underwent a predictable increase or decrease in velocity during the occlusion. Specifically, participants received 12 blocked presentations where the object moved at 12°/s or 24°/s for 400 ms, after which it was occluded for either 400 or 800 ms and then reappeared at either the same (12°/s and 12°/s or 24°/s and 24°/s) or a changed (12°/s and 24°/s or 24°/s and 12°/s) velocity.

As shown in figure 9.2, the results for presentations in which object velocity remained unchanged were consistent with our previous work, with eye velocity decaying after object disappearance and then recovering back toward previous levels in advance of object reappearance. Furthermore, we found clear predictive scaling of eye velocity in the presentations in which

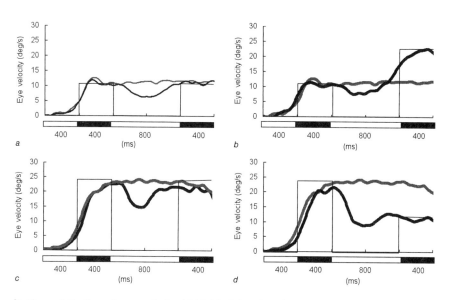

▶ **Figure 9.2** Smooth eye velocity (thick black lines) and pursuit object (thin black lines) versus time (ms) for each motion characteristic. *(a)* Object velocity was initially 12°/s and reappeared at 12°/s. *(b)* Object velocity was initially 12°/s and reappeared at 24°/s. *(c)* Object velocity was initially 24°/s and reappeared at 24°/s. *(d)* Object velocity was initially 24°/s and reappeared at 12°/s. When time bars are black, the pursuit object was visible. Smooth eye velocity (thick gray lines) for control presentations is included for comparison.

there was an expected change in object velocity. Of most importance was the finding that eye velocity initially decayed from approximately 12°/s following object occlusion but then increased to almost 20°/s at object reappearance, far beyond the level that would be expected from a preserved (or decaying) efference copy.

Another situation that requires predictive scaling of eye velocity occurs when tracking an occluded object that undergoes acceleration. Humans experience such situations daily, and the visual system has evolved specific processing mechanisms capable of extracting information about object acceleration, probably via population coding of the velocity signal in MT (Lisberger & Movshon, 1999). However, acceleration is monitored with less precision than the discrimination of direction and speed (Watamaniuk & Heinen, 2003; Werkhoven, Snippe, & Toet, 1992). For example, when an object falls under gravity it undergoes constant acceleration of -9.8 m/s^2. Or, when a car brakes as it approaches a crossing, the driver will decelerate in order to negotiate the obstacle. In both situations, visual feedback of the approaching object could easily be occluded by surrounding surfaces and objects or perturbed by glare (e.g., from bright sun during the day or another car's headlights during the night).

To examine the capacity of the mechanism controlling smooth pursuit during transient occlusion to exhibit predictive scaling of eye velocity in accord with the acceleration of an object, we (Bennett & Barnes, 2006) performed an experiment that required human subjects to pursue an accelerating object (8, 4, or 0°/s^2) undergoing a transient occlusion (800 ms). The presentations were received in both blocked and random order. This manipulation was included because if smooth ocular pursuit is driven primarily by reflexive mechanisms, there should be little or no influence of receiving presentations in a blocked and hence highly predictable order. We also included both a short (200 ms) and long (600 ms) initial phase of object tracking before disappearance in order to determine whether this factor would limit the buildup of an efference copy loop or if it could be overcome using a representation that enabled prediction of the accelerative motion.

As shown in figure 9.3, participants exhibited anticipatory smooth pursuit before object motion onset in both blocked (predictable) and random (unpredictable) presentations. These results indicate that smooth pursuit onset was anticipatory in both predictable and unpredictable presentations and was not reflexively driven by visual feedback received over the first 150 ms of the object motion. We suggest that this occurred because participants expected the object to move with one of three accelerations in a single direction, enabling them to initiate pursuit before motion onset to minimize retinal slip during the ramp. At least with human subjects (for evidence in monkeys, see Tanaka & Lisberger, 2000), the implication is that randomizing the parameters of a limited set of horizontal object motions (e.g., acceleration and duration of the first ramp) does not eliminate the

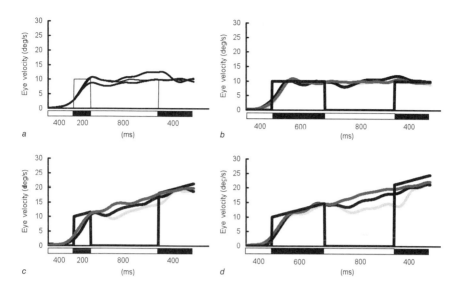

▶ **Figure 9.3**   Smooth eye velocity in random (thick gray lines) and blocked (thick black lines) presentations versus time (ms). The pursuit object is represented by thin black lines. In *(a)* and *(b)*, the object was initially visible for 200 ms, whereas in *(c)* and *(d)*, the object was initially visible for 600 ms. Upper and lower panels show response to object acceleration of $0°/s^2$ and $8°/s^2$. When time bars are black, the pursuit object was visible. Smooth eye velocity for control presentations (thin gray line) is included for comparison.

influence of previous stimuli and the responses to those stimuli, hence creating a situation in which a reflexive response predominates (see also Barnes, Collins, & Arnold, 2005).

For random presentations, the effect of object parameters exhibited in the initial object motion was evident throughout the transient occlusion and at reappearance. Eye velocity when pursuing the $0°/s^2$ object for a short duration (200 ms) was too high at the moment of object disappearance and eventually resulted in eye velocity that was inappropriately high at the moment of reappearance. Conversely, eye velocity when pursuing the $8°/s^2$ object for a short duration (200 ms) was well matched to object velocity at the moment of object disappearance, but it did not quite reach the level of object velocity at the moment of reappearance despite showing a significant recovery after the typical decay. A similar lack of scaling of eye velocity to object velocity at the moment of reappearance was evident in random presentations when the object had initially been pursued for a ramp of longer duration. For example, although participants were able to differentiate object acceleration during the 600 ms ramp and match eye velocity to object velocity, eye velocity underwent a characteristic decay during the occlusion interval followed by a recovery to the level achieved at the end of the initial visible ramp.

For blocked presentations, however, there was evidence of better scaling during the initial object tracking, throughout the transient occlusion, and at reappearance. Eye velocity when pursuing the $0°/s^2$ object was no longer too high as the object disappeared, and it matched object velocity at the moment of reappearance very well. For the $4°/s^2$ and $8°/s^2$ objects, eye velocity at reappearance still undershot object velocity, although it did so to a lesser extent than that observed in random presentations. In fact, having pursued blocked, and hence highly predictable, object motion ($8°/s^2$) for both the shorter (200 ms) and longer (600 ms) duration, the majority of participants exhibited an additional increase in eye velocity at the moment of reappearance over the level achieved at the end of the first visible ramp. This contrasted with the recovery in eye velocity observed during random presentations of $8°/s^2$ objects and showed that the lack of a predictive increase having pursued the longer ramp was not a result of a ceiling effect in which participants were unable to generate higher levels of eye velocity.

Although this study confirmed that participants are able to scale smooth eye velocity during transient occlusion when object motion is predictable, the change in smooth pursuit could have been based on the expected change in object velocity either side of the occlusion and was not necessarily an on-the-fly extraction and representation of the acceleration signal from the initial visible ramp. Therefore, we performed an additional experiment (Bennet, Orban de Xivry, Barnes, & Lefevre, 2007) in which object acceleration and deceleration, initial object velocity, and visible duration before object occlusion were randomized across trials. By maintaining a fixed start position, this combination of parameters enabled us to decorrelate object position and velocity just before occlusion, as well as mean object velocity during the initial visible ramp, from object acceleration. Hence, the design enabled us to determine whether the pursuit response during a transient occlusion was based on a measure of object acceleration or object velocity.

We found that smooth eye movements showed signs of acceleration discrimination when object motion was visible for at least 500 ms. During the initial, visible part of the object motion leading up to the transient occlusion, smooth eye velocity was appropriately scaled to object velocity ($0°/s$ or $8°/s$) generated by the various levels of object acceleration ($-4, -8, -12, -16°/s^2$ or $-8, -4, 0, 4, 8°/s^2$). The smooth eye velocity then deflected from its preocclusion trajectory but recovered to a level that was positively scaled, albeit with some error in absolute magnitude, to object velocity at reappearance. This would not have been expected if smooth eye velocity were controlled using a measure of object velocity taken just before the transient occlusion. Furthermore, the difference in recovery for each level of object acceleration was not consistent with an extrapolation based on a measure of mean object velocity during the initial ramp, which was negatively related to object acceleration. However, even though there was evidence of scaling the oculomotor response to object acceleration, there was still significant retinal slip when object acceleration was $-8°/s^2$ and $8°/s^2$. Thus, it seems that although information related to object acceleration can be extracted on the fly during the initial visible ramp, the process is not sufficient to drive the predictive oculomotor response in the absence of visual input.

The finding that ocular pursuit does not scale to object acceleration following an initial 200 ms ramp indicates that the temporal limits of extracting this information on the fly are longer than those required to extract object velocity (see Lisberger, 1998). Interestingly, though, our finding that 200 ms was not sufficient to scale ocular pursuit to target acceleration is in accord with the temporal limits of acceleration discrimination reported in psychophysical studies (Brouwer, Brenner, & Smeets, 2002). These results indicate that on-the-fly extraction of acceleration might be achieved indirectly through sequential sampling of the velocity signal. This requires a mechanism in which velocity information from the immediate past is temporarily stored so that it can be compared with current velocity. There is evidence for such behavior from tasks requiring motion perception (Greenlee, Lang, Mergner, & Seeger, 1995), and the notion of sampling and temporarily storing velocity information is one that has been put forward previously to explain the ability to make anticipatory smooth pursuit movements (Barnes & Asselman, 1991) as well as the ability to approximate the acceleration and deceleration of sinusoidal target motion (Barnes, 1994).

Coordination Between Smooth Pursuit and Saccades

As noted in the opening paragraphs of this chapter, smooth pursuit and saccades traditionally have been viewed as distinct gaze-orienting eye movements that have different dynamics, underlying substrates, and functional roles. As such, they are typically studied in isolation, or their contributions are separated for analysis (e.g., saccades are removed from smooth eye movement). Still, in everyday situations smooth pursuit and saccades often play complementary roles when tracking a moving object. This is particularly evident when a person attempts to foveate a fast-moving object that follows an unpredictable trajectory (e.g., a pesky house fly or a rugby football bouncing across the pitch). Under such circumstances, the delay in initiating smooth pursuit combined with the dynamics of limited onset would make continuous foveation of the object unfeasible. Therefore, the pursuit system tracks the unpredictable moving object with a combination of smooth pursuit and saccades.

When the moving object is continuously visible and participants are making smooth eye movements, visual feedback is available regarding retinal slip and position error. However, this information is not available during saccades. Although it is accepted that saccade programming is based on position error, it is less well known that saccades also use input related to object velocity. This is most obvious in situations where a participant makes a saccade when tracking a moving object. With a saccade latency of approximately 150 ms during smooth pursuit eye movements, the saccade would always fall short of the moving object if programmed according to position error alone. Therefore, it is necessary to take account of the smooth eye movement (which corresponds well to object velocity) that occurs during saccade programming (for detailed findings, see De Brouwer et al., 2002). Similarly, although it is accepted that smooth pursuit eye movements receive input from velocity error in the form of retinal slip (Robinson et al., 1986), it is less well accepted that smooth pursuit is also influenced by position error.

Several observations, however, indicate a contribution from position error to smooth pursuit. For example, in the Rashbass paradigm (Rashbass, 1961), the step of object position before onset in the direction opposite to subsequent object motion, which was originally developed to eliminate saccades during the initial smooth pursuit response, generates smooth eye movement (Wyatt & Pola, 1987). Furthermore, it has been shown that a sudden change of the position of a moving object causes a change in smooth eye velocity in order to minimize the position error (Carl & Gellman, 1987; Segraves & Goldberg, 1994). Stabilization experiments artificially projecting the object onto the retina at a fixed offset relative to the fovea have also shown that participants exhibit smooth pursuit eye movements in an attempt to correct for position error (Barnes et al., 1995; Morris & Lisberger, 1987; Wyatt & Pola, 1981).

When the moving object undergoes transient occlusion, visual feedback regarding position and velocity error is no longer available. Consequently, the development of position and velocity error that occurs as a result of reduced eye velocity can be corrected only by reference to an internal representation that reflects the trajectory of the moving object. One solution to this problem might be to exhibit a recovery in smooth pursuit that brings eye velocity well above object velocity. We have never observed such a response in any of our studies (Bennett & Barnes, 2003, 2004). Rather, although participants exhibit a predictive recovery in smooth pursuit during occlusion that occurs in anticipation of object reappearance, eye velocity does not exceed object velocity and eliminate the developing position error (see figures 9.2 and 9.3). An obvious reason for not adopting such a strategy is that it would likely result in significant retinal slip at the moment of object reappearance, and such a slip could create more problems than a residual position error creates. Some of our early observations demonstrated that participants respond to the position error resulting from reduced gain of smooth pursuit by releasing saccades that continuously place the eye slightly ahead of the expected trajectory of the unseen object (for qualitative description, see Becker & Fuchs, 1985; Madelain & Krauzlis, 2003).

In another study, we reported more detailed analyses of how saccades and smooth pursuit are combined during object occlusion (Orban de Xivry,

Bennett, Lefèvre, & Barnes, 2006). In this study, participants tracked a moving object that was subject to an independent but predictable change of position or velocity at reappearance. More specifically, the object motion was modified during the occlusion such that the object reappeared at one of three possible positions and with one of three possible velocities. The reappearance positions were computed as if the pursuit object moved from the end point of the first 400 ms ramp at a velocity of 12°/s, 18°/s, or 24°/s during the occlusion. When the object velocity was equal to 18°/s, the reappearance position was a simple linear extrapolation from the first ramp and resulted in no position step. On the other hand, when the occlusion velocity was either 12°/s or 24°/s, the object appeared either closer (negative position step) or farther (positive position step) than what was expected from the extrapolation of the first ramp. By varying the occlusion velocity, we created a position step at the moment of object reappearance of –6°, 0°, or 6°. We used a similar procedure to generate the velocity step, which represented the difference between actual and expected object velocity at reappearance (from the first 400 ms, 18°/s). Modifying object velocity at the moment of reappearance created a velocity step of –6°/s, 0°/s, or 6°/s. This velocity step was independent of the reappearance position and hence the position step.

Using this novel paradigm, we (Orban de Xivry et al., 2006) were able to examine independently the responses of the smooth and saccadic systems to different but predictable combinations of position steps and velocity steps. In line with our previous studies (Bennett & Barnes, 2005b), we found that a combination of smooth pursuit eye movements and saccades was made in response to the disappearance of a moving object. The smooth pursuit component of this response decayed following object disappearance and then recovered to a level that was scaled to the expected object velocity. However, a predictable velocity step had no effect on the discrete measures of the saccadic response.

In addition, we (Orban de Xivry et al., 2006) found that the discrete measures of the smooth pursuit response during the transient occlusion (e.g., minimum eye velocity) were not influenced by the predictable position step and hence change in object reappearance position. Rather, participants modified their saccadic response in order to deal with the predictable position step and thus the change in eye displacement required to align the gaze at the moment of object reappearance. For example, when the object reappeared with a –6° position step, more saccades were made in the direction opposite to the smooth eye movement (backward saccades). In contrast, when the object appeared with a 6° position step, saccadic amplitudes were larger and mainly forward, in the direction of the smooth eye movement.

Initially these results seemed to suggest that given predictable changes in object parameters during the transient occlusion, the resulting smooth eye velocity depends on object velocity but not object position, whereas the saccadic response depends on object position but not object velocity. However, when we further investigated the interaction between the smooth and saccadic eye movements on a trial-by-trial basis, we found that the saccadic and smooth pursuit systems worked in synergy during object occlusion. The saccadic system modified its contribution to the total eye displacement to compensate for changes in the smooth eye displacement resulting from smooth pursuit (see figure 9.4). Whatever the magnitude of the smooth eye movement, corrective saccades tended to allow the overall eye displacement to closely match object displacement. Thus, when smooth pursuit eye movements contributed less to eye displacement during occlusion, the saccadic system increased its contribution. This compensation for the variability of the smooth response occurred without any visual feedback and suggests that extraretinal signals derived from the smooth eye movement are available to the saccadic system. Furthermore, given that there is no retinal position error or retinal slip for the control of saccades or smooth pursuit during transient occlusion, it seems that participants compared the ongoing trajectory of the eye to an internal representation of future object motion.

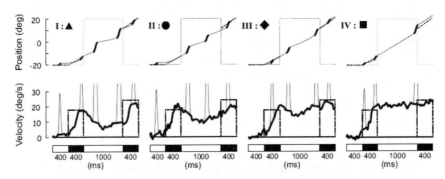

▶ **Figure 9.4**   Eye (solid lines) and pursuit object (dashed traces) position (upper panels) and velocity (lower panels) versus time (ms) for four typical presentations (I, II, III, IV) of the same combination of position step (6°) and velocity step (6°/s). When time bars (bottom of the graphs) are black, the pursuit object was visible. On the position panels, thin solid lines correspond to smooth eye movements and thick solid lines correspond to saccades. On the velocity panels, thick solid lines represent desaccaded smooth eye velocity and thin solid lines correspond to saccades.

Reprinted from J.J. Orban de Xivry et al., 2006, "Evidence for synergy between saccades and smooth pursuit during transient target disappearance," *Journal of Neurophysiology* 95: 418-427. Used with permission.

Model of Ocular Pursuit

As noted earlier, Barnes and Asselman (1991) proposed a model containing a direct (reflexive) loop that receives input from efference copy and an indirect (predictive) loop that accumulates and stores velocity-based information.

This novel arrangement was able to explain both reflexive and predictive influences on smooth pursuit (see also Barnes & Wells, 1999). It was later refined by Bennett and Barnes (2004) to include a local memory structure termed *MEM* within the indirect loop that preserves the visuomotor drive following the loss of visual feedback, as well as variable gain signals that make it possible to simulate the predictive recovery in eye velocity during transient object disappearance (see figure 9.5). In this modified version, the direct loop still represents ongoing efference copy, which perpetuates eye motion when there is only a weak expectation regarding the upcoming stimulus characteristics, and retinal input is also received in the form of a negative visual feedback pathway. As in traditional models of ocular pursuit, the direct loop acts as a positive feedback pathway, but the sampling and holding of a copy of the visuomotor drive signal allows the motion information to be preserved even when the target is extinguished and visual input is cut off. The indirect loop is positioned parallel to the direct loop, and it consolidates motion information obtained by sampling and holding and allows the generation of anticipatory eye movements based on previously experienced stimuli.

In figure 9.5, retinal input is arranged as a negative visual feedback pathway, and extraretinal input comes from either a direct (reflexive) or an indirect (predictive) loop. The direct loop represents ongoing efference copy, which perpetuates eye motion when there is only a weak expectation regarding the upcoming stimulus characteristics. The direct loop is

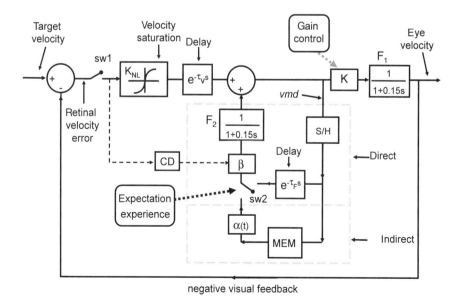

▶ **Figure 9.5** An integrative model of ocular pursuit.

within the negative feedback pathway and acts as a leaky integrator. The indirect loop includes a local memory structure, MEM, which integrates the visuomotor drive signal (vmd) until its output matches the input. The value of MEM is held when the input is reduced, such as during a transient occlusion, which enables eye velocity to be reinstated to its previous level. The signal to modulate β, the output gain of the efference copy loop, comes from a conflict detector (CD) that registers the loss of input when the target disappears. β is also influenced by expectation of whether the target will reappear based on previous experience of stimulus characteristics. The indirect loop includes a variable gain modulator (α), which is tuned to the appropriate magnitude and timing over repeated presentations to minimize pursuit error.

The ability of this model to predict upcoming object trajectory results from the combination of two variable gain signals that act on the visuomotor drive. β is normally unity, but it is reduced when a conflict detector registers the loss of visual input when the object is occluded and then reinstated if there is an expectation that the object will reappear. When the object is not expected to reappear, β is not reinstated and eye velocity continues to decay in accordance with experimental observations. A further variable gain signal, α, acts only on the output of MEM and is tuned over repeated presentations to allow the indirect loop to function as a dynamic memory, changing its output over time to mimic time-changing motion stimuli. In the case where an object moves with constant velocity, MEM reaches a level corresponding to that velocity, whereas α is represented as a step function that, when applied to the output of MEM, generates an eye velocity that approximates object velocity. In addition to explaining the prediction and hence extrapolation of occluded objects moving with constant velocity, this model also is able to represent and produce the trajectory of an accelerating object. As shown in figure 9.6, the combined modulation of gain signals α and β generates a predictive recovery in eye velocity toward the expected object trajectory (thin dashed gray line). Simulated eye velocity for control presentations (thick gray line) is included for comparison; α is modeled as a staircase ramp function but there is no loss of drive from visual feedback because the object does not undergo a transient occlusion. Note that the magnitude of gain signals is not represented to scale in order to aid visual inspection.

This was achieved by modeling the variable gain function, α, as a staircase ramp; a good approximation to the acceleration and deceleration characteristics of sinusoidal object motion can also be achieved by sampling and storing the relevant velocity-based information from a single half cycle at 250 ms intervals (Barnes, 1994). Although α was devised somewhat arbitrarily for the purposes of the simulation, we suggest that the gain function is adapted and tuned over repeated presentations by comparing the object and eye trajectory at relatively coarse intervals to minimize the pursuit error.

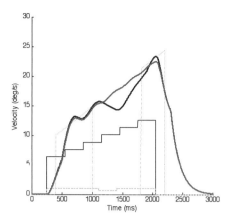

▶ **Figure 9.6**   Smooth eye velocity (thick black line) using a staircase function in which α is initially set at 0.4 and then increased to unity in five equal amplitude steps that each last 300 ms. Normally, β is unity when the eye is pursuing a continuously visible object, but it is set to a reduced level (0.7) 100 ms after the loss of visual feedback (gray line) and then reinstated to unity after a brief delay (300 ms) in expectation of object reappearance.

Experimental Brain Research, Vol. 175(1), pgs. 1-10, 2006, *"Smooth ocular pursuit during the transient disappearance of an accelerating visual target: the role of reflexive and voluntary control,"* M.R. Bennett and G.R. Barnes, fig. 3. © Springer. With kind permission of Springer Science+Business media.

This concept is consistent with the suggestion that long-term adaptation to the pursuit response is achieved by tuning a variable gain function (see Madelain & Krauzlis, 2003).

To account for learning and adaptation, we proposed that the decision to switch between the direct loop and indirect loop, and hence modify the interplay between reflexive and predictive control, depends on the strength of participant expectation regarding the upcoming object parameters. In the first few presentations, when participants do not have any experience of the object motion, they simply react to visual feedback (i.e., demonstrate no anticipatory pursuit before object onset) and elicit a reflexive response based on the direct loop. Following the loss of visual feedback during the occlusion interval, the participants' eye velocity decays exponentially, as reported by Mitrani and Dimitrov (1978). However, once participants develop an expectation that the moving object will appear after a fixed fore-period with particular motion characteristics and subsequently undergo a transient occlusion followed by reappearance, there is a shift in dominance as predictive mechanisms play a role in setting the magnitude of the initial anticipatory response and gating an anticipatory recovery during the occlusion interval. We suggest that this is achieved by switching to the persistent, indirect, velocity-based memory loop. At this early stage, participants are unlikely to have precisely tuned the variable gain function, and thus a significant contribution from visual feedback (part of the reflexive mechanism) is still required. Then, with more experience of past presentations, and hence a strong expectation about the upcoming object parameters, participants are able to scale their recovery in eye velocity while at the same time using saccades to account for the developing position error.

Neural Pathways for Ocular Pursuit

On the basis of electrophysiological recordings in nonhuman primates and more recent functional imaging studies of humans, there is now good understanding of the neural pathways involved in evoking smooth pursuit and saccadic eye movements (for a review, see Pierrot-Deseilligny, Milea, & Müri, 2004). These recent findings have challenged the notion that smooth pursuit and saccades receive input through distinct neural pathways, and it is becoming increasingly evident that there is considerable overlap (see Krauzlis, 2004; Krauzlis & Stone, 1999; Their & Ilg, 2005). It is not our intention to provide an exhaustive account of these neural pathways. Rather, we will briefly describe some of the main findings so that we can later ascertain whether the same pathways remain active when the eye pursues a moving object that undergoes transient occlusion.

For both smooth pursuit and saccades directed toward a visual object, information is initially conveyed from the retina through several networks before finally reaching the oculomotor neurons that stimulate the extraocular muscles. Traditionally, it has been suggested that simple corticoponto-cerebellar connections provide the main pathway to the oculomotor neurons for control of smooth pursuit. From early processing of retinal input at occipital areas (V1, V2, and V3), information is relayed to medial temporal (MT) and medial superior temporal (MST) areas of the visual association cortex (V5 and V5a in humans). Both the MT and MST areas process velocity error signals, whereas the MST area also receives extraretinal inputs (Komatsu & Wurtz, 1989; Newsome, Wurtz, & Komatso, 1988). Importantly, lesion studies have shown that whereas the MT area is largely involved in smooth pursuit onset, the MST area is implicated in the maintenance of smooth pursuit (Dürsteler & Wurtz, 1988). From the MT and MST areas, there are connections to the flocculus and paraflocculus of the cerebellum via the dorsolateral pontine nuclei (DLPN). In addition, there is a second parallel pathway from the MT and MST areas that connects first to the frontal eye field (FEF) and then to the nucleus reticularis tegmenti pontis (NRTP) and the vermis of the cerebellum. It has been suggested that the FEF plays a major role in the control of smooth pursuit onset (Gottlieb, Bruce, & MacAvoy, 1993; Tanaka & Lisberger, 2001) and in the prediction that is required to smoothly pursue sinusoidal trajectories (MacAvoy, Gottlieb, & Bruce, 1991).

Corticopontocerebellar connections also provide a main pathway to the oculomotor neurons for control of saccades. The FEF plays a key role in these networks, with direct projections to the superior colliculus (SC) and brain stem premotor nuclei (PMN), as well as through the basal ganglia (caudate nucleus [CN] and substantia nigra pars reticulata [SNr]) and lateral intraparietal area (LIP). There is also a more direct pathway from the retina and V1 to the SC; this pathway is thought to control saccades of very short latency (express saccades). The classic distinction, therefore, is that whereas the neural pathways for smooth pursuit are arranged to support reflexive control, the neural pathways for saccades bestow some voluntary control. Contrary to this distinction, it is now understood that areas such as the supplementary eye fields (SEF), basal ganglia, and LIP, which are implicated in voluntary control of saccades, are also involved in smooth pursuit eye movements. For example, SEF activation has been implicated in object choice (i.e., decision making) in saccade tasks (Coe, Tomihara, Matsuzawa, & Hikosaka, 2002), but SEF activation is also related to the decision to change smooth pursuit direction (Heinen & Liu, 1997). Also, stimulation in the SEF modifies anticipatory pursuit gain (Missal & Heinen, 2004). Furthermore, areas of the basal ganglia such as the CN receive input from areas of the FEF related to smooth pursuit (Cui, Yan, & Lynch, 2003), and the SNr is involved in initiating voluntary smooth pursuit (Basso, Pokorny, & Liu, 2005).

Neural Pathways for Ocular Pursuit During Transient Occlusion

Given that no retinal input is available during a transient occlusion, extra-retinal signals are required to drive smooth and saccadic eye movements. This has been recognized by many researchers, although there is a difference of opinion regarding the nature of the extraretinal signals. According to the trajectory network model proposed by Grzywacz, Watamaniuk, and McKee (1995), motion detectors aligned with the direction of object motion facilitate activation of similarly tuned motion detectors that fall near or on the motion path, propagating the motion signal. Moreover, it is suggested that the motion signal continues to propagate along the motion detectors when the moving object is occluded or extinguished, which provides a prediction of future object motion.

The implication of this approach is that the same mechanisms that process visual motion are involved in predicting the motion of an occluded object. Evidence that activation in MST areas, the main areas of motion detection, continues when an object is temporarily extinguished is consistent with the propagation of a motion signal (Ilg & Their, 2003; Newsome et al., 1988; Olson, Gatenby, Leung, Skudlarski, & Gore, 2003). However, although MST activation does not differ between tracking an object that remains continuously visible and tracking an object that is temporarily extinguished, activation increases in other neural areas (Lencer et al., 2004). The activation in areas such as the FEF and DLPFC, which cannot be attributed to the initiation of saccades (Nagel et al., 2006), indicates that additional mechanisms are involved in the continuation of smooth pursuit when visual feedback is temporarily unavailable.

As described earlier, there has been much debate about the use of efference copy of the eye movement commands to provide a basic prediction of future object motion, with the main concern being an inevitable decay in the extraretinal signal as eye velocity decreases. It is interesting, therefore, that activation in the MST area, which receives extraretinal inputs (Ilg & Their, 2003), does not correlate with the decrease in smooth pursuit eye velocity that occurs when an object is temporarily extinguished, whereas there is a negative correlation with the increased activation of the FEF and DLPFC (Nagel et al., 2006).

Nagel and colleagues (2006) suggested that the increased activation of the DLPFC and FEF may be due to predictive mechanisms that compensate for the decrease in smooth pursuit velocity. We agree and interpret these findings to suggest that prefrontal areas become increasingly involved in the control of smooth pursuit when there is a greater need to involve predictive mechanisms. It is feasible that the increased activity in the FEF is related to activation of a network that involves a comparison between predicted and current eye position and velocity. These findings also seem to suggest that activity in the MST does not correspond to the efference copy loop because activation in this area might be expected to decrease with the decrease in eye velocity. Further support for this suggestion is evident in the work of Ono and Mustari (2006), who demonstrated that sustained activity in dorsomedial MST (MSTd) neurons associated with smooth pursuit was also evident during suppression of the VOR, but not when making rotational head movements in the dark (VOR dark). They concluded that extraretinal signals present in MSTd neurons likely represent volitional control of smooth pursuit rather than vestibular input or eye movement sensitivity from proprioceptive feedback or an efference copy of eye movements.

Further support for the role of the FEF in predicting a temporarily extinguished trajectory has been reported by Barborica and Ferrera (2003, 2004; see also Xiao, Barborica, & Ferrera, 2007). In the first of these studies, monkeys were required to make a saccade toward the location of an unseen moving object when given a go signal. While the monkeys maintained fixation (and hence before the saccade was initiated), it was found that FEF activity was related to object velocity. Moreover, this relationship between FEF activity and object velocity was preserved when the object was temporarily extinguished. In addition, accurate saccades were made to the extrapolated object position, which led the authors to conclude that the monkeys were able to extract an estimate of future object position using information on object speed and occlusion time. Later studies have shown that the activity in the FEF (e.g., induced by microstimulation in Barborica

& Ferrèra, 2004) is related to the position of the unseen object, which may imply a continuously shifting locus of attention (i.e., a saccade plan) that moves coincident with the unseen object trajectory. The implication is that predictive activity in the FEF is not simply related to motor activity, which is consistent with our suggestion that an internal representation of object-related velocity can be generated in the absence of eye movements.

Although we are gaining a better understanding of the neural pathways involved in tracking an occluded or temporarily extinguished moving object, it is still unknown what comparisons are made and where these comparisons take place. One solution would be to control eye position alone—that is, the brain might sense when the eye is no longer positioned near the occluded trajectory and respond with a corrective movement. Work using object images stabilized on the retina indicates that the decision to respond with a saccadic or smooth eye movement likely depends on the size of the required correction, with smooth eye movement dominating for position error less than 2° to 3° (Barnes et al., 1995; Kommerel & Taumer, 1972).

An alternative approach could be to compare separate representations of extrapolated object position and velocity to the changing eye position and velocity. In other words, the brain might use separate mechanisms of position and velocity control to generate a well-coordinated response. For saccades to be accurately located on the occluded trajectory, this would require the eye velocity to be integrated to give eye position. Orban de Xivry and Lefèvre (2007) have suggested that a comparison for position-coded signals could occur in the LIP (Bremmer, Distler, & Hoffmann, 1997), which is known to be involved in remapping the visual scene when keeping track of saccades (Duhamel, Colby, & Goldberg, 1992; Heide et al., 2001; Medendorp, Goltz, Vilis, & Crawford, 2003) and of smooth pursuit eye movements (Schlack, Hoffmann, & Bremmer, 2003). For the control of smooth pursuit, it is noteworthy that the DLPFC, which has connections with the FEF, has been associated for some time with working memory (Levy & Goldman-Rakic, 2000; Passingham & Sakai, 2004). Therefore, it follows that if the FEF represents the unseen object velocity, this information could be relayed to prefrontal areas for comparison with an estimate on current eye velocity.

Pursuit Against a Background: Suppression of the Optokinetic Reflex

Although we have shown that the combination of smooth eye movements and saccades brings the eye toward an appropriate position and velocity at the moment a moving object reappears, a potential consequence of removing retinal input during a transient occlusion is that the presence of a structured background will likely have even greater negative effect on the ability to maintain smooth pursuit. In young adults pursuing continuously visible predictable object motion, gain is high and there is a negligible effect of the passive (OKR) drive. The implication is that the oculomotor system countermands the conflicting input of passive (OKR) drive by increasing the active (smooth pursuit) drive (Schweigart, Mergner, & Barnes, 1999; Worfolk & Barnes, 1992).

However, when visual input regarding object motion is degraded, such as when the eye tracks objects located in the periphery, the gain of smooth pursuit is reduced, indicating that the potentiated response is still dependent on the visual feedback (Barnes & Crombie, 1985). Furthermore, large OKR-induced reductions in smooth pursuit gain occur when the background suddenly shifts in any direction other than opposite the direction of the eye motion (Lindner, Schwarz, & Ilg, 2001). This occurs even when the shift in background is made before the onset of anticipatory smooth pursuit (i.e., no pursuit-induced background image motion) and when the pursuit object is suddenly extinguished (i.e., no relative motion between the pursuit object and background), confirming the importance of extraretinal input in countermanding the OKR drive (Lindner & Ilg, 2006). Given our finding that extraretinal input drives the pursuit response during transient occlusion of a moving object, it remains important to determine what type of background motion induces OKR effects and how the smooth and saccadic systems respond in countermanding these passive drives.

In addition to the degree of separation between the object and the structured background (Goltz & Whitney, 2004; Masson, Proteau, & Mestre, 1993) and the direction of background motion (Lindner et al., 2001; Lindner & Ilg, 2006) determining the influence of passive OKR drive on ocular pursuit, the depth of background relative to the moving object also mediates the conflicting effect. OKR drive exerts a stronger influence when retinal inputs coincide with the plane of convergence (Howard & Marton, 1992); when the moving object is in a more distant depth plane than the occluder, there is a decrease in the number of saccades and the amplitude of saccadic corrections. At present, however, only a limited type of occluder has been studied, and no direct measurement of the combined smooth and saccadic pursuit response has been made (see Churchland et al., 2003). For instance, it has yet to be resolved whether the influence of an occluder on the ability to maintain smooth pursuit is the result of physical differences in retinal disparities related to OKR or if there is a role for other higher-order perceptual processes. The use of additional cues to depth to discriminate between an occluder and an object becomes particularly important when both are located at large distances (i.e., >10 m) because they produce perceptually irresolvable retinal disparities. In this situation, pictorial cues such as perspective, relative size, interposition, luminance (brightness), and contrast may all contribute to the final perception of object depth. At present, it is unknown how these physical and perceptual cues (alone or in combination) influence the conjugate ocular pursuit response during a transient occlusion and how they are weighted as the information on depth differences provided by retinal disparity is modified.

Oculomanual Pursuit

It is well known that a close relationship exists between movement of the eyes and movement of other effectors of the upper and lower limbs. It is rare for eye movements to occur in isolation because they often provide visual feedback about objects that are the focus of object-directed actions such as reaching and grasping. In addition, eye movements provide extra-retinal information that is used to construct an internal representation of three-dimensional space in eye-centered coordinates (Andersen & Buneo, 2002; Batista, Buneo, Snyder, & Andersen, 1999). By learning to coordinate movements of the hand with movements of the eyes, it is suggested that hand movements can also be represented in eye-centered coordinates, thus minimizing problems associated with performing transformations between different coordinate frames of reference.

When driving (Marple-Horvat et al., 2005; Wilkie & Wann, 2003) and stepping on obstacles (Hollands & Marple-Horvat, 1996), the prevention of eye movements that would normally be coordinated with limb movements leads to impaired motor performance. The suggestion is that the oculo-motor signal from saccadic eye movements that initially place the eye on the object and smooth eye movements that keep the eye on the object as the distance between object and observer is reduced provides information to the neural structures controlling upper- and lower-limb movements. Similarly, it has been shown that synchronous (coordinated) eye and hand move-ments confer a significant advantage to manual tracking performance (i.e., reduced root mean square (RMS) amplitude error) versus hand movement performed alone (Miall, Reckess, & Imamizu, 2001). Increased cerebellar activity was found to accompany the improved performance in the synchro-nous eye–hand tracking, confirming the importance of the cerebellum in coordinating and learning to coordinate neural signals from eye and hand movements. Currently, however, it is unknown how the modified ocular response during a transient occlusion influences concurrent control of the hand. This knowledge will elucidate to what extent participants use motor commands from ongoing eye movement to control their hand movement, or whether they extract the necessary information from a more persistent representation derived from previous or planned attempts.

Although eye movements facilitate accurate performance of concurrent hand movements, there is some evidence that the limits of ocular pursuit can be extended by concurrent hand movements. This may confer an advantage by keeping the object image on the fovea, facilitating the perception of object characteristics. Previous research has indicated that smooth ocular pursuit latency is reduced (Gauthier & Hofferer, 1976) and maximum velocity is increased when participants perform concurrent hand movement (Gauthier, Vercher, Mussa Ivaldi, & Marchetti, 1988) or pursue internally generated limb movement (Leist, Freund, & Cohen, 1987). The main sequence for saccadic eye movements is also modified when performed concurrently with hand movement (Epelboim et al., 1997; Snyder, Calton, Dickinson, & Lawrence, 2002). In terms of smooth pursuit eye movements, it has been suggested that the advantage of performing concurrent upper-limb movements is conveyed by efferent and afferent (i.e., proprioception) signals. Still, it has yet to be examined how efference copy and arm afference from manual pursuit movement influence the continuation of ocular pursuit during transient occlusion. For instance, it remains to be determined if hand movement performed concurrently with eye movement can help offset the potentially negative effect of OKR (i.e., reduced gain of smooth pursuit and increased saccadic eye displacement) during pursuit of a transiently occluded object. This is an important omission because it is known that eye movement control is particularly sensitive to the available visual feedback during transient occlusion (both of the object and background), whereas volitional hand movements can be made in the absence of vision.

Summary and Future Directions

In this chapter, we have discussed the predictive nature of smooth and saccadic eye movements that are observed when tracking a moving object in the absence of visual feedback. In particular, we summarized findings from experiments that have examined the onset and continuation of pursuit when a moving object suddenly disappears or is occluded. Such eye movements are critical to maintaining gaze orientation in our normal surroundings where fast-moving objects, which cannot be pursued with accuracy using retinal input alone, are frequently occluded by other surfaces and objects.

In recognition of this fact, we presented a model of ocular pursuit including a novel arrangement of extraretinal input that can account for both reflexive and predictive eye control required to track simple and complex object motion. This is an important consideration because although predictive eye movements are critical to successful object tracking, they tend to occur only when the participant has a strong expectation based on previous experience or advance cues.

Finally, we described evidence from electrophysiological and imaging studies that have provided some insight as to where in the neural substrate these reflexive and predictive mechanisms are located. The next challenge will be to determine how the interplay between reflexive and predictive mechanisms unfolds when pursuing moving objects in the tasks and visual contexts that have high fidelity with our natural surroundings.

CHAPTER 10

Oculomotor Contributions to Reaching: Close Is Good Enough

GORDON BINSTED, KYLE BROWNELL,
TYLER ROLHEISER, AND MATTHEW HEATH

Whether we are driving a car, hitting a ball, or simply picking up a cup of coffee, our motor systems rely upon our ocular system to search ahead and gather information (Land, 2005). Conventionally, vision of both the effector and the target is used to prepare and execute goal-directed limb movements (for a review see Heath, 2005; see also chapters 1 and 2). However, an equally pervasive feature of manual control is the stark stereotypy of eye–hand coordination: The eye and hand appear tethered in a highly adaptive fashion to optimize task success.

In this chapter, we summarize the characteristic behaviors present during coordinated eye movement and action, the subservient anatomy, and the dominant accounts of the functional role of this coordination. The viewpoints on eye–hand action are clustered into three main themes. First, some theorists view coordination in terms of spatial reference frames, where eye–hand movement arises from the need to express our visual action space (i.e., peripersonal space) in a common eye-centered manner. Others hold that strategic benefit is gained by prepositioning the eye—visually acquiring the target and making hand–target comparisons. Third, common source accounts suggest that coupling is derived from efferent and afferent information shared between motor systems. Finally, we present a number of questions to be addressed in the hope of connecting the extant understanding of eye–hand behavior to more general concepts such as the functional outcomes of neural events.

This work was supported by Natural Sciences and Engineering Research Council of Canada Discovery Grants to GB and MH.

Common Anatomies, Divergent Functions

Before going into any direct discussion of eye–hand action, we need to provide an account of the functional systems underlying both saccadic and manual goal-directed movements. The central issues for both systems can be simplified to specifying the direction and amplitude of the required action; however, each system does this differently. Moreover, despite the sequential presentation of the systems and structures, it is likely that the functions and interactions operate in a highly parallel fashion (see Battaglia-Mayer, Archambault, & Caminiti, 2006).

Eye

Successfully specifying a saccade requires interaction among many cortical and subcortical regions (Girard & Berthoz, 2005). At its lowest level, the amplitude of a saccade is specified by the discharge frequency of the extraocular motor neurons arising from the oculomotor nuclei (oculomotor, trochlear, abducens). The direction of a saccade is predicated on how and what muscles are activated, dictated by premotor burst and omnipause neurons within two separate gaze centers in the brain stem (see figure 10.1). Furthermore, a prerequisite to activity within the brain stem circuitry is a motor command from the superior colliculus (SC) that provides the gaze centers (paramedian pontine reticular formation [PPRF] and rostral interstitial nucleus of the medial longitudinal fasciculus [iMLF]); see Rodgers, Munoz, Scott, & Pare, 2006) with a motor command to move the eye to the intended new foveal location (as determined by the visual

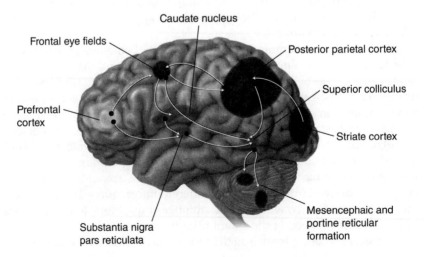

▶ **Figure 10.1**   The subcortical and cortical structure involved in producing volitional saccades. Arrows show hypothesized directional connections during saccade execution.

array). In short, inhibition of omnipause neurons is released via input from saccade-related burst neurons in the SC, leading to activation of excitatory burst neurons (pons and midbrain) and the pulse of neuromotor activity related to a saccadic response.

Although the SC provides the crucial command, its activity is shaped by inputs from the prefrontal cortex (PPC), frontal eye field (FEF), and substantia nigra par reticulata (SNr). The PPC provides visual guidance to saccades by modulating the visual inputs to the SC according to attention locus; that is, by the behavioral relevance of a visual stimulus. Moreover, the FEF and associated prefrontal regions form an executive center that activates SC neurons, selecting the target for voluntary saccades when several potential goals are possible. Using these same connections, the FEF also suppresses reflexive orienting and permits voluntary saccades to nonvisual targets. The basal ganglia subsequently funnel inputs from frontal areas and act as a gate for the voluntary control of saccades. Activity in the SNr prevents unwanted saccades via inhibition of SC while voluntary saccades are permitted by disinhibition arising from the caudate, which is activated by signals from the frontal cortex (Findlay & Walker, 1999).

Hand

Before any action takes place, a person must select a goal, an often demanding process modulated bottom-up by the visual salience of objects or top-down by our behavioral goals and expectations of rewards (see chapter 4). Critical to this process is the manner in which the cortex represents targets for action (i.e., PPC) and for perception (i.e., inferior temporal lobe [IT]; Milner & Goodale, 1995). In brief, output from primary visual areas converges on centers for conscious judgments and determinations (so-called *ventral regions* within IT) and areas for the unconscious control of action (so-called *dorsal regions* within PPC).

Whereas the IT appears to address aspects of conscious perception and feed regions associated with high-level processes, the PPC appears to play a central role in unconscious target localization and updating spatial locations across eye or limb movements (Binsted, Brownell, Vorontsova, Heath, & Saucier, 2007; Heath, Neely, Yakimishyn, & Binsted, 2008; Medendorp, Goltz, Vilis, & Crawford, 2003; Medendorp, Smith, Tweed, & Crawford, 2001; Merriam, Genovese, & Colby, 2003). Arising from this determination, a motor command is prepared via combined parietal input from superior parietal (SPL) and parietal reach regions (PRR) to frontal motor cortices (i.e., supplementary, premotor, and primary motor cortex; see Glover, 2004, for a review). This efference takes into account the difference between the current position of the hand and the location of the target (i.e., motor error; see Buneo & Andersen, 2006). Following movement initiation, this frontoparietal circuit remains active, minimizing motor errors through iterative comparisons between target and hand (inferior parietal lobule

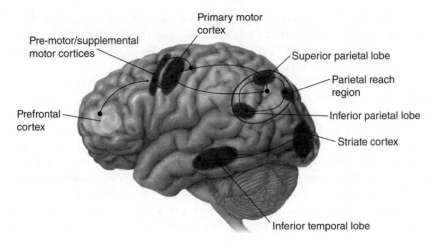

▶ **Figure 10.2**   Schematic depiction of the subcortical and cortical structures involved in goal-directed reaching. Regions of cerebral cortex directly involved in the frontoparietal motor circuit and those involved in decision making (intention and memory; frontal association area) are shown. Arrows represent hypothesized directional connections during movement execution.

[IPL]; see figure 10.2). (See Naranjo et al., 2007, for a detailed account of frontoparietal dynamics.)

Importantly, a number of common regions are subsumed by both the ocular and manual motor systems. The PPC, most notably the IPL and likely the PRR, serves similar purposes in both networks (i.e., target extraction and spatial transformation, as discussed later). Furthermore, frontal motor regions (i.e., premotor cortex and FEF) are active in close proximity, allowing for the tenability of shared or interacting motor commands. Accordingly, it is reasonable to predict temporal convergence of function, suggesting that the areas are not only performing comparable processes but also performing them at the same time.

Eye–Hand Coupling Behavior

Given the heavy reliance of goal-directed movement on visual feature extraction (e.g., target position, size) and the close structural association between the ocular system and the manual system, visual targets are not surprisingly drawn to the fovea during reaches (Carey, 2000; Neggers & Bekkering, 2000). For example, if a person is asked to make a discrete aiming response to a specified target, the eyes normally execute a rapid saccadic response, resulting in target fixation (Carlton, 1981; Fisk & Goodale, 1985). The eyes usually begin moving in advance of the limb and arrive at the target location in concert with early kinematic markers of limb execution (e.g., peak acceleration; Helsen, Elliott, Starkes, & Ricker, 2000).

However, the subsumed spatiotemporal relationships between eye movements and hand movements during such goal-directed action are much more involved than this fixed effector order might suggest (Binsted, Chua, Helsen, & Elliott, 2001; Ehresman, Saucier, Heath, & Binsted, 2008; Furneaux & Land, 1999; Herst, Epelboim, & Steinman, 2001; Land & McLeod, 2000). For example, temporal coupling varies as a function of the availability of optical information (e.g., Fisk & Goodale, 1985; Sailer, Eggert, & Straube, 2005; Thura, Hadj-Bouziane, Meunier, & Boussaoud, 2008). In sequential double-step tasks, the eye advances well ahead of hand foveation (200 ms; Wilmut, Wann, & Brown, 2006), whereas in more natural tasks the eye performs frequent look-ahead fixations to preacquire target features (Mennie, Hayhoe, & Sullivan, 2007). Moreover, reaching kinematics and end-state accuracy are directly influenced by fixation location (i.e., target foveation) such that gaze deviation degrades reach accuracy (Binsted & Elliott, 1999b; Crawford, Henriques, Medendorp, & Khan, 2003; Henriques & Crawford, 2000; Terao, Andersson, Flanagan, & Johansson, 2002), and introduced saccadic bias generates concomitant manual error (e.g., Müller-Lyer illusions: Bernardis, Knox, & Bruno, 2005; Binsted et al., 2001; Thompson & Westwood, 2007; saccadic adaptation: Neggers & Bekkering, 2000, 2001). The stereotypical sequencing between eye and hand, though robust, is also modulated by task instructions and participant strategy. If the task requires high precision, the hand initiation is delayed until complete target acquisition is attained (via fixation), whereas hand response may even precede saccadic response in situations requiring low precision and high response rate (e.g., Carnahan & Marteniuk, 1991).

Although common initiation latency may not be ubiquitous to all eye–hand movements, one omnipresent characteristic of coordination is movement termination (Helsen, Starkes, Elliott, & Buekers, 1998). The eyes always attain the target position before the hand (despite task instructions), arriving at the target (or thereabouts) just after peak acceleration of the limb (Helsen et al., 2000). Pragmatically, this makes sense for limb control; the eyes are in a position to gather information at a time when it is most needed (i.e., when the hand approaches the target; Carlton, 1981; Woodworth, 1899). Such eye positioning facilitates the commonly observed reduction in spatial variability of the hand following peak velocity (Heath, Westwood, & Binsted, 2004; Helsen et al., 2000). Similarly, eye movements and arm movements (and not just end location) mutually influence each other's kinematic profiles (Fisk & Goodale, 1985; Gauthier, Nommay, & Vercher, 1990; Snyder, Calton, Dickinson, & Lawrence, 2002; van Donkelaar, 1998; Vercher, Magenes, Prablanc, & Gauthier, 1994). Both smooth pursuit and saccadic responses achieve higher velocities when accompanying a hand response, and the accuracy of the manual response may be significantly biased by concurrent eye responses. Such coreliance reveals a shared architecture or mutual triggering between oculomotor and manual subcortical and cortical architectures (Miall, Reckess, & Imamizu, 2001; van Donkelaar, Lee, & Drew, 2000, 2002). However, eye and arm movements can also become naturally, and adaptively, decoupled (Crawford, Henriques, & Medendorp, 2003; Steinman, Pizlo, Forofonova, & Epelboim, 2003); for example, consider how you adjust the radio or reach for a drink while averting your eyes to the task of driving. Conversely, eye–hand coupling can reach pathological levels following damage to the SPL and inferior parietal sulcus (e.g., magnetic misreaching; Carey, Coleman, & Della Sala, 1997) such that the hand becomes obligated to follow the eye despite cognitive effort to do otherwise.

Frames of Reference Hypothesis

During the planning of a movement response to an environmental stimulus, visual, auditory, and somatic information must coalesce to form a movement plan. Given a wealth of information from the clinical literature (i.e., literature on ataxia; Milner et al., 2001; Perenin & Vighetto, 1988; Revol et al., 2003), a reasonable speculation is to label the parietal cortex as the primary location for the integration of sensory information.

If we begin by simplifying the task to the integration of visual information arriving from the dorsal stream, it is apparent that the parietal cortex possesses information regarding contrast (delivering edges and textures) and movement in an external frame of reference. In other words, all of the task-relevant information will be referenced to the external environment. Movement plans directed from M1, however, are not planned with respect to a dynamic external world; instead, they must specify the task in terms of effector systems (e.g., agonist–antagonist muscle pairs). Visual information must be transformed into an internal frame of reference before this information becomes usable by the motor system.

Unfortunately for the motor system, it is not possible to simply reduce the production of accurate movement to the interaction between vision and movement—auditory and somatosensory information also arrive in the parietal cortex for integration into a movement plan. This begets a problem of integration (Anderson & Buneo, 2002): Multiple sensory systems ostensibly dump information into the parietal cortex from completely different coordinate maps. Generally, visual information arrives in an external (eye-centered) frame of reference (Mullette-Gillman, Cohen, & Groh, 2005), whereas auditory and somatic inputs tend to be coded in a head-based frame of reference (Avillac, Denève, Olivier, Pouget, & Duhamel, 2005). This information must be rendered useful for not only the manual motor system but also the saccadic system. The theorized solution to this problem lies in establishing a common and disbursed frame of reference from all of these modalities, perhaps within the ventral intraparietal (VIP) area (Schlack, Sterbing-D'Angelo, Hartung, Hoffman, & Bremmer, 2005).

The lateral intraparietal (LIP) area is involved in the planning of saccades based on any environmental stimulus (for a review see Anderson & Buneo, 2002). To demonstrate this, Stricane, Anderson, and Mazzoni (1996) examined how neurons in a monkey's LIP area responded to a task that required a saccade to either an auditory or a visual cue. When compared with neuronal activity based on visual input, neuronal discharge in many recorded cells remained the same in the presence of an auditory cue. Furthermore, neurons responding to the auditory saccade task seemed to be modulated by eye position, presumably due to environmental information arriving at the LIP area in an external or environmental frame of reference. This information is transformed by LIP neurons into an eye-centered frame of reference that is subsequently read out by the saccadic system to drive a saccade.

In predicting the parietal events associated with a reaching movement, it would be reasonable to assume limb-centered referencing for cortical activity associated with the eyes regardless of sensory modality. However, a meta-analysis by Anderson and Buneo (2002) reported that during a visually guided pointing task, many neurons in the PRR did not discharge in a manner consistent with a limb-centered frame of reference but instead discharged in a manner consistent with an eye-centered frame of reference. Due to the limb-centered requirements of frontal motor areas for specifying the limb trajectory, these results were interpreted as evidence of externally referenced visual information arriving at the PRR being transformed to an eye-centered system. Furthermore, Cohen and Anderson (2000) demonstrated corroborating evidence of motor planning in eye-centered coordinates. Specifically, they showed that for a reaching movement based on an auditory cue, PRR neurons discharged in a manner that was heavily modulated by eye position. In fact, PRR population coding was more heavily influenced by eye position than by the location of the hand itself. Cohen and Anderson attributed this finding to PRR neurons preferentially planning movements of limbs in eye-centered coordinates.

Given the mounting evidence from single-cell recordings (e.g., Anderson & Buneo, 2002; Batista, Buneo, Snyder, & Anderson, 1999; Schlack et al., 2005), it is likely that a common, eye-centered coordinate frame of reference serves as the primary output for both the saccadic and the manual motor systems from the parietal cortex. Although the proposed reference frame is retinotopically centered, the general frame of reference can be modified by what is known as a *gain field*—a progressive switch that shifts the firing pattern of neurons in either the LIP area or the PRR in response to changes in eye, body, or limb position (Anderson & Buneo, 2002). Hence, the established parietal frame of reference is not a static construct. Instead, as the position of the eyes changes, so does the retinotopic frame of reference through gain field modulation; the frame of reference in the PRR has also been shown to adapt based on learning (Buneo & Anderson, 2006). This remapping ensures that a movement plan formulated during a change in eye position can be updated via a simple adjustment of the gain field, a mechanism in concurrence with the real-time nature of sensorimotor transformation (see Westwood & Goodale, 2003). A common frame of reference at a parietal level (i.e., between LIP areas and PRR) possesses intuitive appeal on two levels: Human interaction with the environment primarily relies on the visual system, and the common reference frame would certainly abet coordination between the visual and manual motor systems (Batista et al., 1999).

Though the single-cell recording evidence seems to suggest an eye-centered frame of reference in both the LIP area and PRR, only a small percentage of cells within an area are recorded, and the recorded cells do not behave homogenously; inferences on function are due to the relative behavior of some cells. Furthermore, it is always necessary to exert a degree of caution when extrapolating single-cell primate recordings to human behavior.

Fortunately, frame-of-reference transformation studies are not confined to single-cell paradigms. If the saccadic and manual motor systems indeed share a common representation in the parietal cortex, and it is modified by a gain field modulated by eye position, TMS should disrupt coordinated eye–hand behavior. In two complementary studies, van Donkelaar and colleagues (2000, 2002) used an experimental design employing TMS to further document this phenomenon. In the first of these studies, participants completed three conditions of a pointing task. In the first condition, the eye and hand shared the same starting and end position. In the other two conditions, the starting position of the eye was farther from the end position and the starting position of the hand remained the same. Though the saccadic movement and pointing movement shared a common end position in conditions 2 and 3, the saccadic amplitude was progressively increased. Not surprisingly, normal reaching (condition 1) demonstrated hand-path influences of saccadic amplitude. However, when a TMS pulse was applied to the PRR just before the saccade began, the increased saccadic amplitude had no influence on hand kinematics. The gain field representing eye position presumably was not able to update the common representation (Andersen & Buneo, 2002), therefore sparing the limb from saccadic disruption.

Although the contribution of the parietal cortex is substantial, many studies have established that a further frame-of-reference transformation must occur before overt limb movement. Furthermore, the dorsal premotor cortex (PMd) is implicated in this process (Chouinard & Paus, 2006). The second study by van Donkelaar and colleagues (2002) used a paradigm similar to that used in the first study to observe the contributions of the PMd to frame-of-reference transformations. In contrast to their first experiment, disrupting the activity in PMd before the onset of movement resulted in hand movements that reflected an increased amplitude much like the saccadic system. These results can also be interpreted using the model proposed by Andersen and Buneo (2002): The transformation from eye-centered coordinates (PRR) to limb-centered coordinates (PMd) could not take place due to the magnetic disruption. The hand movement, therefore, completely reflected the retinal-based (gain-susceptible) motor program.

The Andersen and Buneo (2002) position holds distinct logical and parsimonious appeal; however, recent evidence suggests that reference frames may be abandoned for a different type of neural encoding. A single-cell recording paradigm developed by Graziano (2006) documents multiple frames of reference in the premotor cortex (PMC). During a reaching task, the firing pattern of each neuron was active during reaches made to a particular response field; that is, each neuron was responsible for coding for a particular region of space. Interestingly, these regions were not dependent on a limb-centered frame of reference or on a retinal frame of reference. The firing rate of each neuron was modulated by the difference vectors: eye and target, hand and target, and eye and hand. Thus, neurons in the PMC appear to be involved in integrating limb-centered coordinates into a reaching plan based on error-related transformations, not simply translating from eye to hand coordinates.

Although the topic of frame-of-reference transformation is far from complete, it seems that the amalgamation of visual and other information takes place within regions of the parietal cortex, and this information is coded in a common frame of reference. Once translated to the PMC, this information undergoes a further frame-of-reference transformation before it is sent to the motor cortex using a frame of reference perhaps unique to the frontal lobes. What remains to be examined is the potential for modulations to occur along any part of this cortical circuitry. Might a gain effect taking place in the parietal cortex update a motor plan in M1 just before movement execution? Would this require neurons within M1 to perform subtle frame-of-reference transformations? Perhaps salient environmental features regarding the position of the eye relative to visual landmarks is passed to the parietal cortex, which translates the information into a common reference frame. This reference frame is then modulated by gain fields representing the current position of the retina and body position before being passed to the premotor cortex. Upon arrival, a movement plan from the frontal lobes is combined with the visually based coordinates and further translated into a new frame of reference.

Common Command Hypothesis

An alternative but not mutually exclusive account of the interaction between ocular and manual systems points to the idea that both systems may simply share a common denominator—efference. That is, eye–hand symbiosis occurs as a result of a common motor command (Bizzi, Kalil, & Tagliassco, 1971; Bock, 1986), only later to be tuned to the effector. Consistent with this hypothesis, electromyographic activity of both the manual and ocular systems appears nearly simultaneously (e.g., 20 ms separation; see Biguer, Jeannerod, & Prablanc, 1982; Biguer, Prablanc, & Jeannerod, 1984; Gribble, Everling, Ford, & Mattar, 2002; Turner, Owens, & Anderson, 1995). This brief advantage in initiation time for the eyes is thought to reflect the greater inertia or motor time associated with limb movements versus eye movements (Biguer et al., 1982, 1984; Binsted et al., 2001).

The spatiotemporal characteristics of eye and hand superficially seem to support the common command hypothesis; however, this does not hold on closer examination. Although both eye movements and hand movements typically undershoot the target position with a secondary corrective movement (or saccade in the case of the eyes), bringing the effector to rest on the target (Helsen et al., 2000), trial-to-trial analyses indicate little relation between the eye position and hand position at the termination of their initial movements toward the target (Binsted & Elliott, 1999b). Furthermore, although strong temporal relationships are present for RT and subsequent kinematic markers (Helsen et al., 2000), positional data suggest that eye and hand movements are unlikely planned together (see also Binsted & Elliott, 1999b; Binsted et al., 2001). Instead, temporal relationships merely occur as a function of variations of detection, volition, and attention before movement initiation.

The impracticality of common coding may be carried further by considering the physical parameters of each system. Specifically, the saccadic movements may be specified in accord with Listing's law (i.e., the eye can only reach positions that can be achieved by a single rotation around the axis lying on Listing's plane, or the frontal plane passing through the center of rotation of the eye), a feature inconsistent with the curved rotation surface regularly demonstrated in gross limb movements (>30°; Hore, Watts, & Vilis, 1992; Miller, Theeuwen, & Gielen, 1992). The eyes also display a linear relationship between saccadic amplitude and velocity that is independent of accuracy requirements. Thus, the failure to reproduce the seminal speed–accuracy trade-offs displayed in limb movements (Binsted & Elliott, 1999a) should be expected and the presence of common code is unlikely.

Afferent Information Hypothesis

A major implication of the common command position is that arm movements are planned before proper foveation of the target. In other words, the motor command initially sent to the upper limb is based on an estimation of the target location derived from peripheral retina input (Biguer et al., 1982; Gribble et al., 2002). An alternative account of this behavior is that sensory-based feedback from the moving limb supports the constituent (late) planning and control processes of action. In an attempt to dissociate eye and hand control along these lines, Binsted and Elliott (1999b) had participants make discrete aiming movements to the vertex of Müller-Lyer figures. Although the illusion robustly influenced saccades (i.e., end points), the illusion did not yield a reliable influence on the hand (see also Bernardis et al., 2005; Thompson & Westwood, 2007), a finding counter to such an afferent account of coupling. These data further indicate that, at least in terms of spatial accuracy, the eye and the hand exhibit independence, potentially due to independent movement preparation, online modulation of the hand movement during its primary trajectory, or perhaps insufficiency of ocular afference (Bock, 1993; Ehresman et al., 2008; Elliott et al., 1999; Heath et al., 2004; Prablanc, Echallier, Jeannerod, & Komilis, 1979; Prablanc, Echallier, Komilis, & Jeannerod, 1979).

Consistent with this idea is the finding that the peripheral retina provides suboptimal estimates of the target location (Bock, 1993; Prablanc, Echallier, Jeannerod, et al., 1979; Prablanc, Echallier, Komilis, et al., 1979). This inadequacy suggests that the motor command sent to the arm (common or otherwise) minimally contains an error signal proportional to the limitations of the peripheral retina. How, then, does the limb successfully attain the target, in many cases in a ballistic (and therefore presumably correction-free) manner? One possibility is that ocular afference associated with target foveation directly influences motor preparation. However, though superficially cogent, such an account is problematic. For example, as previously discussed, the limb is initiated within a few tenths of a second of saccade completion. Thus, even if precise afference (proprioceptive or otherwise) is available, insufficient time exists to utilize the input for manual program preparation, particularly when transmission time, neuromechanical delay, and even cursor processing are taken into account (Biguer et al., 1982; Desmurget et al., 2005; Desmurget, Pélisson, Rossetti, & Prablanc, 1998).

Another feedback-derived account of eye–hand coordination emphasizes the role of final eye position in determining aiming precision. As such, the end of the ocular saccade (after onset of hand movement) is used to relocate target position on the basis of foveal or perifoveal afference. Presumably, such information is used to update visual signals utilized by the manual system to adjust the ongoing hand trajectory (Desmurget & Grafton, 2000; Goodale, Pélisson, & Prablanc, 1986; Grea et al., 2002; Pélisson, Prablanc, Goodale, & Jeannerod, 1986; Prablanc & Martin, 1992; Prablanc, Pélisson, & Goodale, 1986). Anatomically, this account seems viable owing to the convergence of manual and ocular control systems in the PPC (i.e., IPL and PRR). Indeed, in a follow-up to their earlier work (Binsted & Elliott, 1999b), Binsted and colleagues (2001) examined the role of ocular proprioception of target position using illusory Müller-Lyer figures. The relationship between eye and hand was varied both temporally and directionally by staggering eye and hand start times and by having participants begin their saccade either ipsilaterally or contralaterally to the manual response. The finding that the limb was biased toward the absolute eye displacement suggests that manual end-point codes are derived from scalar saccadic amplitude. Furthermore, this transfer is necessarily time constrained—spatial yoking between systems only occurred when eye and hand movements occurred together. Thus, the kinematic features of simple, visually guided movements are influenced by nonvisual ocular feedback. Moreover, the saccadic (position) signal itself may provide critical information to guide the hand and update an ongoing action plan (Binsted et al., 2001; Enright, 1995; Flanders, Daghestani, & Berthoz, 1999; Soechting, Engel, & Flanders, 2001).

In support of this foveation hypothesis, Desmurget and colleagues (2005), among others (Binsted & Elliott 1999a, 1999b; Binsted et al., 2001; Deubel, Wolf, & Hauske, 1982; Prablanc & Jeannerod, 1975), found that goal-directed saccadic responses consist of two phases reminiscent of the two phases reported for manual aiming: an initial saccade undershooting the target by approximately 10% of required amplitude and a corrective saccade (or saccades) attaining accurate foveation. Importantly, the limb demonstrates similar undershooting bias (see Lyons, Hansen, Hurding, & Elliott, 2006, but also see Heath & Binsted, 2007). Furthermore, afference arising from the initial saccade is insufficient; anchoring the eye at the target seems to only yield tangible manual advantage when saccadic updates (i.e., direct target foveation) are available (Desmurget et al., 2005). Though partially substantiating a fixation hypothesis, it is not known why such an information source would only be used to inform aiming amplitude at the cost of directional error. In addition, if fixation coordinates were central to limb control, gaze amplitude variability (central to target location estimation) should have a concomitant effect on hand end-point variability, but this does not appear to be the case (Desmurget et al., 2005). Moreover, how is a benefit yielded from corrective target reacquisition given the already discussed systemic delays compounded by the regularly reported latency of 50 to 100 ms before stable fixation? Finally, evidence from unconstrained movements (Soechting & Lacquaniti, 1981; for a review see Desmurget et al., 1998) provides even more equivocal findings regarding fixation afference as a target source for the manual system (McIntyre, Stratta, & Lacquaniti, 1997).

One possible solution to these unbalanced and contradictory findings is predicated on the use of parafoveal target capture before completion of the primary saccade (Desmurget et al., 2005). Such a scheme skirts the delay problems associated with any requirement of final target fixation while permitting improved target acquisition owing to the previously discussed limitations of the peripheral retinal inputs. Moreover, use of parafoveal cues at this point would permit direct hand–target comparison at a time when online corrections of limb trajectory are known to occur (Heath et al., 2004; Prablanc & Martin, 1992). Consistent with this view, subliminal double-step paradigms repeatedly demonstrate corrections to the hand trajectory that precede the initiation of a corrective saccade (Desmurget et al., 2005; Prablanc & Martin, 1992; Sarlegna et al., 2003).

Strategy Hypothesis

Up to this point, we have focused on relatively mechanistic justifications for the coupling between eye and hand. Although these bases likely exist to some extent (i.e., spatial reference frame transformations must occur at some level), we would be remiss not to consider strategy (i.e., cognition) as a moderating influence. For example, Carnahan and Marteniuk (1991) showed that the synchronization between ocular and manual systems is adjusted as a function of participant instruction. When the experimenter urged accuracy, fixation was achieved well in advance of hand initiation, whereas the hand preceded the eye when speed was emphasized. In addition, the relative precision requirement of the systems are different—"for the eyes, close is good enough" (Binsted et al., 2001, p. 583)—so it would be unreasonable to expect any rigid connections between systems. Furthermore, despite the differences in spatiotemporal performances across experiments and conditions, the eye was ubiquitously in a position to provide visual, if not proprioceptive, information about the relative positions of the hand and target during limb deceleration. Thus, rather than the hand being a slave to ocular efference, or afference for that matter, the eyes appear to serve the feedback needs of the hand on a demand basis.

If we reconsider the previously presented hypotheses within a strategic framework, we might simply suggest that the eye and hand often display shared characteristics due to the sharing of common data—target and task information. For example, the temporal correlations between eye and hand (hallmarks of a common command process) are simply a convenient by-product of a strategy dictating the precise gathering of task information. Though perhaps simply coincidental or serendipitous, such an account would alleviate the corollary impairments of stereotyped function and the limitations of neural conductance. Stated another way, why would we expect two movements arising from the same visual input to not bear strong resemblance to one another (even if they share common neural substrates)?

If we continue to examine the anatomy of the system, once again we see that the parietal cortices serve the function of target extraction for both eye and hand. However, instead of relying on this juxtaposition, the addition of executive strategy (via circuitous connections to the DLPFC) allows context-dependent modulation of both saccades and reaches concurrently (i.e., flexibility). These secondary connections may also permit the involvement of structures within ventral visual pathways, accounting for the relative efficacy of perception on tasks requiring concurrent eye and hand movements (Bernardis et al., 2005; Binsted & Elliott, 1999b; Binsted et al., 2001; Thompson & Westwood, 2007).

Finally, taking a cognitive view to the spatial representation hypotheses, the proposed eye-centered transformations simply become a means to an end: It is easiest to get both the limb and the eye to the same place if they are prepared using common information. Eye and hand motor sequences may be based on a common source (i.e., PPC), but the subsequent anatomical differences associated with execution conceivably influence how environmental information is stored and used (Rolheiser, Binsted, & Brownell, 2006). Thus the role of fixation-derived afference is one of opportunity: When concurrent information is available, it is used; however, if information is too slow, it's irrelevant and ignored.

Conclusions: Close Is Good Enough

The goal of the hand is to hit the target; for the eye, simply being within a degree or two is sufficient (Binsted & Elliott, 1999a; Binsted et al., 2001). The eyes need only to get close enough to the target to supply an estimate of motor error—the relative positions of the hand and object (Binsted et al., 2001; Johansson, Westling, Bäckström, & Flanagan, 2001; Regan & Gray, 2001; Steinman et al., 2003). This general principle is evidenced by the goal-driven, yet plastic, coordination between eye and hand; amplitude signals are used when available, and foveation optimizes but is not critical for the evocation of an accurate limb response. Thus, instead of considering the hand as coupled or yoked to the eye, the eye is better conceived as the subordinate. The eyes lead the way, serving up a volley of visual (or nonvisual ocular) information critical to the hand while also providing a common language (i.e., frame of reference) specific to the movement goal. This performance optimizes the efficacy of the provided afference, regardless of whether the tuning occurs through anatomical necessity or executive machinations.

This perspective, though simple, also aids in understanding the neural substrates that map spatial vision onto overt goal-directed behaviors. Although the neural mechanisms underlying eye–hand coordination are intricate, the brain must perform certain tasks in order to successfully complete a precise goal-directed hand movement. The target must be acquired from the visual scene, both by recognizing it as such and determining its physical parameters. This step is common to both systems, and so are the constituent cortical processing centers. The visual system must then make this information available in a manner that is accessible and useful to the motor system (i.e., eye-centered coordinates in the PPC). Finally, the eye must actively seek additional information due to inadequacies in peripheral retinal acuity. This information is provided in forms such as corollary copy, proprioception, parafoveal or foveal localization, and, of course, direct hand–target comparison.

Future Directions

Investigations into eye–hand coordination have recently taken full advantage of modern techniques such as TMS and fMRI while retaining a strong association with classic behavioral neuroscience. What is needed now is a concerted attempt to integrate the eye–hand behavior and anatomy into the extant knowledge of allied systems to address questions of function in a larger way. Although it's reasonable to make blanket statements regarding yoking and close being good enough, relationships to broader concepts of locomotion and memory, as well as understanding with regard to disease and development, are required.

Thus, although the present discussion provided a framework for understanding the state of knowledge regarding oculomanual coordination, it is difficult not to pose a few questions. How does this system work when the target is no longer present (i.e., during memory-guided action; see chapter 5)? Such a system of communal information usage would be beneficial in situations involving reduced or decayed cues. Similarly, much of the extant literature regarding the online control of movement relies heavily on concepts of feed-forward control (i.e., predicting the outcome of motor commands). How are the internal models for this task integrated into the complex eye–hand circuit? Given the somewhat reconceptualized manner in which the premotor cortex has been reported to encode a movement plan (i.e., error derived), what does this mean for the projections from the premotor cortex (PMC), such as to the primary motor cortex (see Schieber, 2001)? The functions of the reciprocal connections among the supplementary motor, premotor, and primary motor cortices with basal ganglia are also worth revision (Romanelli, Esposito, Schaal, & Heit, 2005). Might all these areas be using the equivalent of a frontal frame of reference? How does the error-derived nature of this coordinate system relate to the goal-achievement role of basal ganglia?

CHAPTER 11

Eye–Hand Coordination in Goal-Directed Action: Normal and Pathological Functioning

WERNER F. HELSEN, PETER FEYS,
ELKE HEREMANS, AND ANN LAVRYSEN

M oving an arm to contact a target is a skill used daily in tasks such as turning on the light, opening a door, or picking up a glass of wine. In addition, we often have to make series of movements that vary in spatiotemporal difficulty, such as dialing a number on a telephone, using a calculator, or entering a security code in a bank terminal. The apparent simplicity of these movements belies the underlying complexity involved in the temporal organization and spatial control of the eye–head–hand system.

A great deal of research has already examined the visual control of upper-limb movements (Proteau & Elliott, 1992). However, because of technological limitations, former studies on the visual control of upper-limb movements were based on performance measures (e.g., reaction time, movement time) and kinematic variables reflecting changes in the limb movement (e.g., primary velocity and acceleration profile, discontinuities in acceleration), without examining eye movements. In 1996, the Motor Behaviour lab of McMaster University in Canada and the Perception and Performance Lab of K.U. Leuven in Belgium were some of the first labs to use synchronous measurements and high-speed sampling of temporal and spatial features of both eye movements and limb movements to examine speeded aiming with multiple degrees of freedom (e.g., Helsen, Starkes, & Buekers, 1997; Helsen, Starkes, Elliott, & Ricker, 1998b). These experiments offered a unique opportunity to study the natural coupling between eye movements and limb movements and to challenge recent models of speed–accuracy relationships in limb control (see Elliott, Helsen, & Chua, 2001). The goal of the present chapter is to highlight the role of visual afference in manual goal-directed movements in normal and pathological functioning.

Retinal Versus Extraretinal Information

When inspecting the outside world, our eyes rapidly travel from one location to the other to gather relevant information for efficient interaction with the world. The main intention of these rapid eye movements, or saccades, is to bring point of gaze (PG), or the spot where the eyes focus, to relevant environmental features. During these fixations, the PG is stably focused on a specific point of the outside world. The eyes are oriented so that the object of interest is projected onto the most sensitive part of the retina. This important spot is called the *fovea*. It is a limited area of only 1° that guarantees the highest possible visual acuity. Around the fovea, peripheral vision provides less detailed information of the surroundings. Retinal visual information is the primary source of information guiding goal-directed movements. In addition, there are several extraretinal visual signals that can be used in the planning and updating of goal-directed movements. These signals arise from the saccades made from one point to the other. They include afferent information from the muscles orienting the eyes and from the oculomotor efferent commands.

Both before and during limb movements, visual afference is processed and used in the planning, updating, and correction of the ongoing movement. In this chapter, we review methodological strategies for studying the role of vision in the planning and control of goal-directed movements. First, we discuss various outcome parameters, such as reaction time (i.e., the time between stimulus presentation and movement onset), movement time (i.e, the time to travel from the initial home position to the target position), and total response time (i.e., the sum of reaction and movement time). The relative time associated with each of these movement components indicates the time spent on movement planning versus online control. Second, we examine kinematic variables in single and repetitive aiming movements. These kinematic variables, such as peak acceleration, peak velocity, and time to peak velocity, provide insight into the typical characteristics of online movement regulation. Specifically, in the absence of visual feedback, the limb movements typically have a bell-shaped velocity profile, suggesting that no adaptations are made online. Alternatively, more time is spent during the movement for updates and corrections when there is opportunity for visual feedback processing (Elliott, Binsted, & Heath, 1999). This results in a skewed velocity profile that is characterized by a relatively greater amount of time spent after peak velocity. Third, we examine the parameters of eye movement to provide additional insight into the processes underlying the interactions between eye movements and hand movements (see Starkes, Helsen, & Elliott, 2002, for a review). Fourth, we present the results of functional imaging of brain regions involved in eye–hand coordination. Finally, we discuss the potential use of eye movements as a mirror of our thoughts in the context of motor imagery. The first part of this chapter focuses on normal functioning, and the second part is dedicated to the study of eye–hand coordination in pathological functioning.

Visuomotor Control in Normal Functioning

In a first experiment, Helsen and colleagues (1997) addressed the coordination between PG and hand movements in a speeded aiming task to predictable targets of three eccentricities (35, 40, and 45 cm). In each condition subjects moved the eyes, head, trunk, and hand freely (see figure 11.1).

Analyses were conducted for the frequencies for initiation order of PG and the hand, the correlation between initiation latencies of PG and the

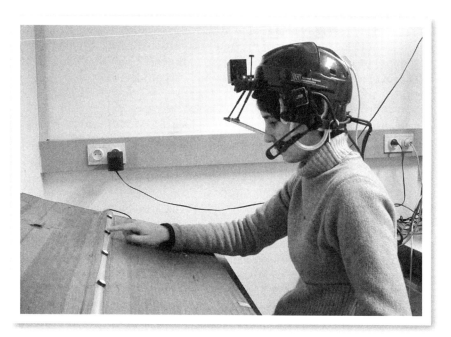

▶ **Figure 11.1**   Experimental setup of a discrete aiming task in which a participant moves as quickly as possible from the home button (in front of the participant) to one or two target buttons. Movement is made in response to a visual stimulus. The participant is wearing a head-mounted gaze tracker ASL-4100.

hand, and initiation, movement, and response times of PG and the hand. Regardless of the distance to be covered, there was a remarkable temporal relationship between the arrival of the eye and the arrival of the limb on the target. Specifically, PG always arrived on the target area first and at roughly 50% of the hand response time. Varying eccentricity increased reaction time of PG but not of the hand. Though hand response time varied by as much as 100 ms, an invariant feature was found for the proportional arrival time across conditions. Both PG and hand movements were fixed with regard to movement end point, and optimization of proportional time across conditions resulted from independent alteration of the individual component effectors.

Regarding the functional importance of proportional time in the visual control of voluntary movements, Helsen and colleagues (1997) speculated that, by PG arriving on the target area first and at roughly 50% of the hand response time, there would be ample opportunity for the eye to provide extraretinal information on the position of the target either through oculomotor efference or proprioceptive feedback resulting from the large primary saccade. In the remaining time before the arrival of the hand, this could readily be combined with ongoing visual and proprioceptive information about the limb position. Given the preponderance of aiming models that propose a dual submovement structure (for a review, see Elliott, 1992), proportional time may be a good way of making the best use of information provided by PG as a result of the first primarily ballistic submovement. In a somewhat similar way, invariant termination of PG and limb movements has also been reported by Carnahan and Marteniuk (1991).

Spatiotemporal Characteristics of Eye Movements and Limb Kinematics During Single Aiming Movements

To further examine the meaning of the invariant relationship between the arrival of the eyes and the arrival of the limb on the target position, Helsen, Elliott, Starkes, and Ricker (1998a) investigated the temporal and spatial coordination of both PG and hand kinematics in a speeded aiming task to an eccentrically positioned visual target. On the majority of trials, PG showed a pattern of a large initial saccade that slightly undershot the target followed by one or more smaller corrective saccades used to reach the target. The hand exhibited a similar pattern of first undershooting the target and then making small corrective movements. As in the work by Helsen and colleagues (1997), an invariant feature was found for the ratio of PG and hand response time (50%). In line with these results, a striking temporal coupling was found between completion of the primary eye saccade and time to peak acceleration for the limb. Spatially, peak hand velocity coincided with completion of 50% of total movement distance. Thus, during the latter portion of the hand movement, the eye is already over the target area and is well placed to provide visual information regarding

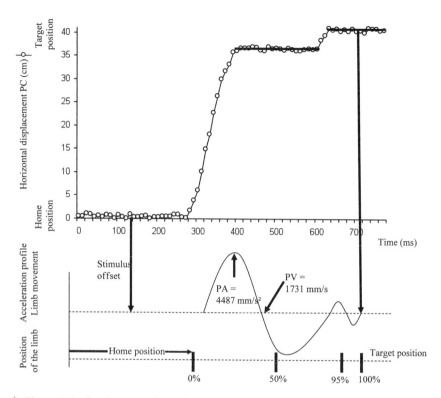

▶ **Figure 11.2**   Spatiotemporal coordination between PG and hand movements. The arrival of the saccade is linked closely to the kinematics of the hand movement.

Adapted, by permission, from W. F. Helsen, et al., 1998a, "Temporal and spatial coupling of point of gaze and hand movements in aiming," *Journal of Motor Behavior* 30: 249-259.

the relative positions of both the hand and the target for closed-loop limb control (see figure 11.2).

In a follow-up study, Helsen, Elliott, Starkes, and Ricker (2000) examined the temporospatial coupling of PG and movements of the finger, elbow, and shoulder during a similar speeded aiming task. On the majority of trials, a large initial saccade slightly undershot the target, and one or more smaller corrective saccades brought the eyes to the target position. The finger, elbow, and shoulder exhibited a similar pattern of undershooting their final position and then making small corrective movements. Eye movements usually preceded limb movements, and the eyes always arrived at the target well in advance of the finger. Again, there was a clear temporal coupling between primary saccade completion and peak acceleration of the finger, elbow, and shoulder. The movement of the limb segment was usually initiated in a proximal-to-distal pattern. Increased variability in elbow and shoulder position as the movement progressed clearly reduced variability in finger position.

Spatiotemporal Characteristics of Eye Movements and Limb Kinematics During Repetitive Aiming Movements

In addition to executing single aiming movements, humans often have to make series of movements that vary in spatiotemporal difficulty, such as using a calculator or entering a security code in a bank terminal. To examine how eye–hand coordination in three-dimensional single movements is different from repetitive one-dimensional aiming movements, we used a paradigm in which participants wore an orthotic on the preferred limb. The orthotic was aligned to the anatomical axis of the wrist joint (Lavrysen, Elliott, Buekers, Feys, & Helsen, 2007) and was built in such a way that it restricted wrist movements to flexion and extension. Wrist angular position was registered by means of nonferromagnetic, high-precision shaft encoders fixed on the movement axis of the orthotic. The orthotic was also designed for future use in an fMRI environment (see figure 11.3).

Participants performed a unimanual wrist flexion–extension aiming task. They were seated in a comfortable armchair with their forearms resting in supports so that their hand movements were made in the horizontal plane only. A cardboard panel prevented direct vision of the forearm. Wrist angular position was presented as a cursor of 10 mm diameter on a 43 cm monitor that was located 50 cm in front of the participants. Flexion of the right hand resulted in a displacement of the cursor to the left. Consequently, extension of the right hand resulted in movements of the cursor to the right. The required wrist angle of 40° corresponded with 200 mm cursor

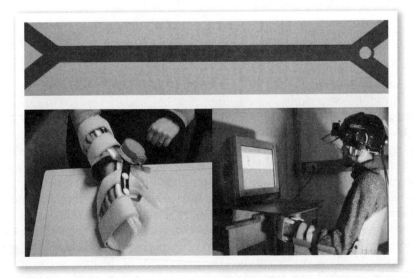

▶ **Figure 11.3** Right-hand orthotic with shaft encoder allowing only flexion and extension movements at the wrist and presenting both visual stimuli and hand representation (movement feedback) on a monitor.

displacement on the screen. Thus, the visual angle to cover the distance was approximately 20°. To facilitate the comparison of wrist and eye positions, the angle corresponding to this distance was normalized to 40° for both effectors. The participants were asked to align the cursor to the left and right end of the line at the rhythm of a metronome.

In this repetitive or cyclical aiming task, saccades were initiated only after the hand had already left the target (see figure 11.4). This reversed initiation pattern as compared with discrete aiming is probably related to the specific task demands. The subsequent saccade was postponed to provide stable visual target information to the ongoing hand movement (gaze anchoring; see Neggers & Bekkering, 2000). Of greater interest was the termination of PG, which always concluded before the hand reached peak velocity (similar to findings by Helsen et al., 1998a, 2000, who used a discrete aiming paradigm). This temporal aspect of eye–hand coordination in a cyclical aiming task has been shown to be consistent and independent of afferent perturbations induced by visual illusions (Lavrysen et al., 2006).

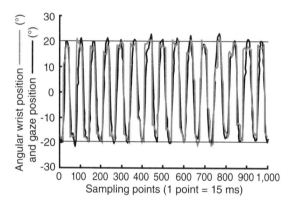

▶ **Figure 11.4** Sample trial for one subject aiming to a pointing-in figure in a saccade cursor condition. The dotted lines depict angular position, while the dashed lines depict PG.

The only factor influencing the timing pattern was the functional disparity between hand and hemisphere systems (see chapter 12 and Buekers & Helsen, 2000; Helsen, Starkes, Elliott, & Buekers, 1998; Lavrysen et al., 2007; Mieschke, Elliott, Helsen, Carson, & Coull, 2001). Specifically, in a group of strongly lateralized right-handers, the execution of fast, continuous wrist flexion–extension movements differed according to the hand used to perform the task (Lavrysen et al., 2007). Not surprisingly, the preferred hand enjoyed advantages in some aspects of movement execution, such as more consistency in MT. More interestingly, peak velocity of the hand and onset of eye fixation both occurred earlier when participants were using the left hand versus the right hand. Surprisingly, strong left-handers exhibited the same pattern of performance (Lavrysen et al., 2007). Thus, the mode of control was different when using the left or the right hand, independent of hand preference. Perhaps the need for more online guidance when using the left hand creates a need for earlier saccade completion. In this way, visual afference is available earlier in the movement so that enough time is available to process visual information and use it to guide the movement.

Neural Architecture

In addition to the examination of behavioral and kinematic eye and limb parameters, in more recent years we have attempted to bridge the gap between the behavioral sciences and the neurosciences. In this context, fMRI is a technique that allows us to use MRI to visualize underlying neural substrates of movement. During scanning, participants are subjected to a strong, homogeneous magnetic field (the MR magnet, conventionally 1.5 or 3 T) that induces an alignment of atomic nuclei—in particular the proton nuclei of hydrogen atoms—parallel with this field. Application of a radiofrequency (RF) pulse changes the alignment of the proton magnetic moments from being parallel with the static magnetic field. The excited protons recover their original alignment within a time called *relaxation time*, and the created magnetization effect induces an exponentially decaying radio signal that can be detected and reconstructed in an image (see Huettel, Song, & McCarthy, 2004).

Functional MRI makes use of the transverse relaxation time (T2), which is especially associated with local field inhomogeneities due to susceptibility differences of tissues or specific particles (e.g., oxyhemoglobin and deoxyhemoglobin). A sensory, motor, or cognitive task produces a localized increase in neural activity. This results in a local vasodilatation followed by a temporary increase of blood flow to compensate for the increased local metabolic demands due to oxygen and glucose consumption. The relative amount of oxygenated and deoxygenated hemoglobin produces relative differences in magnetic properties that can be detected during scanning. This signal is called the *blood oxygen level dependent* (BOLD) contrast. In the present research, the Philips Intera Achieva 3.0 T scanner at the University Hospital of Gasthuisberg (Leuven, Belgium) was used to visualize the brain areas involved in eye–hand coordination. Given the asymmetric visuomotor control strategy that participants adopted in previous work (e.g., Lavrysen et al., 2007), it was hypothesized that the brain processes underlying the movements with the left and right hand might be different. In this context, Lavrysen and colleagues (2008) conducted an fMRI experiment in which right-handed participants performed movements with their right or left hand in isolation or coordinated with saccades (see figure 11.5).

The results showed that there were similarities but also differences between brain areas involved in the specific eye–hand coordination condi-

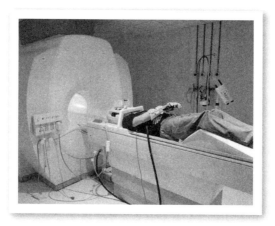

▶ **Figure 11.5** Experimental setup of the cyclical aiming task in the MR scanner of the University Hospital of Gasthuisberg.

tions. The cyclical aiming task was used in an fMRI environment, enabling integrated data recording of eye and hand movements with cerebral activation patterns. The areas involved in eye–hand coordination, inferred by contrasting the coordinated conditions with the isolated eye and hand conditions, revealed a network involving the cerebellum as well as cortical and subcortical structures. Interestingly, for eye–hand coordination using the left hand compared with coordination using the right hand, there were significantly higher activated areas in the ipsilateral cerebellar lobule, the thalamus, and the parietal cortex. Because these areas are all involved with online guidance and feedback processing of movement, the functional activation differences might be related to the differences in specializations of the hands. Using the left hand might engage more regions in order to compensate for greater variability in force production or for the increased demands for coordinated versus independent control of eye and limb movement. Alternatively, the results could simply reflect a difference between the dominant right hand and nondominant left hand of right-handers.

To substantiate that the observed differences were due to a difference in functional specialization between both hand and hemisphere systems and not to hand preference per se, the next step was to evaluate the same patterns in left-handers. Therefore, another study was conducted under identical conditions with 11 extremely left-handed participants (Lavrysen, 2005). First, the behavioral data revealed that the time to peak velocity was earlier when aiming with the left hand (48.9%) than it was when aiming with the right hand (60.3%). Because this was also the case with right-handers (Lavrysen et al., 2008), it appears that the mode of control is different when using the left hand or the right hand. This difference is independent of hand preference. However, eye–hand coordination did not change with the hand used.

When evaluating the functional imaging data (Lavrysen, 2005), again, asymmetries were observed that are consistent with what was described in the right-handed group in Lavrysen and colleagues (2008). The results of the contrast between coordinated and isolated movement conditions are presented in figure 11.6 for both left-handers and right-handers. A remarkable parallel can be drawn between the activated loci for eye–hand coordination using the right hand (two upper panels) or left hand (two lower panels). When using the left hand, activation is more pronounced in ipsilateral cerebellar and contralateral sensorimotor areas, whereas using the right hand produces more bilateral occipital activation.

Visual inspection of these data indicates that the activated network for eye–hand coordination is different according to the hand used. However, a statistical comparison revealed no significant differences between both coordination modes for the left-handers. This suggests that in this group,

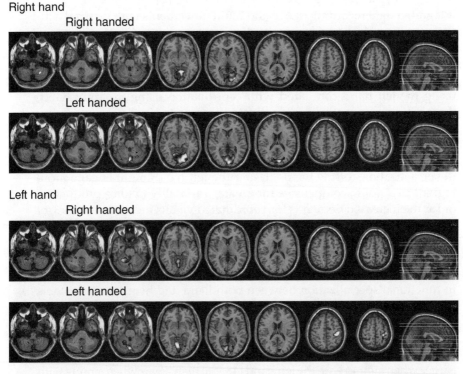

Right hand
    Right handed

    Left handed

Left hand
    Right handed

    Left handed

▶ **Figure 11.6** Group statistical parametric maps (SPMs) for coordinated versus isolated eye and hand movements for the right and left hands of right- and left-handers. The SPMs (thresholded at $z = 4.15$) are displayed on horizontal slices (z-value from left to right: –46, –36, –27, –9, 0, 19, 53, and 63). The right side of the scans corresponds to the right side of the brain.

similar regions are allocated for the coordination of the left and right hand with the accompanying eye movements. This finding suggests that in comparison with right-handers, left-handers do not benefit from the right hand–left hemisphere advantages to the same degree because of lack of practice with this hand. Alternatively, it could be that left-handers already engage more areas with their preferred hand so that it reaches the same level of activation of the less-practiced nonpreferred hand. A third possibility is that left-handers are not a homogeneous group and that between-person variability makes it difficult for any consistent pattern of activation to emerge.

Eye Movements as a Mirror of Our Thoughts: Motor Imagery

Motor imagery can be defined as the mental rehearsal of a motor act in the absence of an overt motor output (Crammond, 1997). It can be performed in different modalities, such as visual, auditory, tactile, kinesthetic, olfactory, gustatory, or any combination of these senses. The visual modality, which is the most well known, can be described as imagining seeing yourself performing the task. This technique, also known as *visualization,* has been used for many years by athletes to improve their performance (Murphy, 1994). Recent studies suggest that mental training based on motor imagery can also be valuable in the training of musicians (Meister et al., 2004), highly skilled manual technicians such as surgeons (Rogers, 2006), and even in the rehabilitation of patients with neurological disorders (Jackson, Lafleur, Malouin, Richards, & Doyon, 2001). As such, motor imagery represents an intriguing additional practice method that can be used in various domains to increase the amount of training without adding to the physical demands. Additionally, it can serve as an alternative practice strategy for people who are (temporally) unable to execute movements physically due to injury, illness, immobilization, or paralysis (see the later sections of this chapter).

When studying these new applications, it is necessary to monitor whether participants are performing the imagery tasks correctly. People may be unable to accurately imagine the required movement in the temporospatial domain and so they use alternative strategies or even fail to suppress muscular activity during imagery (Sharma, Pomeroy, & Baron, 2006). Methods traditionally used to assess the performance of motor imagery are questionnaires, interviews, and mental chronometry. Unfortunately, these methods have the disadvantage of being subjective. In addition, they focus mainly on the global movement instead of offering a detailed monitoring of the ongoing mental process.

Therefore, in a recent study (Heremans, Helsen, & Feys, 2008), we aimed to develop an alternative approach, based on the technique of eye movement registration, to objectively measure and monitor motor imagery processes. This approach was based on two lines of evidence. First, it has been shown that there is a tight temporospatial coupling between eye movements and hand movements during goal-directed single aiming (Helsen et al., 1998a,

2000) and repetitive aiming (Lavrysen et al., 2006). Second, recent studies within the field of imagery research have found that eye movements reflect the content of the imagined stimulus during the imagery of auditory scenes, recently viewed pictures, and moving stimuli (De'Sperati, 2003). Heremans and colleagues (Heremans, Helsen, & Feys, 2008) investigated whether the latter findings can be generalized to the imagery of our own body movements and, more specifically, to goal-directed movements of the arm and hand. Eye movements of right-handed subjects were recorded using electro-oculography (EOG) during both physical execution and visual motor imagery of a cyclical aiming task (identical to the one described earlier) performed at three intertarget distances. We found that 89% of the subjects made task-related eye movements during imagery with the eyes open, and 84% of participants did so during imagery with the eyes closed. Both the number and amplitude of the eye movements during imagery closely resembled those of the eye movements made during physical execution of the task (see figure 11.7).

Given these findings, we suggested that both the motor and visual components of the movement are reenacted during motor imagery of the task, implying that the coupling between eye movements and hand movements remains intact even when hand movements are merely imagined as opposed to being physically executed. We hypothesized that the observed eye movements during imagery are not merely epiphenomenal but instead help participants to correctly position the imagined hand movements within the mental space. This implies that an internal visual representation exists

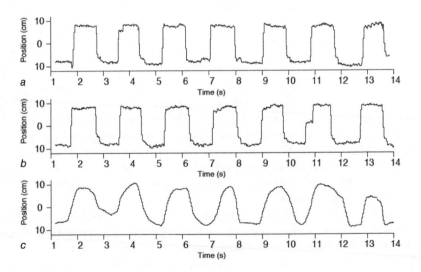

▶ **Figure 11.7** Typical eye movement patterns during (a) physical execution, (b) motor imagery with the eyes open, and (c) motor imagery with the eyes closed.

that is treated similarly to the external world. This interpretation, however, remains speculative and is now being investigated in more detail.

In summary, our observations (Heremans, Helsen, & Feys, 2008) have demonstrated that eye movements provide a unique window into the mind during motor imagery of goal-directed wrist movements. As such, recordings of eye movement can be considered an objective complementary technique to evaluate compliance and imagery ability for the majority of normal subjects.

Summary of Visuomotor Control in Normal Functioning

An integrative methodology linking behavioral, kinematic, and brain imaging techniques provides a unique opportunity to study the natural coupling between eye movements and limb movements. This approach also allows us to update the current models of speed–accuracy relationships in limb control. Our findings are consistent with a two-component model of rapid, goal-directed limb movements (see chapter 1). This model of manual aiming holds that the first portion of an aiming movement is controlled by a centrally prepared set of motor commands that provide the initial accelerative, and perhaps decelerative, impulse that moves the limb into the vicinity of the target. This ballistic portion of the movement typically undershoots the target position, and a second, visually directed phase of the movement brings the limb onto the target. Presumably this second phase is designed to correct any error associated with the initial movement impulse.

Our accomplishments in this regard over the past decade can be summarized as follows:

Regardless of the distance to be covered, there is a remarkable temporal relationship between the arrival of the eye and the arrival of the limb on the target position. Because PG always arrives on the target area first and at roughly 50% of the hand response time, there is ample opportunity for the eye to provide retinal and extraretinal information on target position either through oculomotor efference or visual and proprioceptive feedback resulting from the large primary saccade.

There seems to be an invariant relationship between the spatiotemporal characteristics of eye movements and limb kinematics in goal-directed movement that is optimal for the pickup of visual feedback. Specifically, the end of a saccade toward a target corresponds temporally to the peak acceleration of the hand. Spatially, peak velocity of the hand coincides with 50% of the total movement distance. Thus, during the latter portion of the hand movement, the eye is already over the target area and is well placed to provide visual information regarding the relative positions of both the hand and the target for closed-loop limb control. Along the same lines, a significant relationship has been found between the number of secondary corrective eye movements and finger movements, both temporally and spatially.

In terms of manual asymmetries, a right-hand advantage was found for movement execution and a left-hand advantage was found for movement initiation. Evidence has suggested that right-hand advantages for movement execution can be attributed to the propensity of the left hemisphere for using response-produced feedback during the homing-in phase.

An initial temporal improvement and a decreased variability of response has been found within the first 10 trials of practice. In addition, the arrival of PG on the target is optimized toward 50% of hand response time. This temporal invariant related to end position can also be demonstrated through secondary analyses of earlier data from, for example, Vercher, Magenes, Prablanc, and Gauthier (1994).

Cerebral activation patterns underlying eye–hand coordination might reflect the asymmetries in information processing capacities of the left and right hand independent of hand preference. Finally, the natural coupling between eye movements and hand movements remains intact even when hand movements are merely imagined as opposed to being physically executed.

Visuomotor Control in Cerebellar Pathology

Eye–hand coordination in healthy subjects is, as described in the previous section, characterized by a precise temporospatial coupling that enables accurate execution of goal-directed movements. The temporospatial coupling is adapted to both environmental conditions and limb characteristics (Helsen et al., 2000). The temporal coupling between saccadic and ballistic hand movements is adapted to the type and amount of visual information that is available during movement execution (Lavrysen et al., 2006), regardless of whether the right or left hand is being used (Lavrysen et al., 2008). This underlines the extent to which the neural networks are involved in programming coordinated movements of the eye and hand.

This section focuses on visuomotor control in patients with neurological deficits. In this regard, the cerebellar system is of particular interest because it is involved in the control of eye and hand movements performed separately and in coordination. This was clearly shown by an fMRI study in which there was a greater activation during coordinated eye–hand tracking compared with independent motor activity of both systems (Feys, Maes, et al., 2005; Miall, Reckess, & Imamizu, 2001). Furthermore, the cerebellum is highly involved in the acquisition of novel coordinated eye–hand movement tasks (Miall & Jenkinson, 2005). We first address eye and hand movement deficits in patients with cerebellar dysfunction and then discuss pathological eye–hand interactions during visually guided arm movements. Next, we present a potential mechanism that may explain the increased reliance on visual feedback for accurate motor performance. In this respect, the particular interplay between proprioceptive and visual motor control is of major importance. Finally, we explore the potential use of eye movements in the study of motor imagery in pathological functioning.

Deficits in Eye and Hand Movement in Cerebellar Pathology

Movements of patients with cerebellar pathology are typically characterized by ataxia. Ataxia, or atypical chaos in movement, has multiple characteristics, such as increased RT, delayed antagonist function, prolonged MT, abnormally curved paths, overshooting and undershooting (dysmetria), and tremor (Diener & Dichgans, 1992; Sailer, Eggert, & Straube, 2005). The timing of the activation of muscles involved in movement is a crucial parameter regulated by the cerebellum. The delayed onset of antagonist activity leads to insufficient breaking of the ballistic movement and movement overshoots (Bastian & Thach, 1995; Hore, Wild, & Diener, 1991). Hypermetria resulting in target overshooting is also a common finding in patients with cerebellar deficits and in patients with multiple sclerosis (MS) with tremor (Deuschl, Wenzelburger, Loffler, Raethjen, & Stolze, 2000; Quintern et al., 1999; Topka, Konczak, & Dichgans, 1998). The previously described ataxic features are found in patients with miscellaneous cerebellar deficits with and without the additional presence of tremor (Bonnefoi-Kyriacou, Legallet, Lee, & Trouche, 1998; Day, Thompson, Harding, & Marsden, 1998; Rand, Shimansky, Stelmach, Bracha, & Bloedel, 2000; Topka et al., 1998).

Cerebellar ataxia in general, and tremor in particular, is also observed in people with MS because MS is a chronic progressive disease of the central nervous system characterized by heterogeneous patterns of inflammation, demyelination, and axonal loss. Depending on the location of lesions and atrophy within the brain, MS may occur with a variation of motor symptoms such as muscle weakness, spasticity, and incoordination, leading to severe limitations of activities of daily life (ADL). Limb tremor is estimated to be clinically present in 25% to 50% of patients with MS and is strongly related to impairment and disability (Alusi, Worthington, Glickman, & Bain, 2001; Pittock, McClelland, Mayr, Rodriguez, & Matsumoto, 2004). Tremor in MS is not seen during rest but typically emerges when limb posture is maintained against gravity (postural tremor). In particular, patients experiencing tremor due to MS may also show an increased amplitude toward the termination of visually guided goal-directed movements. This is called *intention tremor* or *cerebellar tremor* (Deuschl, Raethjen, Lindemann, & Krack, 2001).

MS tremor has been associated with disruptions of the cerebellar afferent and efferent pathways such as the cerebello-rubro-thalamocortical tract (Deuschl, Bain, & Brin, 1998). In support of this view, Liu, Ingram, Palace, and Miall (1999) linked the action tremor in a patient with MS with multiple focal lesions in the ipsilateral cerebellar hemisphere, the cerebellar peduncles, the reticular formation, and the inferior olive. An MRI study by Feys, Helsen, Beukers et al. (2006) also demonstrated that the amplitude of intention tremor, measured during the performance of a visually guided goal-directed task, was significantly related to the infratentorial lesion load (i.e., volume of lesions in the brain stem and cerebellum). More specifically, the results of this study demonstrated that MS tremor amplitude correlated with the lesion load in the contralateral pons, and patients with more severe tremor in both arms had a greater lesion load bilaterally in the pons.

About one-third of patients with MS also clinically demonstrate abnormal eye movements such as gaze-evoked nystagmus, saccadic overshooting (hypermetria), fixation instability, and impaired smooth pursuit (Armstrong, 1999; Averbuch-Heller, 2001; Clanet & Brassat, 2000; Eggenberger, 1996). Abnormal eye movements are also related to damage of the brain stem or cerebellum (Bogousslavsky et al.,1986; Downey et al., 2002; Eggenberger, 1996; Serra, Derwenskus, Downey, & Leigh, 2003).

The cerebellum plays an important role in fine-tuning eye movements and eye fixations by means of projections to the brain stem nuclei formation (Averbuch-Heller, 2001; Versino, Hurko, & Zee, 1996). Many abnormalities in eye movement appear immediately after a cerebellar insult and after experimentally induced blocks (Versino et al., 1996). Oculomotor abnormalities such as acquired pendular nystagmus and saccadic intrusions, which occur frequently in MS, interfere with steady fixations on a target. Pendular nystagmus, related to multiple lesions disrupting connections among dentate, inferior olive, and red nuclei (Armstrong, 1999; Lopez, Bronstein, Gresty, Du Boulay, & Rudge, 1996), reflects abnormalities of internal feedback circuits such as the reciprocal connections between brain stem nuclei and the cerebellum (Averbuch-Heller & Leigh, 1996). Saccadic intrusions are involuntary, abnormal, quick eye movements with or without intervals. Macrosaccadic oscillations in cerebellar patients may reflect saccadic dysmetria with continuous overshooting of targets (Averbuch-Heller, 2001). Patients with Friedreich's ataxia show various combinations of cerebellar, vestibular, and brain stem ocular signs, including fixation instability. It appears that both intention tremor and oculomotor incoordination are associated with dysfunction of the cerebellum or its afferent and efferent connected structures (Alusi, Glickman, Aziz, & Bain, 1999; Averbuch-Heller, 2001; Eggenberger, 1996; Versino et al., 1996).

From a clinical point of view, abnormal eye movements such as multiple saccades and saccadic dysmetria are common in patients with limb ataxia (Eggenberger, 1996; Sailer et al., 2005; Serra et al., 2003). Through synchronous measurements of eye movements and limb movements, researchers have investigated the occurrence of deficits in eye movements during the execution of hand movements. The first studies in patients with cerebellar deficits were conducted by Brown, Kessler, Hefter, Cooke, and Freund (1993) and van Donkelaar and Lee (1994). These researchers showed that during tracking tasks, both the eye and the hand movements were characterized by a delayed onset as well as significant inaccuracies that resulted in a series of corrective saccades or submovements needed to achieve the appropriate position. Given these studies, the authors suggested a reciprocal exchange of information between eye movements and hand movements. A candidate for this integration process is the cerebellum and its connected structures, since these receive input from both eye and hand motor commands and, as such, either directly or indirectly influence the efferent commands of both systems (van Donkelaar & Lee, 1994). In a finding supporting this hypothesis, deficits in eye movements such as saccadic dysmetria were observed in more than 75% of patients with MS who were selected based on the presence of cerebellar tremor (Feys, Helsen, Lavrysen, Nuttin, & Ketelaer, 2003). In addition to the study of eye–hand coordination in healthy subjects, extensive research on eye–hand coordination in patients with cerebellar eye and hand deficits related to MS is relevant to better understanding the interactions between eye and hand movements.

Eye–Hand Coordination and Interactions in Cerebellar Pathology

Cerebellar dysfunction has often served as a pathological model for studying visuomotor control in eye–hand coordination (Day et al., 1998; Sailer et al., 2005; van Donkelaar & Lee, 1994). MS intention tremor can also serve as a pathological model for investigating eye–hand coordination during visuomotor control. This approach was supported by the following observations.

▶ The severity of intention tremor in the arm correlates with the lesion load in the infratentorial brain (Feys, Maes et al., 2005; Liu et al., 1999; Nakashima, Fujihara, Okita, Takase, & Itoyama, 1999).

▶ The infratentorial brain controls oculomotor function. Therefore, it is not surprising that oculomotor deficits such as saccadic dysmetria and unsteady gaze fixation are present in patients with MS tremor (Feys, Helsen, Lavrysen, et al., 2003; Feys, Helsen, et al., 2005; Nakashima et al., 1999).

▶ Patients with MS tremor are more dependent on visual feedback of their performance for the online control of hand movements, as discussed later (Feys, Helsen, Liu, et al., 2003; Liu et al., 1997). This is probably a result of their reduced capacity for predictive control, which may be associated with the cerebellar system (Miall, Weir, Wolpert, & Stein, 1993).

Studies of patients with MS and arm intention tremor demonstrated abnormal eye movements during discrete goal-directed hand movements (Feys, Helsen, Lavrysen, et al., 2003; Feys, Helsen, et al., 2005). The amplitude and speed of the primary saccades were enlarged (saccadic dysmetria) and prolonged, and the ballistic hand movement was also characterized by target overshoot and slower execution. However, the temporal coupling between the primary saccadic and hand movements was largely preserved during the performance of a wrist step-tracking task. As in healthy subjects, eye and hand reaction times were highly related, and the saccadic completion time corresponded with peak velocity of the hand. The latter relationship indicated that patients' hand initiation and antagonist muscle activity were also delayed during the discrete goal-directed tasks since saccades were prolonged (Feys, Helsen, et al., 2005). In other words, the unfolding of the ballistic hand movement was adapted to the characteristics of the saccade. In the spatial display, both the saccadic and ballistic hand movements of patients with cerebellar disorders were larger than those of healthy controls. Therefore, although deficits in eye and hand movement were observed, the coordination between goal-directed eye movements and hand movements is well preserved in patients with cerebellar deficits related to MS. A similar conclusion was made for planned movements in patients with other cerebellar lesions (Sailer et al., 2005).

During the homing-in or target phase of aiming movements, patients with MS also showed deficits in gaze fixation on the target (Feys, Helsen, Lavrysen, et al., 2003; 2005). Both patients with MS and healthy controls made fixational eye movements, indicating that these are normal behaviors used to refresh the image with visual information on the retina (Hotson, 1982). However, the amplitude of the fixational eye movements was greater in the group with MS, indicating an unsteady target fixation, and an association was found between the number of fixational eye movements and the number of hand oscillations (Feys, Helsen, et al., 2005). Therefore, further studies were performed to differentiate between these relationships on the programming level versus interactions on the perception–action level.

The eye movements in patients with MS tremor were found to have a substantial effect on hand movements. The comparison between coordinated eye–hand tracking and isolated eye or hand tracking revealed that the target overshoot of the hand was reduced or even similar to normal target undershoot when patients fixated the target continuously (i.e., when they did not make an enlarged saccade toward the target; see figure 11.8). This clearly suggests that the saccadic dysmetria (overshoot) contributed to target overshoot of the primary hand movement.

In the target phase, the overall amplitude of both fixational eye movements and arm intention tremor was greater during a coordinated eye–hand tracking condition than it was during an isolated hand tracking condition with continuous target fixation (Feys, Helsen, et al., 2005). On the one hand, this may suggest that the amplitude of fixational eye movements was enlarged during coordinated tracking due to the preceding (deficient) saccades. An unsteady gaze fixation is likely to compromise the accuracy of

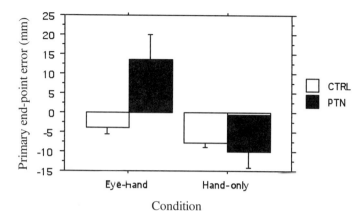

▶ **Figure 11.8**   Time to mean end-point error (and standard error) of the hand after the ballistic hand movement in conditions with simultaneous eye and hand movement (eye–hand
condition) and isolated hand movement with continuous target fixation (hand-only condition) for both healthy controls and patients with MS tremor.

the visual afferents about the precise hand position relative to the stationary target position. The subsequent corrective hand movements may then
be less accurate and require additional voluntary error correction, thereby
enhancing the overall amplitude of intention tremor.

On the other hand, the amplitude of hand tremor in the target phase
may be modulated by the size and the speed of the preceding ballistic
hand movements in the transport phase and may be independent of the
enlarged fixational eye movements. Therefore, in a follow-up study, factors contributing to deficits in eye and hand movement were disentangled
(Feys et al., 2008). Specifically, magnitudes of the primary saccadic and
hand movements were modified to differentiate the effects of the primary
saccadic and hand movements in the transport phase on fixational eye
movements on the one hand and hand tremor amplitude in the target
phase on the other. An important finding in patients with MS, but not in
healthy controls, was that the amplitude of fixational eye movements at the
target depended on the amplitude of the preceding saccade, whereas the
overall tremor amplitude increased when the amplitude of fixational eye
movements was greater. This demonstrated that the size of the fixational
eye movements influenced MS intention tremor. It is hypothesized that
the unstable target fixation in patients with MS tremor compromised the
accuracy of the visual information about the precise location of the target
relative to the hand. This impeded motor performance thereby elicits more
voluntary correction movements and involuntary tremor by means of a
perception–action cycle.

In contrast to the profound effect of eye movements on hand tremor,
hand tremor did not significantly influence the fixational eye movements,

as revealed by comparing coordinated eye–hand movements with isolated eye movements and eye movements accompanying the left and right hand in patients with asymmetric tremor severity. The postsaccadic deficits in eye fixation were observed regardless of whether intention tremor was present and independent of tremor severity. However, there was no relationship between the deficits in eye movement and the deficits in hand movement during coordinated action. Patients with MS and mild oculomotor deficits may have marked hand tremor and vice versa. However, regardless of whether patients with MS exhibited mild or severe oculomotor deficits, experimental manipulations induced similar changes in both the size of fixational eye movements and the severity of hand tremor (Feys, Helsen, Lavrysen, et al., 2003; Feys, Helsen, et al., 2005; Feys et al., 2008).

A similar one-way influence of eye movements on motor behavior has been reported in patients with various cerebellar dysfunctions. Crowdy, Hollands, Ferguson, and Marple-Horvat (2000) demonstrated that oculo-motor deficits had a negative influence on visually guided stepping. These patients were able to improve their locomotor stepping performance after rehearsal of accurate eye movements (Crowdy et al., 2002). Thus, patients with MS tremor may also show reduced hand tremor amplitude if the saccadic amplitude is reduced by sequentially executing eye and hand movements to reach an object.

Visual Movement Control in Cerebellar Pathology

It is well known that patients with cerebellar deficits show a specific dif-ficulty (independent of unsteady gaze fixation) in using visual information to control arm and hand movements (Cody, Lovgreen, & Schady, 1993; Day et al., 1998; Liu et al., 1997; Stein & Glickstein, 1992). In addition, growing evidence suggests that this patient group has difficulties in the online pro-cessing of kinesthetic information even though no manifest sensory deficits are present (Grill, Hallett, & McShane, 1997; Shimansky et al., 1997). An abnormality associated with online processing of proprioceptive informa-tion regarding the hand position during aiming or reaching tasks may explain the enhanced reliance on visual feedback (Cody et al., 1993; Liu et al., 1997; Rand et al., 2000). The cerebellar system may be heavily involved in the online control of visually guided goal-directed movements since the cerebellum is regarded as the neural locus of internal models that connect sensory information and motor actions (Debaere, Wenderoth, Sunaert, Van Hecke, & Swinnen, 2003; Glickstein, 2000; Liu, Robertson, & Miall, 2003; Wolpert, Miall, & Kawato, 1998). To provide further support for the previously mentioned hypothesis, we investigated the tracking behavior of patients with MS tremor during both visual movement control and pro-prioceptive movement control (without vision). In this section, we discuss the effects of visual information on both movement accuracy and severity of involuntary cerebellar tremor.

In healthy subjects as well as in patients with MS tremor, a decrease in performance accuracy is observed in the absence of visual information about hand position. However, the decrease in accuracy is greater in patients with tremor than in healthy controls (Feys, Helsen, Liu, et al., 2003). The increased movement error in the absence of visual feedback is not regarded as an artifact of tremor since tremor amplitude is significantly smaller during memory-guided compared with visually guided tracking (Feys, Helsen, Liu, et al., 2003; Liu et al., 1997). In other words, patients with MS are more reliant on visual feedback of the hand position for accurate motor performance.

To better understand the mechanism of increased reliance on visual feedback, the processing of proprioceptive information was studied through artificial stimulation of the muscle spindles by means of tendon vibration (Feys, Helsen, Buekers, et al., 2006). Tendon vibration is a strong stimulator of muscle spindle afferents, thereby biasing the information about muscle length and resulting in predictable movement illusions. During memory-guided movements, tendon vibration typically reduces movement amplitude and causes target undershoot (Verschueren, Cordo, & Swinnen, 1998). To differentiate between possible additional effects caused by tremor and the disease of MS, patients with MS and tremor were compared with patients with MS without tremor and with healthy controls. As expected, the application of tendon vibration during memory-guided movements reduced movement amplitude. However, the vibration-induced decrease of movement amplitude was significantly smaller in the tremor group than it was in the groups without tremor. The results indicate that proprioceptive information was used for the online control of movements, but to a lesser extent in patients with MS and tremor compared with patients with MS without tremor or with healthy controls.

The behavior of patients with MS with and without intention tremor suggested that patients with tremor have specific deficits in using proprioceptive information. It is also possible to argue that the decreased use of the muscle spindle afferent information is directly related to the MS lesions causing intention tremor, considering the role of the cerebellum in sensorimotor integration (Desmurget et al., 2001; Jueptner et al., 1997; Wolpert et al., 1998). Brain lesions in the cerebellar system may have caused proprioceptive deficits since the cerebellum has been attributed a role in sensory discrimination (Feys et al., 2006; Gao et al., 1996; Jueptner et al., 1997).

However, although patients with cerebellar degeneration exhibit a dysfunction in perception of movement velocity and duration, no difficulties in perceiving the limb position or movement amplitude have been reported (Grill, Hallett, Marcus, & McShane, 1994; Maschke, Gomez, Tuite, & Konczak, 2003). Therefore, it is hypothesized that patients with cerebellar deficits may have adopted strategies to cope with the noise in the proprioceptive input signals that compromises the accuracy of the perceived hand position.

The compensatory strategy may be to reduce the weight of noisy propriocep-tive input during online movement control to avoid excessive movement errors (Liu et al., 1999). As such, patients with cerebellar deficits are more reliant on visual feedback for accurate motor performance when compared with people who can fully benefit from their proprioceptive information.

Use of Eye Movements to Study Motor Imagery in Pathological Functioning

In healthy subjects, partially overlapping neural networks, including bilateral premotor and parietal areas, basal ganglia, and cerebellum, were activated during both real and imagined hand movements (Gerardin et al., 2000). During real movements, the consequences of dysfunction in one of these areas are clearly expressed in motor behavior. Due to the concealed nature of imagery, it is far less clear to what extent imagery of a movement is also affected by impaired function of one (or several) of these areas, as is the case in patients with neurological disorders. For example, patients with a hemiplegic upper limb after stroke have the ability to imagine movements of the paralyzed arm even after years of limb disuse (Johnson, Sprehn, & Saykin, 2002). However, this ability is compromised in patients with lesions in the parietal cortex or putamen (Danckert et al., 2002; Li, 2000). In patients with Parkinson's disease, which is caused by deficits in the basal ganglia, motor imagery ability showed contrary results depending on the design that was used (Frak, Cohen, & Pourcher, 2004; Tamir, Dickstein, & Huberman, 2007).

Although there have been promising results regarding the use of motor imagery as an additional therapy within the field of neurological rehabilita-tion, the success of this therapy depends on the patient's imagery ability. Therefore, it is absolutely necessary to test the imagery ability of patients with neurological deficits before implementing imagery techniques in their rehabilitation. As mentioned previously, we recently developed a method to monitor motor imagery in our lab (Heremans, Helsen, & Feys, 2008). This method is based on the similarities in eye movements made during physical execution and imagery of goal-directed movements. Up to now, this monitoring method was validated only in young, healthy people. Follow-up studies are now being conducted to examine whether it can also be used to evaluate the imagery ability of patients with neurological deficits.

In a related study (Heremans, Helsen, De Poel, Alaerts, Meyns, & Feys, 2009), we investigated whether the use of external cues might facilitate sub-jects' motor imagery performance. In healthy subjects, visual and auditory cues during imagery increased vividness and accuracy of eye movements. A study by Helsen, Tremblay, Van den Berg, and Elliott (2004) showed the importance of making accurate eye movements while practicing a motor skill. As such, it seems that accurate eye movements may have a similar facilitating effect during imagery. We speculate that imagery practice may benefit from the use of external cues eliciting accurate eye movements. The use of cues might be even more important when imagery is used in the rehabilitation of certain groups of patients with neurological deficits. In patients with Parkinson's disease, for example, external cues enhance motor performance during physical execution of a task (Brown & Marsden, 1988; Siegert et al., 2002). Also, in patients with MS tremor, the use of additional (visual) cues during imagery might be useful since, as mentioned earlier, these patients are more reliant on visual feedback for accurate motor performance. It remains to be seen whether the positive effect of cuing found during physical practice in these groups also generalizes to mental practice in pathological functioning.

Summary of Visuomotor Control in Cerebellar Pathology

Patients with cerebellar dysfunction not only demonstrate deficits in limb motor function but also manifest abnormal eye movements. Patients with MS tremor were selected as a pathological model to study eye–hand coordination and interactions. Interestingly, an invariant coupling between the saccadic completion time and the peak velocity of the hand was found, suggesting that the temporal coupling was preserved in these patients during predictable goal-directed movements (Feys, Helsen, et al., 2005).

Interactions between eye movements and hand movements, however, occur during visually guided movements, with deficits in eye movement having a one-way negative effect on hand motor performance. This is observed during the ballistic phase as well as the homing-in phase of the movement of the hand toward the target. Near the target, enlarged fixational eye movements induce an unsteady gaze fixation that leads to inappropriate movement corrections.

Despite experiencing abnormalities in eye movement that disturb the accurate perception of the target and hand position, patients with cerebellar dysfunction show an increased reliance on visual feedback for accurate motor performance. This paradoxical finding may be explained by studies demonstrating a decreased capacity in the online processing of proprioceptive feedback.

Conclusions and Future Directions

Over the past several decades, an increased reliance on the visual control of voluntary movement has emerged in daily life (e.g., when reading and typing text messages) and in many professional settings (e.g., when using a mouse with a computer). The apparent simplicity of these eye and hand movements in healthy adults belies the underlying complexity involved in the temporal organization and spatial control of the movements. From the study of pathological functioning, however, it becomes clear that even mild brain damage may have a detrimental effect on the smooth execution of goal-directed aiming movements. The goal of the present chapter was to examine the role of visual afference in normal and pathological functioning to gain a better understanding of the acquisition and performance of goal-directed aiming movements.

Surprisingly, the behavioral, kinematic, brain imaging, and motor imagery data presented in this chapter are still consistent with a two-component explanation of the control of rapid, goal-directed limb movements. This model of manual aiming (for a review, see Elliott et al., 2001) holds that the first portion of an aiming movement is controlled by a centrally prepared set of motor commands that provide the initial accelerative (and subsequent decelerative) impulse that moves the limb into the vicinity of the target. The ballistic portion of the movement typically undershoots the target position, and a second, visually directed phase of the movement brings the limb onto the target. Visuomotor control thus consists of a versatile process that is flexible enough to adopt a strategy that will make the most use of the information available while meeting the demands of the task and the cues at hand. Though some may think that these observations mean that we should view the hand system as a slave to the ocular system, it may be more appropriate to consider the eyes as the servants of the hand (see chapter 10).

In this chapter, we attempted to provide a basis for future research in the area of eye–hand coordination, bridging the gap between the behavioral sciences and the neurosciences. We may look ahead and expect the following outcomes in the near future:

▶ The theoretical and empirical emphasis on the acquisition and performance of rapid visual control, combining measurements of eye and limb movements, may further moderate the current infatuation with open-loop processes.

▶ The study of both normal and pathological functioning may result in new insights into the neural plasticity associated with the learning of motor skills.

▶ The integration of neuroimaging data with behavioral and kinematic parameters may provide new insights into the cooperative interaction of the two cerebral hemispheres, as well as into the sensory (parietal) and motor (prefrontal) brain areas in the acquisition and performance of goal-directed movement.

Although our research interests were primarily theoretical, we may also anticipate practical and clinical implications:

▶ The optimization of human–machine interactions (e.g., interactions at bank terminals), especially in special circumstances (e.g., eye–hand coordination under magnification used by surgeons) and for improving robots (e.g., grasping tasks)

▶ A better understanding of pathologic functioning, especially with respect to movement disorders in which closed-loop control takes precedence over open-loop control (e.g., parkinsonism, stroke), with the potential to reveal new rehabilitation treatments that may improve functioning in daily life

CHAPTER 12

Lateralization of Goal-Directed Movement

ROBERT L. SAINBURG

This chapter discusses the neural foundations of motor lateralization, or handedness. First we examine lateralization, a phenomenon that has been described for a variety of neural systems. Next, we discuss evidence for both cultural and genetic determinants of handedness and the important interaction between these two determinants. The critical role of genetics is exemplified by the recent identification of a gene related to handedness. The importance of activity-dependent processes in genetically guided development of the corticospinal system is exemplified as a model of interaction between genetics and behavior. After reviewing the origins of handedness, we discuss the specific neurobehavioral processes that have become lateralized. We emphasize recent evidence indicating that the dominant and nondominant systems have become specialized for independent but complementary functions.

For the sake of clarity, a particular arm and its contralateral hemisphere are referred to as a *hemisphere–arm system*. We review evidence that the dominant hemisphere–arm system has become specialized for predicting and controlling limb and task dynamics, as required to achieve coordinated arm trajectories, whereas the nondominant system has become specialized for controlling limb impedance, as required to stabilize the limb in a given position. We next review evidence that both hemispheres are used when performing movements with a single arm, suggesting a role of each hemisphere in unilateral control. Then we demonstrate that damage to the ipsilateral hemisphere in patients with stroke leads to motor deficits in the arm previously thought of as intact with regard to sensorimotor coordination. The fact that these deficits can be predicted by motor lateralization provides strong evidence that each hemisphere contributes complementary processes to the control of each arm. However, the question of why each hemisphere does not provide equal contributions to each arm, leading to symmetrical coordination, remains unanswered.

Neural Lateralization

Before the seminal research of Gazzaniga and colleagues on disconnection syndrome in split-brain patients (Gazzaniga, 1998), neural lateralization was viewed predominantly through the Liepmann model (Derakhshan, 2004; Geschwind, 1975; Liepmann, 1905). Liepmann described a major (or master) hemisphere and a minor (or slave) hemisphere. Gazzaniga's research on split-brain patients emancipated the minor hemisphere, revealing that each hemisphere has advantages for different functions. In most people, the left hemisphere mediates semantic and lexicon features of language, whereas the right hemisphere mediates an array of complex functions, including speech prosody, nonverbal communication, specific types of visuospatial analysis, and certain types of memory (Grimshaw, 1998; Hauser, 1993; Bowers et al., 1985; Hellige, 1996; Reeves, 1985; Tompkins & Flowers, 1985). Thus, lateralization of systems such as cognition, perception, and language is now understood as a fundamental organizational feature of the human nervous system (Anzola, 1980; Boles & Karner, 1996; Heilman, Bowers, Valenstein, & Watson, 1986). Gazzaniga proposed that the advantage of such lateralization might be to reduce redundancy of neural circuits, thereby allowing each hemisphere more neural substrate for its functions. Thus, during evolution, each function was allowed to expand in complexity without the cost of developing new neural tissue. Gazzaniga's research on disconnection syndrome elegantly supported this view of neural lateralization, revealing specialization of each hemisphere for different but complementary functions.

Motor Lateralization

The emancipation of the right hemisphere brought about by split-brain research has not yet been fully realized for motor functions, which still tend to be viewed from the master–slave perspective. Even the terminology associated with handedness is essentially different from that used to refer to lateralization in other systems. The terms *hand preference* and *handedness* indicate a view of motor lateralization as a personal inclination rather than a reflection of neural organization. This view might arise from the practical observation that humans can use either arm to perform virtually any task, as long as we are not concerned with accuracy or efficiency. For example, we might use our nondominant arm to toss our keys to a friend while our dominant arm is preoccupied with scribbling a note. However, this does not suggest that the nondominant arm should be used as the lead manipulator in skilled tasks, such as targeted throwing or dexterous manipulations. It has been argued that the inclination to use a particular hand is established early in life and becomes consolidated during skill development. This presumably results in the adult expression of handedness (Perelle & Ehrman, 2005). From this perspective, handedness emerges from cultural and behavioral influences, which perpetuates the view that handedness is unique among neural lateralizations.

Role of Culture in Determining Handedness

If handedness reflects an individual predilection for using one hand more often for specific tasks, we might expect a fairly equal distribution of left-handers and right-handers among the greater population. However, it is also plausible that the strong bias toward right-handedness that persists across cultures (Medland, Perelle, De Monte, & Ehrman, 2004) and time (Corballis, 1983) could be perpetuated by purely social transmission. The factors that have been proposed to produce this bias are many, including in utero positional asymmetries, the side of feeding the mother chooses, preferences of adults for carrying children, and a bias in parental modeling of eating, drawing, and writing behaviors (Blackburn & Knusel, 2006).

From an opposing perspective, the strong prejudice against left-handedness that has persisted for many years across many cultures contradicts the hypothesis of a cultural origin for handedness and begs the question of why left-handers seem to persist in our population. In his 2005 book, *A Left-Hand Turn Around the World*, David Wolman describes a long history of religious, political, and social persecution that left-handers have endured over the ages. Perelle and Ehrman (1994) point out that in one East Asian culture, as late as 1994, toddlers showing a preference for the left hand had that hand tied behind their back. If tying the hand was unsuccessful in discouraging left-handedness, the left arm might even be broken to discourage its use. Perelle and Ehrman (2005) state that even this extreme measure did not succeed in eliminating left-handers from that population, and children continued to emerge as left-handers even without adult models. Thus, the persistence of left-handers in the population provides evidence against a purely cultural origin for handedness.

However, the public expression of handedness is clearly subject to cultural modification. Medland and colleagues (2004) conducted a cross-cultural survey and concluded that in cultures with formal restrictions on left-handed writing, people report lower rates of left-handedness (e.g., in Mexico 2.4% of the population are left-handers, whereas in Canada left-handers make up 12.4% of the population). This measure of handedness is based on reports of hand preference rather than on actual motor performance. The willingness to use the limb that is optimal for a given task and to report hand preference accurately might vary with the mores of the surrounding culture. Thus, while culture appears to influence the willingness to claim left-handedness or right-handedness, it is unlikely that manual performance asymmetries are established through cultural factors alone. In fact, the strong cultural bias against left-handedness that has persisted across history strongly argues against the idea that handedness reflects a culturally induced preference. Consistent with this idea, Vallortigara and Rogers (2005) recently proposed that the persistence of left-handers in the population might be attributed to evolutionary factors associated with game theory. According to this idea, left-handed genes might benefit from a right-handed population bias. For example, if a shoal of fish all turn right due to a population bias of the escape reflex, this may draw attention from the few left-handers who can escape unscathed. Whatever the influence of culture on handedness, it is unlikely that a person can choose handedness any more than a person can choose the cerebral hemisphere that will mediate syntactic components of verbal language.

Dependence of Handedness on Other Lateralizations

In contrast to the hypothesis that handedness is transmitted through culture, other hypotheses attempting to explain the development of handedness could be referred to as "piggyback" theories. These ideas attribute handedness to an artifact of lateralization in other systems, such as language. Thus, left-hemisphere lateralization for language leads to left-hemisphere, and thus right-hand, preference for language-related motor function, including manual gestures (Corballis, 1997, 2003; Gentilucci & Corballis, 2006) and writing (Perelle & Ehrman, 1983, 2005). Such advantages in right-hand use are hypothesized to result from a reduced processing cost when both motor functions and language functions are processed in the same hemisphere. The resulting motor preference for language-related movements is then thought to entrain all other motor skills toward a right-hand bias.

However, substantial empirical evidence indicates that the side of the brain that is considered dominant for language processing does not predict handedness. An early study (Loring et al., 1990) tested whether amobarbital injected into one carotid artery initially affects language function by anesthetizing the ipsilateral hemisphere. Most people showed left-hemisphere dominance for lexicon-related language functions, but some showed right-side language dominance, and some even showed a reliance on both cerebral hemispheres. Whereas right and bilateral language function was more common in left-handers, the relationship was not strong enough to justify a causal relationship between language dominance and handedness. Studies using fMRI have since supported these findings; Pujol, Deus, Losilla, and Capdevila (1999) showed that most left-handers process verbal information in the left hemisphere, strong evidence against a language determinant of handedness.

Possibly the strongest evidence that handedness is not simply a by-product of language lateralization, however, is the expression of handedness in nonhuman primates. Due largely to the research of Hopkins at Emory University, we now know that chimpanzees, as well as other nonhuman primates, demonstrate strong individual handedness and substantial population-level biases for right-handedness (Hopkins, 2006; Hopkins, Russell, Cantalupo, Freeman, & Schapiro, 2005; Hopkins, Stoinski, Lukas, Ross, & Wesley, 2003; Lonsdorf & Hopkins, 2005; Vauclair, Meguerditchian, & Hopkins, 2005). Motor lateralization does not appear limited to primates and has correlates across the animal kingdom, as detailed in the book edited by Rogers and Andrew (2002), *Comparative Vertebrate Lateralization*. In summary, it is clear that handedness is not a casual preference, and it does not emerge as an artifact from lateralization in other systems, such as language.

Role of Genetics in Determining Handedness

It may appear that this discussion is leading toward a nature rather than nurture explanation for handedness. However, this distinction in biology appears ill-posed due to the intricate interactions between genetics and experience. A number of genetic models have accurately predicted the distribution of handedness in families, communities, and monozygotic twins and their offspring (Annett, 2003; Corballis, 1997; Levy, 1977; Levy & Nagylaki, 1972; McManus, 1985). Some of these models promote handedness as an artifact of lateralization in language and thus are subject to the criticisms discussed previously. However, more recently, Klar (1999, 2003) proposed a single-gene model that accounts for both direction of handedness and the orientation of hair whorl. The interesting feature of this model is that hair whorl is clearly independent of cultural influences but nevertheless seems well correlated with handedness. It should be noted that this model has been criticized by studies that have questioned the strength of the correlation between these two variables (Jansen et al., 2007). Smoking-gun evidence has recently been demonstrated in the form of a gene *(LRRTM1)* that increases the likeliness of being left-handed (Francks et al., 2007). This is the first concrete evidence for a genetic determinant of handedness. Interestingly, previous genetic models have proposed two genotypes: right-hand dominance and non-right-hand dominance. According to this idea, the non-right-handed genotype can result in a mixed-handed, right-handed, or left-handed phenotype. This might correspond to the *LRRTM1* gene recently identified by Francks and colleagues. However, even with such evidence, the origin of handedness is unlikely to be resolved as purely nature or nurture.

As seems to be the rule for neural systems, genetic factors lead to permissive conditions that require activity-dependent processes to facilitate development in a particular direction. An example of the intricate interaction between genetics and experience in determining structure–function relationships in neurobehavioral function is the activity-dependent neural apoptosis in the anterior corticospinal system, recently shown in developing kittens (Friel, Drew, & Martin, 2007; Friel & Martin, 2005; Martin, 2005; Martin, Friel, Salimi, & Chakrabarty, 2007). In adult cats, the pattern of corticospinal terminations in the spinal gray matter is quite different from that in early postnatal development. The pruning of corticospinal axon growth in kittens requires cortical activity during a critical time of postnatal development some 3 to 7 wk after birth. If such activity is prevented by injection of muscimol to the motor cortex, corticospinal axons do not develop the necessary connectivity to support mature coordination. As a result, substantial coordination deficits occur in adult life (Friel et al., 2007). Similar interactions between genetically determined processes and behaviorally driven neural activity likely underlie the establishment of other neurobehavioral functions, such as handedness in human and nonhuman primates.

Biological Correlates of Handedness

If handedness is not a choice and is not dictated by lateralization in other systems, what are its neural correlates? The landmark studies by Kuypers and colleagues established that muscles of the trunk and limb girdle are controlled through bilateral projections, whereas control of arm musculature for reach and prehension arises primarily from descending projections originating in the contralateral cortex and brain stem (Brinkman, Kuypers, & Lawrence, 1970; Holstege & Kuypers, 1982; Kuypers, 1982; Kuypers, Fleming, & Farinholt, 1962; Kuypers & Laurence, 1967; Kuypers & Maisky, 1975; Lawrence & Kuypers, 1968). However, more recent electrophysiological and neuroimaging studies have shown substantial activation of the ipsilateral motor cortex during unilateral hand and arm movements, indicating a role for both hemispheres in controlling each limb (Chen, German, & Zaidel, 1997; Dassonville, Zhu, Uurbil, Kim, & Ashe, 1997; Gitelman et al., 1996; Kawashima, Roland, & O'Sullivan, 1994; Kim et al., 1993; Kutas & Donchin, 1974; Macdonell et al., 1991; Salmelin, Forss, Knuutila, & Hari, 1995; Taniguchi et al., 1998; Tanji, Okano, & Sato, 1988; Viviani, Perani, Grassi, Bettinardi, & Fazio, 1998). Some studies have shown that the hemisphere contralateral to the dominant arm tends to reflect higher levels of activity than its nondominant counterpart demonstrates when unilateral movements of the left and right arm are compared (Dassonville et al., 1997; Kim et al., 1993; Viviani et al., 1998). It is not known whether this asymmetry that favors the dominant hemisphere may be a function of the tasks employed in the imaging studies. Nevertheless, it is clear that unilateral movements of either arm recruit substantial activity in the ipsilateral cortex, a finding that suggests the involvement of both hemispheres during unimanual movements. This idea has been supported by studies of ipsilesional deficits in patients with unilateral lesions due to stroke, a topic covered later in this chapter.

The functional asymmetries just described might arise from behavioral factors that modify central nervous system representations of the peripheral effectors. Merzenich and colleagues have established that practicing certain patterns of finger coordination can alter the representation of the digits in the motor cortex (Buonomano & Merzenich, 1998; Nudo, Milliken, Jenkins, & Merzenich, 1996; Recanzone, Merzenich, Jenkins, Grajski, & Dinse, 1992). Thus, the cortical activation asymmetries might result from rather than produce handedness. However, asymmetries in the gross morphology of neural structures such as the motor cortex (Amunts et al., 1996), basal ganglia (Kooistra & Heilman, 1988), and cerebellum (Snyder, Bilder, Wu, Bogerts, & Lieberman, 1995) are less likely to result from movement experience alone. In summary, it is clear that asymmetries in both brain structures and activations are associated with handedness and that both cerebral hemispheres appear to contribute to unilateral arm and hand movements.

Neurobehavioral Processes Lateralized in Handedness

Although asymmetries in neural structure and function verify the biological foundations of handedness, the neural processes mediated by these asymmetries have yet to be precisely defined. The largest body of research in this area has quantified RT, MT, and final position accuracy during rapid reaching movements in order to differentiate closed-loop from open-loop mechanisms of control. This distinction originates from serial planning and execution models of control. According to these models, open-loop and closed-loop control processes are independent and serial. Closed-loop mechanisms are mediated by sensory feedback during the course of movement, whereas open-loop mechanisms are unaffected by feedback. This distinction was inspired by Woodworth (1899) and was experimentally operationalized by Fitts (1954, 1966; Fitts & Radford, 1966).

Attempts at using this model to differentiate the role of sensory feedback on movements of the dominant and nondominant arm have been largely equivocal. Flowers (1975) and others (Carson, 1993; Elliott, Lyons, Chua, Goodman, & Carson, 1995; Roy, Kalbfleisch, & Elliott, 1994; Todor & Cisneros, 1985; Todor & Doane, 1977) suggested that manual asymmetries emerge from differences in the use of visual feedback that arise when the precision requirements of aiming tasks become high, as reflected by the index of difficulty of the task (Plamondon & Alimi, 1997). However, studies that failed to alter interlimb differences in accuracy by manipulating visual feedback conditions brought this hypothesis into question (Carson, Chua, Elliott, & Goodman, 1990; Chua, Carson, Goodman, & Elliott, 1992; Elliott et al., 1993; Roy & Elliott, 1986). Demonstrating that dominant-arm advantages do not depend on visual feedback conditions, Carson and colleagues (1993) suggested that such advantages result from more effective somatosensory-based error corrections. However, in direct contrast to this suggestion, findings by Bagesteiro and colleagues recently demonstrated that the nondominant arm shows substantial advantages for compensating unexpected loads using somatosensory information (Bagesteiro & Sainburg, 2003, 2005). Thus, neither arm shows a consistent advantage for using sensory information to correct movements. It remains possible, however, that the planning of movements might be lateralized, an idea originated by Liepmann (1905) more than 100 years ago. Consistent with this idea, a number of studies have proposed a dominant-arm and dominant-hemisphere advantage for movement planning, initiation, or sequencing (Annett, Annett, & Hudson, 1979; Elliott et al., 1995; Todor & Kyprie, 1980; Todor & Smiley-Oyen, 1987). Other studies, however, have interpreted nondominant-arm advantages in RT as evidence for nondominant-hemisphere advantages in motor planning (Elliott et al., 1993; Mieschke, Elliott, Helsen, Carson, & Coull, 2001). Overall, this body of research has not yielded consistent data that can be used to differentiate the control processes that underlie motor lateralization.

Lateralization of Costs and Goals

The idea that movement control can be temporally compartmentalized into open-loop and closed-loop processes is a rather simplistic view that reflects early methods in control systems engineering. Recently, more integrative control theories have been proposed for which a strict dissociation between open- and closed-loop processes is difficult. For example, optimal feedback control has recently been incorporated into a theory of biological motor control (Todorov, 2004; Todorov & Jordan, 2002), which proposes that control signals continuously modify feedback gains during the course of movement. These ideas are consistent with experimental studies that have shown modulation of reflex gains in accord with differences in task goals and environmental conditions (Haridas & Zehr, 2003; Kimura, Haggard, & Gomi, 2006; Lacquaniti, Carrozzo, & Borghese, 1993; Prochazka, 1981; Yamamoto & Ohtsuki, 1989). Due to neural delays, early movement conditions (50 ms after movement onset) result from open-loop processes. However, after this initial interval, modulation of feedback gains by descending signals precludes a distinction between open-loop and closed-loop processes. We now suggest that the differences between the hemisphere–limb systems might best be understood from the perspective of optimal control of goal-directed movements (Hasan, 1986; Liu & Todorov, 2007; Scott, 2002, 2004; Todorov, Li, & Pan, 2005). To minimize certain cost functions, estimates of the current state of the limb must be compared with those costs. Such estimates should depend on limb-specific experience, as well as the quality of sensory information available to each system. It is plausible that such state estimates could be differentially tuned for different cost functions for each hemisphere–limb system. For example, the dominant system appears to be tuned to optimize dynamic parameters such as energy expenditure and trajectory shape, whereas the nondominant system appears to be better adapted for achieving and maintaining static positions.

Dominant-System Specialization for Coordination of Limb Dynamics

Recent evidence suggests that each hemisphere–limb system might be differentially tuned to stabilize different aspects of task performance (Sainburg, 2002, 2005). We initially termed this hypothesis *dynamic dominance* because of evidence that control of the dominant-arm trajectory entails more efficient and accurate coordination of muscle actions with the complex biomechanical interactions that arise between moving limb segments. Prominent among these are interaction torques, which are produced when the end of one segment pushes on the end of the other segment through the joint connecting the two. For example, it is possible to hold the right upper arm with the left hand and move the arm back and forth. If the muscles about the right elbow are relaxed, the forearm will flop back and forth. The torque that produces this motion is referred to as an *interaction torque.* For any given segment, motion of attached segments will impose interaction torques that vary with the velocities and accelerations of those segments, which will also vary with the instantaneous configuration of the limb. During limb movements, these interactions produce large torques that often exceed the amplitude of muscle actions on the segments (Ghez & Sainburg, 1995; Gribble & Ostry, 1999; Sainburg, Ghez, & Kalakanis, 1999; Sainburg, Ghilardi, Poizner, & Ghez, 1995). Previous research confirmed an essential role of proprioception in such coordination (Ghez, Gordon, Ghilardi, Christakos, & Cooper, 1990; Sainburg et al., 1995; Sainburg, Poizner, & Ghez, 1993). Thus, patients with proprioceptive loss due to large-fiber sensory neuropathy through the arms and neck are unable to efficiently coordinate muscle actions with interaction torques, even when vision of movement is available.

To test whether the two limbs coordinate the motion of multiple segments differently, we designed a reaching task that would elicit progressively greater interaction torques at the elbow joint (Bagesteiro & Sainburg, 2002; Sainburg & Kalakanis, 2000). The general experimental setup for these experiments is shown in figure 12.1*a*. The arm was supported on a frictionless air-sled support while the subject viewed a virtual environment projected above the arm. After aligning a finger within a start circle, the subject made rapid reaching movements to projected target positions. All targets required the same elbow excursion (20°) but different shoulder excursions (5°, 10°, and 15°). As shown in the sample trajectories of figure 12.1*b*, final positions were slightly more accurate for the nondominant arm. However, the hand trajectories and joint coordination patterns were systematically different. Dominant-hand paths showed curvatures with medial convexities for all target directions, whereas paths of the nondominant arm showed curvatures with oppositely directed lateral convexities that increased in magnitude across directions.

Analysis of limb segment torques revealed substantial differences in coordination; dominant-arm trajectories reflected more efficient coordination. This is illustrated in figure 12.1c, which shows the elbow torques of the dominant and nondominant arm, corresponding to the dashed trials toward target 1 in figure 12.1b. Because the dominant arm employed greater shoulder motion (not shown), the elbow interaction torque was larger,

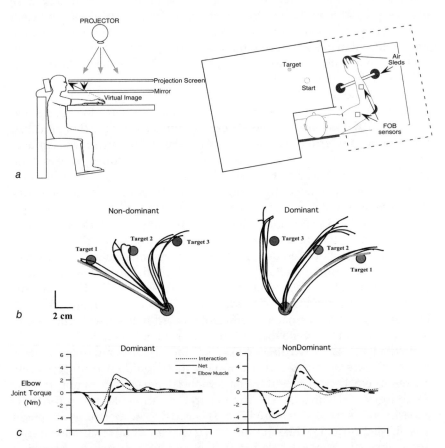

▶ **Figure 12.1**   (a) Experimental setup for the planar reaching studies reviewed in the text. Left: Subjects sit in a chair with the arm resting on a table. Above the arm, a mirror reflects the game display. Right: A start position and target are presented simultaneously on the display. Air sleds support the arm in the horizontal plane, minimizing the effects of friction and gravity on joint torque. Flock of Birds (Ascension Technology Corporation) six degrees-of-freedom sensors are attached to each limb segment. (b) Sample hand paths for the nondominant (left) and dominant (right) arms. (c) Elbow joint torques, segmented into interaction, net, and muscle terms.

requiring smaller muscle torque (dashed line) to produce movements of the same speed and accuracy as those of the nondominant arm. In this way, the dominant-arm system consistently takes advantage of intersegmental inter-actions to make movements that are more torque efficient (Sainburg, 2002, 2005; Sainburg et al., 1999; Sainburg & Kalakanis, 2000). When the mean squared muscle torque at both joints for movements of the nondominant and dominant arm are matched for speed and displacement, dominant-arm movements consistently use less than half the torque used in nondominant movements. This emphasizes the fact that the coordination differences between the limbs are not simply a result of strength differences. In our tasks, nondominant-arm movements demonstrate greater torque production but less efficient movements. These findings have been corroborated by EMG recordings, which revealed corresponding differences in normalized EMG activities between the limbs (Bagesteiro & Sainburg, 2002).

Nondominant-System Specialization for Control of Limb Impedance

Because few functional advantages have been identified in non-dominant-limb performance, the nondominant system traditionally has been viewed as a naive, unpracticed analog of the dominant hemisphere–limb system. In contrast to this view, recent findings have revealed sub-stantial nondominant-limb advantages in positional accuracy (Bagesteiro & Sainburg, 2002; Sainburg, 2002; Sainburg & Kalakanis, 2000) as well as in somatosensory-based load compensation responses, a reflection of imped-ance control (Bagesteiro & Sainburg, 2003, 2005). These findings indicate a nondominant-system advantage for achieving and maintaining stable limb positions. This advantage is not only important for stabilizing the limb at the end of a reaching movement but also for stabilizing an object that is acted on by the dominant arm. For example, when slicing a loaf of bread, the dominant arm tends to control the knife that produces shearing forces on the bread. The nondominant arm impedes these forces in order to hold the bread still. Maintaining a stable posture in the face of varying forces requires active motor output that is specifically adapted to the imposed loads. Nondominant-system specialization for impedance control is con-sistent with anthropological data indicating that the specialized use of the nondominant arm for stabilizing objects evolved to support tool-making functions in early hominids (Marzke, 1971, 1988, 1997).

Dominant and Nondominant Controllers May Be Adapted to Minimize Costs

To test the hypothesis that each hemisphere–limb system might be optimized for different features of performance, two recent studies examined interlimb differences in adaptation to novel dynamic conditions. Schabowsky, Hidler, and Lum (2007) investigated adaptation to an artificial Coriolis force field imposed by a robotic manipulandum. Subjects adapted to the force field while executing reaching movements within a horizontal plane toward targets arranged in four radial directions from a central start location. The experimental setup and target arrangement are shown in figure 12.2*a*. The applied force fields for the left (nondominant) and right (dominant) arms are also depicted in figure 12.2*a*, right. Figure 12.2*b*, top, shows typical trajectories for the right and left arms when subjects were initially exposed to the velocity-dependent force field. As shown, the trajectories are deflected in the direction of the applied force. However, after adaptation, both limbs make comparatively straight movements toward the targets, as reflected by the sample paths in figure 12.2*b*, middle. This adaptation process is shown across subjects in figure 12.2*c* for the target depicted in figure 12.2*b* and across the initial six trials made toward this target. Both the right and left arms were comparable in the time course and extent of adaptation to the force field.

One method of adapting to such a force field is to anticipate the applied forces during the course of movement. This type of adaptation has been demonstrated by unexpectedly removing the force field on occasional catch trials. During such trials, the extent to which the previously applied forces are anticipated is reflected by the aftereffects, or errors that are directed opposite to those forces. Examples of catch trials are shown in black in figure 12.2*b*, bottom, along with a typical adapted trial shown in gray. As can be seen in the figure, when the force field is suddenly removed, subjects make errors that are directed opposite to the direction of the previously applied force, reflecting the anticipation of the forces. However, the amplitude of aftereffects is substantially smaller for the nondominant arm, which indicates a fundamental difference in the way the two arms adapted to the force field. Dominant-arm adaptation led to specific prediction about the applied forces, but nondominant-arm adaptation did not. Instead, adaptation of the nondominant arm appeared to occur by a less specific form of control that involved impeding the effects of the forces through mechanisms that were not direction specific.

A study with a similar design (Duff & Sainburg, 2007) examined adaptation to novel inertial dynamics and showed substantial differences in how each arm adapted accuracy of the final position and initial direction. Whereas initial direction reflects anticipation of the effect of the inertial condition on the arm, final position is independent of such anticipatory mechanisms. Over the course of adaptation, accuracy in final position improved to the same extent for both arms. However, accuracy in initial direction improved only for the dominant arm. As in the previously described study, aftereffect trials showed lower errors for the nondominant arm compared with the dominant arm. In addition, as subjects adapted to the inertial load, aftereffect trials showed progressively larger errors, again only for the dominant arm.

Taken together, these studies support the hypothesis that each hemisphere–limb system employs different cost functions during adaptation

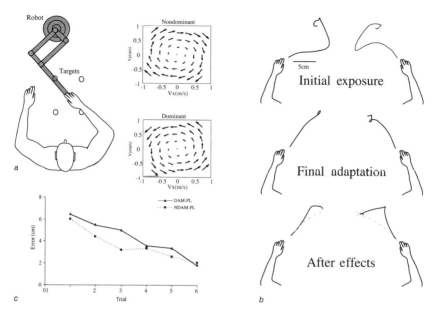

▶ **Figure 12.2** *(a)* Experimental setup for the adaptation study of Shabowski et al (2007). Subjects held a robotic manipulandum that produced programmed velocity-dependent force fields (shown on right). *(b)* Sample performance of left and right hands, shown as hand paths, when first exposed to the force (top), when adaptation has occurred (middle), and when the force field is unexpectedly removed following adaptation (bottom). The latter condition shows the aftereffects of adaptation and is systematically greater for the dominant arm. *(c)* Peak error ± standard error of the dominant and nondominant arms during the early learning phase averaged across all subjects. Only reaches in the anteromedial (AM) and posterolateral (PL) directions are shown. There was no significant difference between arms when reaching in the AL or PM directions.

Experimental Brain Research 182, 2007, pgs. 567-577, "Greater reliance on impedance control in the nondominant arm compared with the dominant arm when adapting to a novel dynamic environment" C.N. Schabowsky, J.M. Hidler, and P.S. Lum, ©Springer. With kind permission of Springer Science+Business Media.

to novel dynamic conditions. The dominant system adapts through progressively more accurate anticipation of the applied forces. In contrast, the nondominant system employs impedance mechanisms that allow progressively more accurate final positions. These findings support the view that each hemisphere–limb system might be differentially tuned for different sets of cost functions: The dominant system is better adapted to dynamic parameters that determine trajectory features, whereas the nondominant system appears better tuned for controlling impedance in order to maintain stable positions.

Predictions for Unilateral Stroke

The research on motor lateralization just described has direct implications for understanding the motor deficits resulting from unilateral stroke. Specifically, damage to the left or right hemisphere should result in distinct deficits that depend on the side of the lesion and that are expressed in the ipsilesional limb. This prediction is based on the hypothesis that each hemisphere is specialized for controlling different aspects of task performance. However, both hemispheres, ipsilateral and contralateral, are normally used to control unilateral arm movements. Therefore, while lesions of the sensorimotor cortices or associated fibers of passage in one hemisphere will produce hemiparesis in the contralesional arm, they should also produce predictable movement deficits in the ipsilesional arm.

Studies in both animals (Gonzalez et al., 2004; Grabowski, Brundin, & Johansson, 1993; Vergara-Aragon, Gonzalez, & Whishaw, 2003) and patients with unilateral brain damage have confirmed substantial deficits in the ipsilesional arm following unilateral brain injury (Carey, Baxter, & Di Fabio, 1998; Desrosiers, Bourbonnais, Bravo, Roy, & Guay, 1996; Haaland & Delaney, 1981; Haaland & Harrington, 1996; Haaland, Prestopnik, Knight, & Lee, 2004; Harrington & Haaland, 1991; Sainburg & Schaefer, 2004; Sunderland, 2000; Wetter, Poole, & Haaland, 2005; Winstein & Pohl, 1995; Wyke, 1967; Yarosh, Hoffman, & Strick, 2004). Haaland and colleagues employed perceptual motor tasks, which require rapid reciprocal tapping between two targets that vary in size and target distance, to examine movement deficits in the ipsilesional arm of patients who have experienced stroke. These experiments employed horizontal movement in the ipsilesional hemispace with the ipsilesional arm (e.g., movement in the right hemispace and arm for patients with right-hemisphere damage) to rule out the confounding effects of motor weakness, visual field cuts, and visual neglect. Lesions in the dominant hemisphere (hemisphere contralateral to the dominant arm) produced deficits in the initial, ballistic component of reaching but not in the secondary, slower component (Haaland, Cleeland, & Carr, 1977; Haaland & Delaney, 1981; Haaland & Harrington, 1996; Haaland, Temkin, Randahl, & Dikmen, 1994; Hunt et al., 1989; Prestopnik, Haaland, Knight, & Lee, 2003). Patients with nondominant-hemisphere lesions showed no deficits in this task. However, in other studies with greater precision requirements, patients with nondominant lesions showed deficits in accuracy of the final position (Haaland et al., 1977; Haaland & Delaney, 1981; Haaland & Harrington, 1996; Haaland et al., 1994; Hunt et al., 1989; Prestopnik et al., 2003; Winstein & Pohl, 1995). These results support the idea that the dominant hemisphere is specialized for controlling the initial trajectory phase of motion, whereas the nondominant hemisphere becomes more important when decelerating the arm toward a stable posture.

In another study demonstrating results consistent with those findings, Winstein and Pohl (1995) showed that nondominant lesions slowed the deceleration phase of rapid aiming movements, whereas dominant lesions slowed the initial, acceleration phase of motion. In a more recent study, Haaland and coworkers (2004) directly tested the idea that dominant lesions produce trajectory deficits and nondominant lesions produce deficits in the final position of targeted reaching movements. In that study, right-handed patients with left-hemisphere lesions showed distinct deficits in movement speed, whereas patients with right-hemisphere lesions showed substantial errors in final position. Such ipsilesional deficits have been associated with impaired performance on functional assessments, including simulated ADLs (Desrosiers et al., 1996; Sunderland, 2000; Wetter et al., 2005), which emphasizes the functional significance of these deficits in patients with chronic stroke.

Schaefer, Haaland, and Sainburg (2007) recently tested the hypothesis that motor lateralization might predict the nature of ipsilesional motor deficits that result from unilateral stroke. Healthy control subjects and patients with either left- or right-hemisphere damage performed targeted single-joint elbow movements of different amplitudes in their ipsilateral hemispace. All subjects were right-hand dominant. Patients with left or right stroke were matched for demographic data, including age, educational level, and gender, as well as size and extent of lesion. All patients were hemiparetic in their contralesional limbs. Figure 12.3 shows the lesion overlap data between patients with left- and right-hemisphere damage. Subjects performed a reaching task restricted to the elbow joint and directed at each of two targets: (1) a short target requiring 15° of elbow excursion and (2) a long target requiring 45° of elbow excursion. Keep in mind that the task was performed with the arm that was ipsilesional to the damaged hemisphere and typically considered unaffected in terms of motor function. However, in our model of motor lateralization, left-hemisphere damage was predicted to produce deficits in the features of the initial trajectory, and right-hemisphere damage was expected to produce deficits in accuracy of the final position.

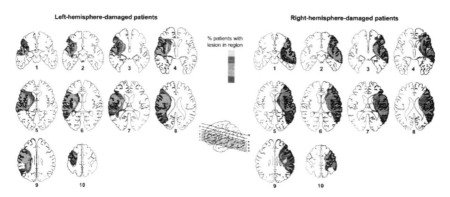

▶ **Figure 12.3**   Lesion locations based on tracing lesions from MRI or computed tomography (CT) scans were superimposed on axial slices separately for patients with left-hemisphere (displayed on left) and right-hemisphere (displayed on right) damage. Colors of shaded regions denote percentage (20%, 40%, 60%, 80%, or 100%) of patients with lesions in the corresponding area.

Adapted, by permission, from S.Y. Schaefer, K.Y. Haaland, and R.L. Sainburg, 2007, "Ipsilesional motor deficits following stroke reflect hemispheric specializations for movement control," *Brain* 130(Pt 8): 2146-2158. © R.L. Sainburg.

In figure 12.4a, representative distributions of the final position are shown for age-matched control subjects and for patients with either right- or left-hemisphere damage. Data from control subjects are shown at the top and data from patients with stroke are shown at the bottom. A comparison of the distributions of final position to the 45° targets between the two groups of patients with stroke (circled) clearly indicates that patients with right-hemisphere damage show substantially more error than their counterparts with left-hemisphere damage show. The graphs of figure 12.4b display the mean and standard errors of these findings across subjects. Note the crossed interaction indicated by substantially lower errors (when compared with control subjects) in the left arm of patients with left-hemisphere damage and the substantially higher errors in the patients with right-hemisphere damage. The fact that MT (figure 12.4b, right) did not show this interaction but was prolonged for patients in both groups confirms that the pattern of errors across our subject groups was not related simply to changes in movement speed, or speed–accuracy trade-offs.

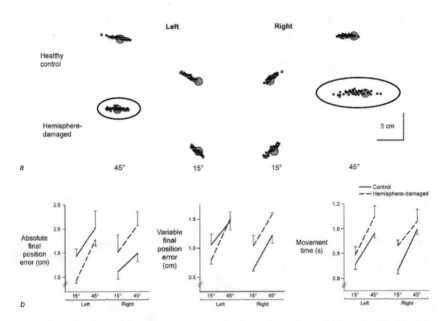

▶ **Figure 12.4** The results of the study by Schaefer et al., 2007, in which patients with right and left hemisphere damage (RHD/LHD) made reaching movements with the ipsilesional (non paretic) arm. (a) Final positions at movement end for each trial (dot) are displayed relative to gray targets for a representative subject from each experimental group. Circled data emphasize the difference between right- and left-hemisphere damage. (b) Mean absolute final position error, mean variable final position error, and MT for each target is displayed for the left and right arms of control subjects and the ipsilesional arms of patients with left- and right-hemisphere damage. Bars indicate standard error of mean.

Adapted, by permission, from S.Y. Schaefer, K.Y. Haaland, and R.L. Sainburg, 2007, "Ipsilesional motor deficits following stroke reflect hemispheric specializations for movement control," Brain 130(Pt 8): 2146-2158. © R.L. Sainburg.

Though right-hemisphere damage resulted in larger errors than those demonstrated by control subjects, left-hemisphere damage resulted in smaller errors. This improvement in select features of performance in patients with stroke suggests that unilateral brain damage may relieve the intact hemisphere from competitive processes previously imposed by the contralateral hemisphere. Note that such interhemispheric competition is a hallmark of disconnection syndrome, as revealed by Gazzaniga (1998) in his research on split-brain patients.

Though neither patient group differed from controls in terms of movement speed, the mechanisms by which speed was specified, through modulation of torque amplitude or torque duration, were differentially affected by left- and right-hemisphere damage. Normally when subjects make movements to a range of distances, movement speed scales with movement distance and peak joint torque scales with movement speed. Because peak torque tends to occur in the first 50 to 100 ms of movement, it is thought to reflect planning mechanisms. Schaefer and colleagues (2007) asked whether patients with left- and right-hemisphere damage show normal planning of movement distance through scaling of peak joint torque. Interestingly, peak joint torque was scaled to movement speed only in patients with right-hemisphere damage. Patients with left-hemisphere damage scaled movement speed by altering torque duration across target amplitudes. Thus, planning of movement distance was intact only when the left hemisphere was intact, a finding consistent with the hypothesis that this system is better adapted for controlling dynamic parameters that determine trajectory features. In summary, ipsilesional deficits in patients with stroke are differentially affected by unilateral stroke in a manner consistent with the idea that each hemisphere is better adapted for controlling certain aspects of movement. Furthermore, these findings support the hypothesis that both hemispheres are necessary for accurate unilateral arm control.

Conclusions

Gazzaniga's (1998) seminal research on disconnection syndrome in split-brain patients provided a robust model for understanding neural lateralization. This research showed that each hemisphere has advantages for different but often complementary functions. Gazzaniga proposed that the advantage of such lateralization might be to reduce redundancy of neural circuits, thereby allowing each hemisphere more neural substrate for a reduced number of functions. Unfortunately, research on motor lateralization, or handedness, has appeared at odds with this model. As a result, handedness has been either attributed to culturally derived preferences or described as an artifact of lateralization in language. However, strong cultural biases against left-handedness, combined with concrete evidence for genetic determinants for handedness, diminish the probability that culture plays a strong role in determining motor lateralization. The idea that handedness is an artifact of lateralization in the language system is also not a viable explanation because of evidence against a strong correlation between hand dominance and language dominance as well as because of the recent identification of handedness in nonhuman primates. Instead, handedness, like other neurobehavioral lateralizations, probably emerged during the course of evolutionary development as an adaptive mechanism to support more complex neurobehavioral functions.

This model of lateralization predicts that each cerebral hemisphere has become specialized for different neurobehavioral functions during the course of evolutionary development. However, many early attempts to identify the specific neurobehavioral processes that might underlie handedness have been elusive and controversial. Most of these studies unsuccessfully endeavored to associate hemisphere specialization with either motor planning or error correction. This endeavor was based on early serial models of motor control. More current models, such as optimal feedback control, propose that during a movement task-relevant goals are continuously tracked by modifying control signals relative to specific cost functions. Recent experimental evidence suggests that the differences between the hemisphere–limb systems might be best understood from this perspective. The two hemisphere–limb systems may have become specialized for stabilizing different aspects of movement: The dominant system appears to adopt cost functions related to dynamic parameters such as energy expenditure and trajectory shape, and the nondominant system is better adapted for achieving and maintaining static positions.

The idea that each hemisphere–limb system might be differentially tuned to stabilize specific aspects of task performance has been supported by experimental evidence that associates the dominant system with more efficient and accurate control over the effects of limb and task dynamics and the nondominant system with more stable and accurate control of steady-state position through modulation of limb impedance. This hypothesis was recently tested in studies of adaptation to novel mechanical environments. The studies confirmed that each limb employed fundamentally different adaptation mechanisms. Whereas the dominant system progressively developed more complete anticipation of the direction and magnitude of applied forces, the nondominant system progressively modified limb impedance in a non-direction-specific manner. Taken together, the studies described in this chapter provide evidence that each hemisphere has become specialized for different but complementary aspects of motor control.

This hypothesis suggests that the hemispheres might cooperate in controlling unilateral movements, an idea consistent with recent evidence for ipsilateral motor and premotor cortex contributions to arm movement. This idea leads to specific predictions for unilateral sensorimotor stroke: Damage to the left and right hemisphere should result in distinct deficits that depend on the side of the lesion and that are expressed in the ipsilesional limb. Studies of ipsilesional motor function in patients with stroke have indeed indicated that ipsilesional deficits are differentially affected by unilateral stroke in a manner consistent with our hypothesis. These findings not only support the idea that both hemispheres are necessary for accurate unilateral arm control but also indicate that there are different but complementary roles for the two hemispheres. Altogether, the evidence provided in this chapter indicates that handedness is not unique among neurobehavioral lateralizations. Instead, handedness reflects the same type of hemispheric separation of function that has been demonstrated for other systems. Thus, it is likely that handedness evolved as requirements for more dexterous and differentiated arm function arose, which was probably related to the emergence of tool use.

Future Directions

A number of important questions regarding motor lateralization remain unanswered. First, little research has examined the role of manual asymmetries in bilateral tasks. Although some studies have suggested a significant effect of handedness on coordination (Swinnen et al., 1998; Treffner & Turvey, 1996; Viviani et al., 1998; Westergaard, 1993), other research suggests that coordination patterns become more symmetric in bilateral movements, leading to speculation that such movements employ a single synergy for both arms (Domkin, Laczko, Jaric, Johansson, & Latash, 2002; Kelso, Southard, & Goodman, 1979a, 1979b). If bilateral movements reduce interlimb differences in coordination, the nature of the resulting coordination could provide critical information about the contribution of each limb's controller. For example, the nondominant arm becoming better able to adapt to novel dynamic conditions would suggest exploitation of its ipsilateral hemisphere during bilateral movements. Such findings could be important in designing rehabilitation protocols for patients with hemiparesis due to stroke, and a number of studies have attempted to exploit this idea in stroke rehabilitation (Cauraugh & Summers, 2005; Harris-Love, McCombe Waller, & Whitall, 2005; Whitall, McCombe Waller, Silver, & Macko, 2000). However, it remains unclear whether asymmetries in performance, measured by careful kinematic and kinetic analysis, are reduced during bilateral movements.

Another important area of investigation that has clinical implications concerns the reversal of handedness through practice. The studies of patients with stroke reviewed in this chapter indicate that the nondominant arm of such patients does not become an effective dominant controller even after years of practice as the major or even sole manipulator. However, in the case of stroke, the control system has been damaged. It remains unknown whether it is possible to reverse handedness through extensive practice with an intact nervous system. Patients with unilateral hand and arm amputations might provide a critical test for this question. Patients with dominant-arm amputations would most likely use the remaining intact arm for dominant-arm functions, even when using a prosthesis. A question of particular interest is whether such intense practice might increase the neural activation of the contralateral hemisphere (previously nondominant) or whether such practice draws more extensively on the ipsilateral hemisphere (previously dominant). In either case, careful kinematic and kinetic analysis of arm coordination over the months and years following amputation might reveal whether dominance can be reversed through practice.

Finally, the question of why a particular arm becomes specialized for certain features of performance remains puzzling. There is no a priori reason to assume that hemispheric lateralization should result in motor asymmetry. Because of extensive bilateral connectivity between the hemispheres, it is plausible that each hemisphere could be equally adept at controlling both the contralateral and ipsilateral arms. In addition, it would appear functionally advantageous to be able to use either arm for any function. Throwing and hitting with the left and right arms could be a great advantage in battle, as well as in sport. The fact that hemispheric specialization appears to lead to asymmetry in movement control suggests that the more extensive and direct sensorimotor connectivity of each hemisphere to its contralateral limb confers essential elements necessary for handedness. In turn, this suggests that lateralization might be reflected in corticospinal, spinothalamocortical, and brain stem–spinal connections. Further research into the physiological asymmetries associated with handedness might help determine why hemispheric asymmetry for motor control leads to arm asymmetry in motor coordination.

CHAPTER 13

Visual Illusions and Action

DAVID A. WESTWOOD

Visual illusions have a rich heritage in experimental and popular psychology. Most people can relate to the concept of an illusion and are familiar with the idea that a person can be tricked into seeing things in a way that differs from the objective reality. Most likely we have all participated in a conversation that begins with, "Look at these two objects and tell me which one is larger," and invariably ends with, "In reality, the two objects are exactly the same size!" Of course, illusions are more than just an interesting parlor trick or conversation starter. The study of illusions holds the promise of unlocking the nature of human perception and conscious awareness, since the very existence of an illusion implies that the perceptual system is influenced by more than just the patterns of stimulus energy that make contact with its array of sensory receptors. Indeed, it is well established that perception, defined for the purpose of this chapter as conscious interpretation of a sensory event, is influenced by both bottom-up (afferent input) and top-down (cognitive) sources of information.

The purpose of this chapter is not to review the rich and complex history of the scientific study of perceptual illusions but to focus on a more recent trend in which illusions are used as a tool to study the sensory processing associated with movement control. In recent years, illusions have been used extensively to study the relationship between perception and action in research motivated by Goodale and Milner's (1992) proposal that the visual control of action is mediated by a system that is separate from the one responsible for visual perception. This chapter discusses the rationale for studying the effects of visual illusions on action and organizes key findings from the literature into coherent themes. It then provides a critical analysis of the logic behind using visual illusions in the study of motor control and makes some suggestions for future research in the field.

Historical Context: Perception and Action

The control of movement depends critically on sensory information. From the simplest reflexes to the most complex voluntary actions, the control of body movements is informed by afferent information about the external environment and the body. Indeed, a comprehensive understanding of the afferent system is not possible without taking into consideration an organism's capacity for movement. After all, a sophisticated afferent system would not have evolved if it did not have direct, or indirect, influence on behaviors leading to survival or reproductive success.

Few would disagree with the idea that afferent information is important for both perception and movement control. However, few systematic attempts have been made to understand the similarities and differences between afferent processing involved in perception and movement control. A quick perusal of many introductory textbooks in cognitive or perceptual psychology or in human movement control gives the impression that the two forms of afferent processing are essentially the same. In other words, the afferent information necessary for the control of movement is provided by the perceptual system; an organism's perception guides its action.

The discussion about perception and action in this chapter is focused on the control of voluntary, rather than reflexive, movements. Few would suggest that the afferent processing in a reflex control circuit, which takes place at the spinal or supraspinal level, is perceptual. Perception—the conscious interpretation of a sensory event—is a product of cortical processing, and the afferent information in a reflex control pathway elicits an efferent response well before the afferent signal reaches the cortex. Unlike reflex control circuits, however, the control of voluntary movement requires cortical processing. It is reasonable to suppose that at this level of control a single afferent processing system might be sufficient for perceptual and motor functions, since this would be an efficient use of cortical resources. Indeed, it is possible to imagine that having separate afferent processing systems for perception and action would be maladaptive because the two systems could interpret the same event in different ways, leading to incongruent or unwanted behaviors.

Consider the example of a worker collecting chocolate bars from a conveyor belt and stacking them into cartons. The worker is engaged in both a perceptual task and a motor task. The perceptual task requires the individual to discriminate the target item, which is the chocolate bar, from the nontarget items such as the conveyor belt, the coworkers, and the carton. The motor task requires the worker to use the upper limbs to move the target item from its original location to a new location in a timely manner.

In one respect, the two tasks require different afferent information. Spatial information is necessary for the motor task but not for the perceptual discrimination task. Likewise, color information may be necessary for the perceptual discrimination task but not for the motor task. To the extent that different types of information are necessary for the two tasks, it seems clear that separate afferent systems are required for perception and action, since it is well established that sensory processing in the cortex is organized into feature-specific modules (Sincich & Horton, 2005).

However, in many cases perceptual and motor tasks require the same information. For example, the size of the object is relevant for the perceptual and motor tasks alike, since this information is used to distinguish the target object from many other competing objects in the environment (i.e., the chocolate bar is smaller than a conveyor belt and smaller than a carton), and size information is also necessary to shape the hand as it grasps and manipulates the object. In cases where perception and action require the same information, independent afferent analysis systems seem unnecessary. In other words, a single computation of object size might be sufficient to allow the worker to discriminate a large object from a small object and to scale an action such as grasping to the size of a target object.

Though the notion that perception and action are guided by a common afferent processing system is intuitively appealing, a number of examples suggest that this is not so. The work of Weiskrantz and colleagues (Weiskrantz, Warrington, Sanders, & Marshall, 1974) on cortical blindness showed that conscious perception of a stimulus is not necessary to make a movement to that stimulus. Patients with a lesion in V1 fail to perceive or otherwise acknowledge a stimulus located in the affected region of visual space but nevertheless retain some ability to point or saccade accurately toward the stimulus when encouraged to make an attempt; this phenomenon is commonly referred to as *blindsight*. The predominant explanation for blindsight holds that conscious perception is mediated by cortical visual areas that receive afferent input from V1, and so conscious perception is disrupted when a lesion is located in that area. However, the control of arm and eye movements can be mediated by subcortical regions (e.g., the SC) or cortical regions (e.g., the PPC via the tectopulvinar projection system) that do not receive input from V1, so these functions remain intact following a lesion to that area. Although intriguing, this line of evidence does not necessarily indicate that the control of voluntary movement is separate from conscious perception. First, the movements of patients with blindsight are less accurate than those of control participants, which suggests that conscious perception might contribute to the control of movement in the intact nervous system. Second, the movements of patients with blindsight can hardly be considered voluntary, since these patients do not spontaneously move toward targets located in the affected region of space; indeed, they require considerable encouragement to do so.

The work of Melvyn Goodale and David Milner with patient D.F., who demonstrated visual form agnosia, provided more convincing evidence that the control of voluntary movement does not depend on conscious perception (Goodale, Milner, Jakobson, & Carey, 1991). D.F. experienced bilateral damage to cortical tissue at the junction of the occipital and temporal lobes subsequent to an anoxic episode, an event which left her with an apperceptive visual agnosia. D.F. was unable to recognize black-and-white drawings of common objects, and she could not judge whether two objects were the same or different. Her performance improved dramatically when texture and color were added to the images, a finding suggesting that her apperceptive agnosia was largely restricted to the perception of form (i.e., shape; Milner et al., 1991; see also chapter 14).

Despite the fact that D.F. could not judge or otherwise indicate the orientation of a high-contrast, tilted slots, she showed a remarkable ability to reach out and place wooden cards into those slots (Goodale et al., 1991). A kinematic analysis of her reaching movements showed that the orientation of the card was correlated with the orientation of the target slot very early in the movement trajectory, well before the card made physical contact with the slot, and well before visual feedback could be used to align the card to the slot as the distance between the two was reduced. In other words, D.F.'s inability to perceive the orientation of the slot had no demonstrable effect on her ability to scale her movement to the orientation of the slot. Unlike patients with blindsight, D.F. did not require encouragement to interact with objects in the surrounding environment, suggesting that her movements were truly voluntary. Also unlike patients with blindsight, D.F.'s movements were indistinguishable from those of control participants, suggesting no visuomotor impairment.

A common interpretation of D.F.'s performance holds that the visual control of voluntary movement is guided by a dedicated visuomotor system located in the PPC, which is located in the dorsal visual stream. This system transforms afferent visual input from the target stimulus into motor commands necessary to implement the intended action. Because D.F.'s lesion was located at the occipitotemporal junction, which is in the ventral visual stream, her visuomotor abilities were not compromised. However, her perceptual abilities were disrupted because the ventral stream is home to the visual systems that support the perception and recognition of objects.

This interpretation is supported by evidence from patients with optic ataxia due to bilateral lesions to the PPC. Optic ataxia is characterized by an inability to make accurate movements to visible targets despite otherwise normal visual perception and motor capacity (Perenin & Vighetto, 1988). Patients with optic ataxia can discriminate among objects of different sizes and shapes but cannot use size or shape information to control accurate reaching or grasping actions toward those objects. In many ways, patients with optic ataxia are the mirror image of patient D.F., since these patients have intact perceptual abilities but impaired visuomotor abilities. In an elegant study directly contrasting patient D.F., who had visual form agnosia, and patient R.V., who had optic ataxia, Goodale and colleagues

(Goodale, Meenan, et al., 1994) showed that D.F. grasped irregularly shaped objects by placing her fingers at appropriate and stable positions on the object surface, whereas R.V. showed a more random distribution of finger contact positions. In a perceptual discrimination task, R.V. was able to differentiate among objects of different shapes, whereas D.F. was unable to do so. These observations demonstrate a striking double dissociation between the perception of object form and the ability to interact with objects on the basis of their form, suggesting that the two functions are independent even though both depend upon the same afferent information.

Milner and Goodale (1995) gathered data from a variety of experimental paradigms supporting the idea that the dorsal visual stream is responsible for the visual control of action and the ventral visual stream is responsible for visual perception. According to their idea, the dorsal and ventral streams receive similar visual inputs from V1, but the two streams transform this information in different ways. The dorsal stream transforms afferent information from the target stimulus into voluntary motor commands, preserving the absolute metrics of the target so that movement will be accurate. The ventral stream transforms afferent target information into an abstract format that is suitable for accessing stored object representations from long-term memory. Absolute metrics are undesirable for this purpose because objects must be recognized across a broad spectrum of conditions in which the exact size, location, shape, luminance, and color of the particular exemplar vary considerably (Goodale & Humphrey, 1998). Milner and Goodale's two–visual streams hypothesis generated a tremendous amount of research designed to address the relationship between conscious visual perception and the control of action, leading to a number of important insights into the operating characteristics of the motor control system.

Visual Illusions as a Tool for Studying Perception and Action in the Intact Brain

The strongest evidence in favor of Goodale and Milner's (1992) two–visual streams hypothesis came from patients with lesions in the dorsal or ventral streams. At the time of the publication of *The Visual Brain in Action* (Milner & Goodale, 1995), it was not clear that the two–visual streams hypothesis had much relevance for the control of behavior in individuals with intact brains, since the two visual streams are heavily interconnected. Dissociations between action and perception in healthy participants had been reported, but it was not clear that these dissociations were related to the dorsal and ventral stream distinction.

For example, Goodale, Pelisson, and Prablanc (1986) found that healthy participants could adjust their reaching movements in response to a change in target location that occurred during a concurrent saccadic eye movement, even though the participants were unaware that the target had moved. Similarly to the case of blindsight described earlier, this finding of Goodale and colleagues is consistent with the idea that conscious perception of a target's features is not necessary to guide an accurate movement to that target. Whereas this conclusion agrees with the main tenet of the two–visual streams hypothesis, the result could be explained by a distinction between cortical and subcortical processing, in which the conscious awareness of target location requires cortical processing that depends on input from V1, whereas the control of arm movements can be mediated by subcortical or cortical systems that do not receive input from V1. In other words, the study by Goodale and colleagues supports the idea that some control of action can occur without conscious perception of the target's features (i.e., like a reflex), but it does not indicate that the same object feature is processed by different systems depending on whether the task is to perceive the object or interact with it.

Visual illusions provide a potentially useful tool for studying the relationship between perception and action in the intact nervous system because these stimulus configurations influence the individual's conscious perceptual experience without altering the physical characteristics of the target. This is an attractive characteristic because, as discussed earlier, it is clear that perception and action each depend on afferent information about the target object. Simply changing the physical characteristics of the target would therefore affect both perception and action, regardless of whether the two functions are mediated by a single system or two different systems. However, changing the properties of the context surrounding the target stimulus—which is what is done in visual illusions—could affect perceptual and motor functions differently if the functions depend on distinct systems that utilize different afferent processing mechanisms. If perception and action are mediated by a single afferent processing system, then illusions should affect perception and action equally.

Wong and Mack (1981) appear to be the first authors to study the effects of a visual illusion on motor behavior. For this study, participants viewed a Duncker illusion, in which a stable visual target is presented within an oscillating frame, creating the perceptual illusion that the target rather than the frame is oscillating. Participants could accurately saccade to the target stimulus when it remained visible, suggesting that the oculomotor system was not influenced by the illusion. Interestingly, when the stimulus was extinguished after the saccade and the participant was asked to look back to the original starting location, the amplitudes of the resulting movements reflected the perceptual illusion that the target rather than the background frame had moved. Although Wong and Mack did not interpret their results in terms of a dissociation between perception and action, the data from the target-visible condition are consistent with Goodale and Milner's two–visual streams hypothesis. Whereas the previously described results of Goodale and colleagues (1986) showed that sensorimotor processing of target location can occur without perceptual awareness of the sensory event, the data of Wong and Mack suggest that qualitatively different representations of target location can exist simultaneously in the sensorimotor and perceptual systems. This finding is consistent with the two–visual streams hypothesis.

In the first study using a visual illusion specifically to address the relationship between perception and action, Aglioti, DeSouza, and Goodale (1995) asked participants to view an Ebbinghaus illusion in which two plastic discs were placed within adjacent annuli composed of either large or small two-dimensional circles. In half of the trials the two discs were the same physical size, which leads to a perceptual illusion that the disc in the annulus of small circles is larger than the disk in the annulus of large circles. In the other half of the trials the disc in the annulus of large circles was physically larger than the disc in the annulus of small circles, so that the two target discs were judged to be of similar sizes. The positions of the two annuli were alternated so that the annulus of small circles was on the left side and right side an equal number of times. Participants were instrumented with infrared-emitting diodes so that the spatial locations of the index finger, thumb, and hand could be tracked as the discs were grasped. To confirm that the perceptual illusion was effective, participants were instructed to pick up the disc in the left annulus if the two discs were judged to be equal in size and to pick up the disc in the right annulus if the two discs were judged to be different in size. The choice of disc thus indicated the participant's perceptual judgment of the relative sizes of the two discs. The maximum separation achieved between the index finger and thumb (i.e., the maximum grip aperture) during the grasping movement was calculated and analyzed to characterize the effect of the annuli on the grasping action.

Participants' perceptual judgments were consistently affected by the illusion, as indicated by which disc they picked up. However, when the two discs were of different sizes, maximum grip aperture was different for the disc in the small annulus and the disc in the large annulus, even though the perceptual experience in this case was that the discs were the same size. In other words, the size of the grasp was scaled to the actual size, and not the perceived size, of the target disc. Likewise, maximum grip apertures were similar for the discs in the small and large annuli when those discs were the same physical size, even though the perception in this case was that the disc in the small annulus was larger than the disc in the large annulus.

Aglioti and coworkers (1995) suggested that object size is processed separately for perception and action, an idea consistent with Goodale and Milner's (1992) proposal that these two functions are mediated by separate systems that utilize different afferent processing mechanisms. The action system, which presumably resides in the dorsal visual stream, computes the exact size of the target disc regardless of the sizes of the circles in the surrounding annulus because the circles in the annulus are irrelevant for the production of an accurate grasping posture. The perceptual system, which presumably resides in the ventral visual stream, represents the size of the target object in relation to the sizes of the circles in the surrounding annulus because the contextual information surrounding the object of interest is usually relevant for understanding its nature and identity. Thus the results of Aglioti and colleagues are often held up as evidence in favor of Goodale and Milner's proposal that perceptual and motor aspects of vision are mediated by distinct processing systems.

Aglioti and colleagues' interesting finding led many to believe that visual illusions—specifically, pictorial illusions—would be a useful tool for exploring the relationship between conscious perception and the control of action in individuals with intact visual and neurological systems. In the few years since its publication, Aglioti and colleagues' 1995 study has been cited an incredible 265 times. It is clearly beyond the scope of this chapter to discuss and synthesize all the findings from this massive body of literature; several review articles have already been written on the topic (Bruno, Bernardis, & Gentilucci, 2008; Carey, 2001; Franz, 2001; Smeets & Brenner, 2006). Instead, this chapter selectively discusses interesting themes and issues that have emerged from the study of visual illusions and action and draws attention to key theoretical and methodological issues that should be kept in mind when reading, or indeed contributing to, this literature.

Illusions and Action: Emerging Themes and Issues

There are many themes and issues that could be discussed in this area, but for this section I have chosen a few that I consider to be of particular interest for the study of human sensorimotor control. Broadly speaking, the themes can be divided into those that are related to the nature of the illusion and its underlying mechanisms, and those that are more closely related to the characteristics of the movement that is directed toward the stimulus array.

Illusion Modality

Some illusions operate in a single sensory modality, such as vision, audition, or somatosensation. Most of the illusions that have been studied in the context of perception and action are unimodal and visual, which is not surprising for a number of reasons. First of all, the psychophysics of visual illusions, versus illusions in other sensory modalities, have been studied in great detail and are reasonably well understood. Second, vision is arguably the most important source of afferent information for the control of movement because it provides spatially and temporally precise information about objects that are at a distance from the body. Third, theoretical interest in the relationship between perception and action has been spurred on by evidence derived from studies of the visual system that converge on the idea that there are significant differences between perception and action in the visual domain. Similar evidence from other sensory systems is scarce.

Interestingly, a few studies have investigated unimodal illusions in the auditory and somatosensory domains. Bridgeman, Aiken, Allen, and Maresh (1997) employed an auditory version of a Roelofs illusion in which the perceived location of an auditory event was altered by the relative location of an auditory background. In this study, participants' verbal judgments of sound location and the accuracy of their open-loop pointing movements were equally affected by the illusion. These findings led the authors to suggest that, in contrast to the apparent situation in the visual domain, the perceptual and sensorimotor systems use a common auditory representation of location.

Westwood and Goodale (2003a) studied a haptic variation of a size-contrast illusion in which participants used their left hand to feel an unseen flanker and target object in sequence and then indicated the size of the target object by adjusting the distance between their right index finger and thumb. The haptic sense is not exclusively somatosensory, since it requires the active control of the body part that experiences somatosensory feedback from the object of interest. In any case, perceptual judgments were affected by the relative size of the flanking object, such that a larger flanker resulted in a smaller size judgment. However, when the right hand was used to reach out and grasp the target object, the size of the peak grip aperture was not affected by the size of the flanking object. This finding suggests that there is a common processing principle in the visual and somatosensory domains, whereby the sensorimotor system computes the metrics of the target object without regard for other objects in the surrounding context, whereas the perceptual system computes the metrics of the target object in relation to other objects in the nearby environment.

The size–weight illusion is an interesting and extremely robust phenomenon that occurs when a person sequentially lifts two objects with equal masses but different sizes (Murray, Ellis, Bandomir, & Ross, 1999). Participants invariably report that the smaller object feels heavier than the larger object, even after lifting the objects many times. This illusion is multimodal in that it depends on visual information, somatosensory information, and proprioceptive information (i.e., sensory feedback about the consequence of the lifting attempt is available from stretch receptors in the engaged muscle groups). The size–weight illusion is an unusual case in which to explore the relationship between perception and action because the perceptual effect emerges only when the individual interacts with the target stimuli.

Flanagan and Beltzner (2000) measured the forces that participants used to grasp and lift two objects in a classic size–weight illusion and found that on the first lifting attempt participants used too much force to manipulate the large object and too little force to lift the small object. However, the forces used for subsequent lifting attempts were identical for the two objects, suggesting that the sensorimotor system obtained, and indeed retained, accurate information about object mass from the initial lifts. Nevertheless, participants continued to report that the smaller object felt heavier than the larger object, indicating a curious dissociation between perception and action. In an effort to rule out the possibility that participants simply regress to a common motor program when lifting objects that are perceived to be of similar heaviness, Grandy and Westwood (2006) studied a variation of the size–weight illusion in which a smaller object was perceived to be heavier than a larger object when in fact the larger object had significantly more mass than the smaller object. In this study, we showed that the perceptual and sensorimotor systems had opposite responses to the two objects; participants used significantly greater forces to lift the large object despite the fact that they continued to report that the small object felt heavier. We suggested that the perceptual experience of heaviness is an amalgamation of sensory and cognitive cues about both mass and density, since both characteristics are relevant to a person's understanding of the material properties of that object and thus the object's composition and identity. In contrast, the sensorimotor system scales manipulation forces to the mass of the object, regardless of its density, since only the mass of the object is relevant for this task. In a finding consistent with this hypothesis, we (White & Westwood, 2009) have recently observed that the perceptual size–weight illusion is not eliminated when participants are trained to correctly anticipate the density of the large and small objects through the use of a color–density associative learning session in which the actual target objects are never seen or manipulated. In other words, we eliminated the mismatch between expectation and feedback that typically occurs with the initial lifting attempt in the size–weight illusion, in which the densities of the large and small objects are discovered to be dramatically different than expected. Even though we eliminated this initial surprise, the densities of the two objects continued to influence participants' judgments of heaviness—presumably because density is an integral component of the perceptual experience of object heaviness.

Locus of the Illusory Effect

Illusions occur because the inducing stimulus influences the processing of information at some level of the sensory system. Thus illusions can originate at any stage of processing, from the sensory receptor all the way through to the sensory association areas in the cerebral cortex. Illusions that affect an early stage of sensory processing should, in principle, affect all subsequent components of the sensory (or motor) system that receive input from that process. The implication of this notion for the two–visual streams hypothesis is relatively straightforward: Illusions that influence sensory processes that occur before the separation of the perceptual and sensorimotor pathways (i.e., between the retina and V1) should affect perceptual judgments and motor responses alike, whereas illusions that affect processing in only one of the two pathways should affect only the corresponding behavior (perceptual judgments in the case of the ventral stream and motor responses in the case of the dorsal stream).

In an elegant set of experiments motivated by this idea, Dyde and Milner (2001) studied the effects of two different categories of orientation illusion on perception and action. In the simultaneous tilt illusion (STI), a target grating with a specific orientation is presented against a background grating that is rotated in a clockwise or counterclockwise direction relative to the target. There is no physical separation between the boundaries of the two gratings. Stimuli of this type induce the perceptual experience that the grating in the foreground is tilted in the direction opposite to that of the background grating. It has been suggested that the STI arises from local processing that occurs early in the visual system, possibly in V1 (Sengpiel, Sen, & Blakemore, 1997). Consistent with the prediction that illusions arising from early stages of visual processing affect later processing in both the ventral and the dorsal streams—and thus penetrate action and perception systems alike—it was found that the STI affected not only judgments of line orientation but also hand orientation as participants reached out to stamp the target grating with a wooden card. Dyde and Milner also studied a rod-and-frame tilt illusion (RFI). In the RFI, a single line with a specific orientation is presented within a much larger rectangular frame that is rotated in a clockwise or counterclockwise direction relative to the target, creating the perceptual illusion that the target is tilted slightly away from the direction of the frame. Unlike the STI, the RFI occurs late in visual processing, probably within the ventral stream, because it requires the decomposition of a complex stimulus into figure and ground elements (Witkin & Asch, 1947). It was predicted that the RFI, like other types of pictorial illusions in which geometrical cues in the background create a false sense of depth or distance, would not affect motor responses because the illusory effect occurs in the ventral stream whereas the action is guided by the dorsal stream. This prediction was borne out, since participants' judgments of line orientation were affected but the orientation of the hand during the posting action was not.

Dyde and Milner's (2001) study provides a crucial caveat to the notion that action systems should resist perceptual illusions, since this prediction is based on the assumption that the locus of the perceptual illusion is within the ventral stream, whereas the control of action is within the dorsal stream. Illusions that originate early in the visual system should penetrate the control of action, since the dorsal stream receives its inputs from these earlier stages of processing. Indeed, illusions that occur in visual areas located in the dorsal stream could well exert a greater influence on action systems than on perceptual systems. Yamagishi, Anderson, and Ashida

(2001) provided some preliminary support for this possibility, showing that the effect of a motion–position illusion—which likely influences processing in the motion-sensitive MT area located in the dorsal visual stream—was three times greater for a visuomotor response compared with a perceptual judgment of stimulus location. However, the effects of the illusion were equal for perception and action when a delay was introduced between the offset of the stimulus and the onset of the response.

The idea that illusions can influence early versus late stages of visual processing is relevant when considering the results of the many studies using the Müller-Lyer figure, or variations thereof, to examine the link between perception and action. A common explanation of the Müller-Lyer illusion is that the inducing arrows are interpreted as geometric perspective cues that signal a protruding or recessed edge in a rectilinear, or built, environment. Thus the arrows create a false impression of depth and a corresponding misperception of stimulus size (Coren & Porac, 1984). According to this notion, the illusory effect of the Müller-Lyer stimulus arises from processing that occurs within the ventral stream, since the interpretation of geometric cues requires access to previous knowledge about the relationship between figural scene elements and depth. However, it is also possible that the inducing arrows create a center-of-mass effect in early stages of visual processing. That is, the end of the target line segment is not disambiguated from the inducing arrow, resulting in a net spatial representation of the vertex region that is shifted in the direction of the arrow. Such an early center-of-mass effect would be expected to penetrate all subsequent stages of visual processing, thus influencing both the ventral and dorsal streams. If these arguments are correct, different predictions could be made about the expected effects of the Müller-Lyer figure; the geometric properties would not be expected to influence actions, whereas the center-of-mass properties would.

Interestingly, many studies using Müller-Lyer figures find small but significant effects of arrow orientation on motor responses, although these effects are typically smaller than those seen in perceptual judgments (e.g., Binsted & Elliott, 1999; Daprati & Gentilucci, 1997; Elliott & Lee, 1995; Gentilucci, Chieffi, Daprati, Saetti, & Toni, 1996; Westwood, Heath, & Roy, 2000; Westwood, McEachern, & Roy, 2001). As discussed earlier, these effects could be attributed to the influence of the Müller-Lyer illusion on early stages of visual processing that penetrate both the dorsal and ventral streams. This possibility is supported by a study that used the hoops version of the Müller-Lyer figure, in which the arrows are replaced with hollow circles, thus eliminating (or at least minimizing) the illusion's geometric property while preserving its center-of-mass property (Wraga, Creem, & Proffitt, 2000). The results of the study—which looked at stepping behavior—are consistent with a similar study that used the conventional form of the Müller-Lyer illusion (e.g., McCarville & Westwood, 2006). This suggests that the center-of-mass property of the figure may be at the root of the effects on motor behavior. Since the two forms of the illusion have not been compared directly in a single study, further work in this area is necessary. In any case, the results of studies using Müller-Lyer figures should be interpreted with appropriate caution.

Object Features Affected by Illusion

There are a number of object features that are relevant for both perception and action, including size, shape, motion, orientation, and location, all of which are therefore logical candidates for illusory manipulation. Generally speaking, most studies of illusions and action have tended to employ displays affecting the perception of stimulus location or stimulus size.

Studies looking at pointing movements (gesturing toward the target), reaching movements (reaching out to physically touch the target), and saccadic eye movements have tended to use illusions of target location, although Lee and van Donkelaar (2002) and van Donkelaar (1999) have used a size-contrast illusion to study reaching movements. Rod-and-frame (also known as *Roelofs)* configurations appear to be ideal for this type of study because they affect the perceptual interpretation of stimulus location, and the actions in question are guided by information about stimulus location. However, a number of studies on pointing, reaching, and saccadic eye movements have used Müller-Lyer figures in which the target of the movement is one of the vertices where the primary line segment intersects the inducing arrowhead. Unlike the Roelofs illusion, however, the Müller-Lyer figure alters the perception of the length of the primary line segment rather than the location of the vertices (Glazebrook et al., 2005; Mack, Heuer, Villardi, & Chambers, 1985). This may render the Müller-Lyer stimulus unsuitable for direct comparisons between perception and pointing, reaching, and saccades, since these actions are guided by location rather than extent information. The situation becomes even more complex in studies that use disembodied Müller-Lyer figures in which there is no primary line segment but simply a point target embedded within an arrowhead pointing toward or away from the movement's starting location (e.g., Bernardis, Knox, & Bruno, 2005; Binsted, Chua, Helsen, & Elliott, 2001; Thompson & Westwood, 2007). Although these studies confirmed that perceptual judgments of stimulus location are affected in the direction predicted by a standard interpretation of the Müller-Lyer stimulus, extensive psychophysical work has not been carried out.

Many studies of illusions and action have used grasping as the behavior of interest. Based on Jeannerod's (1986) important work showing that the peak grip aperture (i.e., the maximal separation between the index finger and the thumb during an object-directed grasping movement) is tightly correlated with the size of the target stimulus, many studies have sought to determine if perceptual size illusions influence grip aperture during prehension. An attractive feature of this approach is that peak grip aperture occurs during the course of the grasping action, before the hand makes physical contact with the target object. Therefore, the measure is relatively uncontaminated by the veridical somatosensory feedback that occurs at the completion of the action. Another appealing feature of grasping is that it is a natural action, in that humans often use the hand to pick up and manipulate objects, whereas some other types of actions, such as reaching to touch a target or pointing to a target, are somewhat unnatural or uncommon.

Most studies of illusions and grasping have used three-dimensional target objects embedded within a two-dimensional size-contrast illusion, such as the Ebbinghaus illusion or Titchener circles, or a two-dimensional Müller-Lyer display. These illusions appear justifiable since it is generally accepted that they affect the perception of object size or length, which is the object feature thought to be used to regulate the size of the grasping aperture (although see Smeets & Brenner, 1999, for an alternative point of view). More recently, in response to concerns that traditional size-contrast illusions may induce obstacle-avoidance strategies (discussed further later in this chapter), some authors have begun using modified size-contrast displays in which a target object is presented beside a single flanking object (e.g., Hu & Goodale, 2000; Westwood & Goodale, 2003b). Whereas these studies have taken steps to demonstrate that the modified displays create the expected effects on size perception, additional psychophysical work is desirable to more clearly establish the mechanisms of the underlying perceptual effect.

Some studies of grasping have used orientation illusions (e.g., Dyde & Milner, 2001; Glover & Dixon, 2001a, 2001b) and measured the orientation of the grasping digits rather than the grip aperture. Again, this strategy appears defensible given that the illusions affect the perception of orientation, and orientation information is presumably required to control the posture of the grasping hand. Potentially problematic are those studies that have required participants to pretend to grasp two-dimensional objects embedded within various pictorial illusions (e.g., Bruno & Bernardis, 2002; Vishton, Rea, Cutting, & Nuñez, 1999). Participants may adopt a very different approach to the control of a pretend grasping movement compared with a true grasping movement (Westwood, Chapman, & Roy, 2000). This change in approach might increase the sensitivity to the perceptual illusion.

Movement Types

As alluded to earlier, humans have an extensive repertoire of movement skills. Of course, movements differ on a number of important dimensions, including the effector system involved (e.g., eye, upper limb, lower limb), the goal of the movement (e.g., to achieve a spatial or temporal outcome or to produce a specific movement pattern), the timescale (e.g., brief, long), and the periodicity (e.g., discrete versus continuous). For the most part, the literature on illusions and action has explored discrete, brief movements that are focused on a spatial goal. The most common movements studied are grasping, reaching, and saccadic eye movements, although there are many studies that look at other types of movements; for example, a number of recent studies have investigated the effects of illusions on lower-limb movements such as stepping (Harris, Weiler, & Westwood, 2009; McCarville & Westwood, 2006; Wraga, Creem, & Proffitt, 2000) and hopping (Glover & Dixon, 2004). The choice of which type of movement to study has been driven by factors ranging from the pragmatic to the theoretical.

Much of the original evidence in support of Goodale and Milner's (1992) model of visual function was based on discrete movements with spatial outcomes, and much of the fundamental neurophysiological research in sensorimotor control has studied these types of movements. Thus it seems appropriate to continue this trend in the illusion domain. The fundamental control principles underlying grasping, reaching, and saccadic eye movements have been studied and characterized extensively at various levels ranging from kinematic description to neurophysiology, the result of which is a rich literature in which to ground the studies of illusions and action. In addition, discrete, rapid movements with spatial outcomes are arguably more stereotyped than other types of movements, which increases the statistical power to detect subtle differences in performance that may be correlated with illusory perceptual experiences. Sophisticated motion-capture systems are available for collecting precise spatial and temporal information from the eyes and limbs, making it a relatively straightforward task to derive kinematic (and in some cases kinetic) indexes of movement performance. Various kinematic indexes have been shown to be correlated tightly with key features of the target object, such as size and location, in rapid, discrete, spatially oriented movements, providing a useful framework for measuring and interpreting psychophysical relationships in the sensorimotor realm. Although the preceding points are all important, they have dramatically restricted the range of actions that have been studied. Few studies have focused on actions that are extended in either time or space beyond a single discrete movement involving one effector system. As a consequence of this narrow focus, we know little about the relevance of the literature on illusions and actions for everyday human behavior, since such behavior incorporates a variety of effector systems and a complex sequence of sensory and motor tasks with a variety of spatial and temporal goals.

It is not possible to succinctly summarize or synthesize the literature on illusions and saccadic, reaching, and grasping movements given the large, and ever-growing, number of studies on each topic. Moreover, there are a large number of methodological issues that must be taken into consideration before reasonable statements can be made about whether a particular type of action is affected by an illusion; some of these issues are discussed later in the chapter. Whereas the first studies in this field began with the relatively simple question of whether perceptual illusions influence action, it has become clear that a simple *yes* or *no* answer is not possible given the number of factors modulating the effects of illusions on action (Bruno & Gentilucci, 2008).

Visual Conditions for Movement

In natural behavior, the targets of our actions often are visible both before and during a movement. As such, visual information can be used to guide action in both a feed-forward and a feedback mode. A number of investigations have examined the role of target visibility in the resistance of action to perceptual illusions, drawing on research showing that the control of action is quite different when the target is removed from view either before or during the response.

It has been known since the early work of Woodworth (1899) that movement accuracy and precision suffer when vision of the target is removed at the onset of the response. This finding paved the way to the widely accepted view that vision of the target or limb during the movement is used to correct errors that occur during movement programming or execution (e.g., Elliott, Helsen, & Chua, 2001). In addition to vision during movement execution, vision of the target before the onset of the response is also important for movement accuracy and precision. For example, Elliott and Madalena (1987) showed that reaches to targets that were removed from view before the onset of the response were less accurate and more variable than were reaches to targets that remained visible, even if the interval between target occlusion and movement onset was as short as 2 s. Westwood, Heath, and Roy (2001) extended Elliott and Madalena's work, showing that movement accuracy and precision deteriorate even if the movement is initiated immediately after the occlusion of the target. This finding suggests that the visuomotor system has no ability to retain accurate target information in memory, although some form of target information is clearly available in memory and accessible to the motor system.

Interestingly, Goodale, Jakobson, and Keillor (1994) found that D.F., a patient with visual form agnosia, could not shape her grip aperture to the size of a target object when she reached to grasp an object 2 s after it had been physically removed, even though her grip scaling was perfectly normal when the target remained present. In light of her known perceptual deficits, Goodale and colleagues proposed that the control of action to remembered objects depends on a perceptual representation of the object that is stored in the ventral stream and that the dorsal stream does not itself retain information about previously viewed targets. Consistent with this idea was the finding by Wong and Mack (1981) that in healthy humans saccades to remembered target stimuli are affected by a Duncker illusion while saccades to visible targets are not.

We have carried out a number of studies (Westwood, Heath, et al., 2000; Westwood, Chapman, et al., 2000; Westwood & Goodale, 2003b; Westwood, McEachern, & Roy, 2001) to determine whether target visibility before movement onset modulates the effects of visual illusions on grasping. Our studies have consistently found that peak grip aperture is more sensitive to pictorial illusions when the target is removed from view before the onset of the response, regardless of whether the target is visible during movement execution. Analogous findings have been obtained by a number of other groups using other types of illusions and other types of movements (e.g., Bridgeman, Peery, & Anand, 1997; Elliott & Lee, 1995; McCarville & Westwood, 2006; Gentilucci, Chieffi, Daprati, Saetti, & Toni, 1996; Hu & Goodale, 2000; Rival, Olivier, Ceyte, & Ferrel, 2003; Wong & Mack, 1981; Yamagishi et al., 2001).

In the most sophisticated of our studies on illusions and target visibility (Westwood & Goodale, 2003b), we used a size-contrast target array that presented rectangular target objects beside larger, smaller, or same-size flanking objects, inducing the perceptual experience that the target object was slightly smaller or larger than its actual size. One group of participants performed in a delay condition in which they viewed the target array for 500 ms, waited through 2,500 ms of complete visual occlusion, and then initiated a grasping movement upon being given an auditory signal. In half of the trials, vision of the target array was restored from the time of the auditory signal until the time of movement initiation (vision trials), and in the other half of the trials vision was not restored at all (occlusion trials). These vision trials and occlusion trials were randomly mixed. Results showed no effect of the flanker size on peak grip aperture in the vision trials but demonstrated a robust effect in the occlusion trials. In addition, an overall larger peak grip aperture was seen in the occlusion trials. A second group of participants took part in a no-delay condition, in which the target array was visible for 500 ms followed immediately by an auditory initiation signal. In half the trials, vision of the array was not occluded until the onset of the grasping movement (vision trials), whereas in the other half of the trials vision was occluded simultaneously with the auditory initiation tone (occlusion trials). Against, these trials were mixed randomly. As in the delay group experiments, the no-delay group studies evidenced no effect of flanker size on peak grip aperture in the vision trials but did demonstrate a robust effect in the occlusion trials. Note that the difference between the vision and occlusion trials was simply the visibility of the target array during the time between response cuing and response initiation (i.e., the RT, or programming phase). In neither type of trial was vision available during the execution of the movement. As such, we proposed that the visuomotor system that mediates the direct transformation of target vision into motor commands operates in real time, at the moment the response is required. If the target is visible at this moment, this system can extract the absolute metrics of the target object (independent of the surrounding visual context) and generate a grasping movement that resists the pictorial illusion. If the target is not visible at this moment, the motor system is forced to access a stored representation of the object that is generated and maintained by the perceptual system. This representation is sensitive to the context in which the target was seen and thus falls prey to the size-contrast illusion. In short, the control of action rests with distinct systems when the target is visible versus occluded at the time of response programming.

The role of target visibility during movement execution in modulating the effects of pictorial illusions is less clear. In Aglioti and colleagues' (1995) original study, vision of the target array was available before and during the grasping movement, leaving the door open to the possibility that online visual feedback available during the response allowed participants to correct for any illusory biases that may have been originally present in their action. However, in a carefully designed follow-up study, Haffenden and Goodale (1998) found no effect of an Ebbinghaus illusion on peak grip aperture even when vision was removed at the onset of the grasping movement. Indeed, Westwood and Goodale (2003b) found no effect of a size-contrast illusion on peak grip aperture in trials where vision of the target array was available before but not during the response. As such, these studies suggest that visual feedback of the target or limb during the response is not necessary for action to remain insensitive to pictorial illusions. In contrast, other studies have found significant effects of illusions in open-loop movements (e.g., Franz, Gegenfurtner, Bülthoff, & Fahle, 2000; Franz, Fahle, Bülthoff, & Gegenfurtner, 2001; Glover & Dixon, 2001a, 2001b; Heath, Rival, & Neely, 2006; Heath, Rival, Westwood, & Neely, 2005; Westwood, Heath, et al., 2000; Westwood, McEachern, et al., 2001). However, many of these studies did not directly compare open-loop and closed-loop movements using the same stimulus array, so it is not clear that visual feedback per se had anything to do with the sensitivity of the action to the illusion. As discussed earlier, illusions operating at early stages of visual processing exert significant effects on actions, such as in the case of the Müller-Lyer illusion, which was used in some of these studies (Heath et al., 2006; Heath et al., 2005; Westwood, Heath, et al., 2000; Westwood, McEachern, et al., 2001), or in the case of the STI as used by Glover and Dixon (2001a, 2001b).

Heath and colleagues (2006) carried out an important study in which they compared the effects of a Müller-Lyer illusion on peak grip aperture in open-loop and closed-loop trials. In one experiment, open-loop and closed-loop trials were presented in blocked order, whereas in a second set of trials the visual conditions were randomly intermixed. The results from the blocked trials showed that effects of the illusion were significant only in the open-loop trials, suggesting that visual feedback may indeed be important for resistance to this type of illusion. However, in the randomly mixed trials, significant effects of the illusion were seen for both the open-loop and closed-loop trials. As such, it seems clear that it is not the availability of visual feedback during movement that determines the effect of the illusion on the action—rather it is the strategic approach that participants take toward the task. In other words, when participants know that visual feedback will be unavailable during the response, they may engage a control strategy in which the target array is committed to memory to guard against the perceived difficulty associated with the loss of visual feedback. This approach may shift the control of the action from a typical real-time mode of control to a more off-line or memory-guided mode of control that makes use of the participants' perceptual understanding of the target object. Indeed, even the threat of losing visual feedback, such as occurs in the randomly mixed open-loop and closed-loop trials, may be sufficient to encourage participants to adopt an off-line mode of control. Analogous results have been obtained in studies that simply compare the spatial accuracy and precision of reaching movements in blocked versus random presentation orders of open-loop and closed-loop trials; the results indicate differences in accuracy for open-loop and closed-loop trials in blocked but not randomly mixed trials (Khan, Elliott, Coull, Chua, & Lyons, 2002; Zelaznik, Hawkins, & Kisselburgh, 1983). Thus, strategic or cognitive factors may figure prominently into the way that actions are controlled and, as a consequence, influence the types of visual information that are used.

Another line of inquiry has focused on the role of binocular vision in the sensitivity of action to pictorial illusions. Presumably binocular vision evolved to enable organisms to extract precise information about the locations of objects in three dimensions, primarily for the purpose of guiding accurate interactions with the environment. Indeed, it has been suggested that the ability of the visuomotor system to extract accurate information about the target objects contained in pictorial illusions is due to the use of localization algorithms that make use of accurate cues about object size and distance (Marotta, DeSouza, Haffenden, & Goodale, 1998)—cues that are primarily binocular in nature. Of course, a common explanation for many pictorial illusions is that the perceptual system is biased toward the processing of monocular depth cues, which are readily tricked by carefully designed visual displays that create the false impression of depth and distance. According to this logic, it might be expected that the ability of action to resist pictorial illusions would be eradicated when the target display is viewed monocularly. Certainly, there is considerable evidence pointing to the role of binocular visual cues in the spatial accuracy of pointing movements and grasping movements outside the context of illusory displays (e.g., Bradshaw et al., 2004; Servos & Goodale, 1994; Servos, Goodale, & Jakobson, 1992). Surprisingly, however, there have been few studies that have directly studied the effect of monocular (versus binocular) vision on the sensitivity of action to illusions.

Marotta and colleagues (1998) compared the effects of an Ebbinghaus illusion on grasping movements made with binocular or monocular vision under conditions in which the height of the visual display (which was presented in the picture plane) was either fixed or randomly varied between trials. In the fixed-height and variable-height trials, participants showed no sensitivity to the illusion when the displays were viewed binocularly. However, in both the fixed-height and variable-height trials, the illusion affected the peak grip aperture when the displays were viewed monocularly. Marotta and colleagues suggested that binocular visual cues are required for the visuomotor system to calibrate the size of the target's retinal image, and when these cues are unavailable, the system must rely on unreliable monocular distance cues that are tricked by pictorial illusions. In a finding consistent with this idea, Dijkerman, Milner, and Carey (1996) observed that patient D.F. (who demonstrated visual form agnosia) was able to orient her hand to the orientation of tilted objects when grasping them with binocular vision but not with monocular vision. Healthy participants, however, perform this task equally well in the two visual conditions. The authors suggested that D.F.'s actions, which are thought to be exclusively under the control of the dorsal stream, require binocular visual input to operate. When binocular cues are unavailable, healthy observers can switch the control of action to the ventral or perceptual stream, whereas D.F. cannot due to the location of her brain lesion.

Otto-de Haart, Carey, and Milne (1999) compared the effects of a Müller-Lyer illusion on peak grip aperture in monocular and binocular conditions and failed to find a difference between the two conditions. Their results showed no significant effect of the illusion in either viewing condition, leading them to question the importance of binocular vision for the resistance of grasping to pictorial illusions. Unlike the study of Marotta and colleagues (1998), however, the study of Otto-de Haart was designed so that the target displays were always shown at a fixed viewing distance and height. As such, it is possible that participants learned that the image size of the target object alone was sufficient information to guide accurate grasping movements. Since image size is a monocular cue, perhaps it is not surprising that grasping performances did not differ between the monocular and binocular conditions.

In a recent study, we (Harvey & Westwood, 2009) examined the effects of a size-contrast display (i.e., a rectangular target presented beside a single flanking rectangle of larger or smaller size) on grasping movements made under monocular and binocular viewing conditions. Target displays were presented at one of two viewing distances, and those distances were presented in blocked order for one set of trials and in random order for another set of trials. Similarly to Marotta and colleagues (1998), we found a significant interaction between flanker size and viewing condition in which the flanker size affected peak grip aperture in the monocular viewing condition but not in the binocular viewing condition. Interestingly, this interaction was seen for both the fixed-distance and variable-distance conditions. Our results add strength to the idea that binocular visual cues are important to the ability of the visuomotor system to compute the accurate size of the target object and that monocular visual cues are utilized for this purpose when binocular vision is unavailable. We are currently carrying out follow-up studies in patients who lack stereopsis in order to determine the specific role of this source of binocular distance information in the ability of the visuomotor system to resist pictorial illusions.

Future Directions

As outlined earlier in the chapter, the majority of research in the field of illusions and action was originally motivated by Goodale and Milner's (1992) hypothesis that distinct visual processing systems are associated with conscious perception and the control of action. It is a particular strength of Goodale and Milner's two–visual streams hypothesis that it is based on findings from diverse methodological approaches, including structural and functional neuroanatomy, neurophysiology, neuropsychology, and psychophysics. Although the observation by Aglioti and colleagues (1995) that grasping was unaffected by an Ebbinghaus size-contrast illusion is consistent with that hypothesis, it was not part of the original body of evidence on which the hypothesis was built. Since the publication of Aglioti and colleagues' study, the link between the findings from studies of visual illusions and action and the two–visual steams hypothesis has become increasingly complex and indeed questionable.

Many studies in the field have been guided by the deceptively simple question, "Is action affected by perceptual illusions?" As discussed previously, the answer to this question must be qualified in terms of the type of action, the effector used, the type of illusion, the sensory modality, the participant's expectations about the availability of sensory feedback, the type of sensory information available both before and during the execution of the action, and presumably other factors that have not yet been explored. Although there are other theoretical reasons for asking this question, the primary motivation behind most studies has been to address the validity of the two–visual streams hypothesis. Note that the two–visual streams hypothesis does not predict that actions should be immune to perceptual illusions. Whereas a finding that an action is insensitive to a particular type of illusion can readily be accommodated by the hypothesis, there are several reasons why evidence to the contrary does not refute the hypothesis.

First, illusions that operate at an early stage of visual processing, before the divergence of the perception and action pathways, should affect perceptual and motor responses alike (Dyde & Milner, 2001). Little is known about the locus of most illusions within the central nervous system, so it is difficult to predict a priori the effect of a specific type of illusion on a specific type of action. This is an area in which more research is desperately required.

Second, a stimulus that affects both perception and action could do so for completely different reasons. For example, the effect on perception could be due to the processing of information from both the target and the surrounding context, capitalizing on typical associations that exist in the world between certain types of contextual cues and distance, whereas the effect on action could arise because the contextual cue is treated as a potential obstacle to avoid (Haffenden, Schiff, & Goodale, 2001; although see also Franz, Bülthoff, & Fahle, 2003). Actions may be affected by visual displays that contain multiple target and nontarget objects because the motor system plans a movement to several stimuli before selecting the single intended action by suppressing the unwanted movement plans, inhibiting some aspects of the intended response as a consequence (e.g., Castiello, 1996). Given the existing literature on distractor interference in goal-directed action (e.g., Tipper, Howard, & Jackson, 1997; Welsh, Elliott, & Weeks, 1999), it is somewhat surprising that this idea has not been pursued with any fervor. In general, a logical way to approach the question of whether an illusion-inducing stimulus affects perception and action for the same reason is to correlate the perceptual and motor effects within subjects. Apart from the studies of Franz and colleagues (2001) and Westwood, Pavlovic-King, and Christensen (2009), surprisingly few studies have attempted this. Whereas Franz and colleagues (2001) reported significant correlations between the perceptual and motor effects of illusory stimuli, Westwood and colleagues found no significant correlation at any point in time during the movement. It seems clear that more studies should employ designs with sufficient statistical power to permit such correlational analyses.

Third, the illusion could exert a significant effect on action that is out of proportion to the effect on perception (Franz et al., 2001). This is a difficult possibility to evaluate, because it requires reliable psychophysical data regarding four relationships: (1) the scaling of the perceptual measure to true changes in the stimulus feature in question (e.g., object size), (2) the scaling of the motor measure to true changes in the stimulus feature in question, (3) the sensitivity of the perceptual measure to the illusion-inducing stimulus (e.g., a size-contrast array), and (4) the sensitivity of the motor measure to the illusion-inducing stimulus. A comparison of (1) and (2) provides a baseline point of reference for the relative sensitivities of the perceptual and motor responses to true changes in the underlying stimulus feature. If the perceptual and motor responses are differentially sensitive to object size, for example, it would not be surprising to find different sensitivities to illusions of object size—in other words, the comparison of (3) and (4). Only if the comparison between (3) and (4) is different from the comparison between (1) and (2) can it be concluded that action and perception are disproportionately sensitive to the illusion. Although this recommendation is reminiscent of Glover and Dixon's (2001a, 2001b) scaled illusion effect (SIE) procedure, it is somewhat different since it does not involve the formation of composite measures that can be misleading. Very few studies have employed the necessary psychophysical procedures to test the hypothesis of proportionate effects in action and perception, with the careful work of Franz being a notable exception. In fact, Franz's studies consistently demonstrate proportionate effects of illusions on action and perception, contrary to the original conclusion reached by Aglioti and coworkers (1995).

Fourth, the measures used to characterize the performance of the action and perception tasks may not bear a simple relationship to the nature of the underlying processing. Early studies of illusions and action gave little consideration to the measure chosen to quantify motor performance, often choosing one simply because past studies had shown it to be associated with changes in a specific object feature such as size or location. Glover and Dixon (2001a) were the first to report that the same measurement taken at different points in time during the unfolding action may show different sensitivities to perceptual illusions. Indeed, Glover and Dixon went so far as to propose that the feed-forward and feedback control phases of action utilize distinct visual processing mechanisms that are differentially sensitive to contextual sources of target information. Although this controversial idea has met considerable resistance from contrary findings (e.g., Danckert, Sharif, Haffenden, Schiff, & Goodale, 2002; Franz, Scharnowski, & Gegenfurtner, 2005; Glover, 2004; Heath et al., 2005; Mendoza, Elliott, Meegan, Lyons, & Welsh, 2006; Westwood, Pavlovic-King, & Christensen, 2009), Glover and Dixon brought much-needed attention to the question of how to quantify action performance. The situation is similar for the perceptual side of the story, since many studies of illusions and action have given insufficient consideration to the method used to assess perceptual sensitivity to illusions. For example, Haffenden and Goodale (1998) developed a novel method for assessing participants' perceptions of object size by having participants adjust the separation between the index finger and thumb to indicate the apparent size of a target stimulus. The rationale was to obtain an interval-scale perceptual measure using the same effector system that would be used to perform a grasping movement, thereby facilitating comparisons between the perception and action tasks. This procedure had face validity in the sense that participants were asked to report their perception of the size of the target object. The procedure also had construct validity in the sense that the measurements showed the typical effect of the perceptual illusion. Haffenden and Goodale's procedure has been used in a number of studies comparing the effects of visual illusions on grasping and size perception (Otto-de Haart et al., 1999; Westwood, Chapman, et al., 2000; Westwood, Heath, et al., 2000; Westwood, McEachern, et al., 2001; Westwood & Goodale, 2003b). However, Franz (2003) and Amazeen and DaSilva (2005) have recently demonstrated that the manual report procedure is not necessarily correlated with other, more traditional, measures of perceptual sensitivity, such as magnitude estimation or the method of constant stimuli (Coren & Girgus, 1972). Indeed, the effects of illusions on manual reports are consistently greater than the effects observed by more traditional perceptual measures (Franz, 2003). Although it remains unclear why manual reports differ from other methods of assessing perceptual experience, this observation calls attention the importance of understanding the psychophysical properties of the measure used to quantify perception.

Fifth, the action under investigation may not be controlled by the visuomotor mechanisms that reside in the dorsal stream. This is among the most intriguing and important issues that have emerged from the study of illusions and action and from the two–visual streams hypothesis. Earlier, I discussed two themes that support the idea that task characteristics can modulate the way that visual information is used to control action:

1. When the target is visible until the onset of the response, the action is less likely to be influenced by a pictorial illusion than it is when the target is occluded before response onset.

2. If the target is viewed binocularly, the action is less likely to be influenced by a pictorial illusion than if the target is viewed monocularly.

These observations, among others, suggest that illusions may be a useful tool to study how the visual control of action changes in different situations. However, a task-dependent increase in the sensitivity of an action to a perceptual illusion does not necessarily mean that the control of that action has shifted from the dorsal stream to the ventral stream. Conclusions about the locus of control in the central nervous system require independent evidence from other techniques capable of localizing regions that are (1) engaged during the performance of a particular task (e.g., ERP, fMRI, positron emission tomography [PET]), (2) necessary for the performance of a particular task (e.g., TMS, permanent or reversible inactivation of a region of tissue), or (3) associated with altered performance of a particular task (e.g., naturally occurring lesions). Considerably more research of this type is needed, since it has become commonplace in this field to assume that effects of illusions on action are attributable to an increased reliance of the motor system on processing that takes place in the ventral stream. Indeed, the results of a TMS study (Lee & van Donkelaar, 2002) and human lesion study (Coello, Danckert, Blangero, & Rossetti, 2007) with visual illusions suggest that the effects of visual illusions on action do not map onto a simple dorsal–ventral dichotomy of visual control.

The visual illusion paradigm can be a useful method for exploring questions about the relationship between perception and action if appropriate methods are used. In particular, more emphasis needs to be given to carefully mapping the psychophysical relationships between the properties of the stimulus array used and the perceptual and motor measures taken during task performance. In addition, studies should include data from sufficient numbers of participants to permit the performance of statistically powerful tests of the association between the perceptual and motor effects of the illusion-inducing array. Additional research using tools such as fMRI and TMS is important to begin mapping the observed processing characteristics of perceptual and motor responses onto the appropriate neural substrates.

Aside from the question of whether perceptual illusions are a useful technique to explore the validity of the two–visual streams hypothesis, illusion-inducing stimuli provide an important tool for studying the nature of the visual processing that is used in the control of action. Before the advent of this paradigm, few studies had systematically considered the nature of the visual processing used by the motor system to plan and execute skilled movements. Emphasis was given to the mere presence or absence of target information at different stages of the movement or to the timing of visual information. If nothing else, the visual illusion paradigm has been useful for exploring changes in the way that nontarget (i.e., contextual) sources of visual information are used to control action in different situations, thus providing a richer understanding of the fundamental mechanisms that underlie the control of skilled action.

CHAPTER 14

Two Visual Streams: Neuropsychological Evidence

DAVID P. CAREY

The science of goal-directed movement has always been multidisciplinary. Recently, scientists from motor control and kinesiology have developed substantial interest in the neurobiology of reaching in nonhuman primates and in patients with brain damage and deficits in looking and reaching. The two–visual systems model of posterior neocortex has enjoyed considerable popularity outside of clinical neuropsychology and certainly has generated substantial praise (in parallel with criticism) within it. After more than 15 years, a reappraisal of one variant of the model is well overdue. This particular variant is especially relevant for scientists interested in sensorimotor control and its interface with cognition. In this chapter I argue that early concerns about the overreliance of the model on one patient with visual agnosia have been addressed through new work on optic ataxia. Some of this latter research on dorsal stream function and dysfunction, inspired by the two–visual systems theory, is now extending beyond the limits of the model.

Two Visual Pathways in the Cerebral Cortex

Work in the 1960s by Trevarthen, Ingle, Schneider, and others anticipated the heavily cited two visual systems hypothesis of Ungerleider and Mishkin (1982) and its subsequent revision by Milner and Goodale (1995; Goodale & Milner, 1992, Milner & Goodale, 2008).[1] In fact, several works from clinical

---

[1]Jeannerod (1994) also suggested a variant of the model that differs from that of Milner and Goodale mainly in how much action representation is represented in the dorsal stream (see Jeannerod, 1994). In addition, Glover and Dixon have a variant that subdivides motor functions into planning and control (see Glover, 2004; Glover & Dixon, 2001).

neurology (e.g., Kleist, 1934, cited in Grüsser & Landis, 1991) and neuro-anatomy also suggested a distinction between spatial and object vision (e.g., Glickstein, May III, & Mercier, 1985). Nevertheless, the Ungerleider and Mishkin and in particular the Milner and Goodale models have become the most influential. The purpose of the present chapter is to review these alternatives in terms of the two decades of research on patients with brain damage that have passed since the initial formulations.[2]

The two visual streams (see figure 14.1) have been discussed so extensively in visual neuropsychology that only a brief précis is provided here. The ventral chain of areas in the occipitotemporal cortex plays crucial roles in the processing of perceptual information about form, faces, color, and other visual attributes crucial for recognition and perception of visual stimuli. The distinction between the two variants of the two–visual systems hypothesis is in what the dorsal stream of the occipitoparietal cortical regions is specialized for. In Ungerlieder and Mishkin, spatial vision, including judgments of spatial attributes (such as which of two targets is closer to a landmark) and the use of spatial information to guide movement, is crucial, where as in the Milner and Goodale account, the use of any visual attribute (not just spatial position such as distance or orientation) for the guidance of sensorimotor acts is crucial.

Early Arguments Against the Milner and Goodale Account

Critics of any two–visual systems account frequently argue that cross talk between visual cortical areas in both streams invalidates these simple dichotomies. However, these critics often ignore much of the excellent anatomy performed by Ungerleider and colleagues (e.g., Boussaoud, Desimone, & Ungerleider, 1992; Ungerleider & Mishkin, 1982), which has stood the test of time. The two pathways are relatively independent of one another—they are interconnected much more heavily within stream than across stream (e.g., Catani, Jones, Donato, & ffytche, 2003; Felleman, Xiao, & McClendon, 1997; Galletti et al., 2001; Shipp, Blanton, & Zeki, 1998) and mainly communicate with one another via the superior temporal polysensory area, the frontal eye fields, and a few other subdivisions of the premotor and prefrontal cortex (Boussaoud, Ungerleider, & Desimone, 1990; Young, 1992). The two streams also have relatively distinct targets in the frontal lobes (Grol et al., 2007; Petrides & Pandya, 2007; Tomassini et al., 2007).

---

[2]Many neuroimaging and behavioral studies that speak to these issues will not be addressed in this chapter (see Culham, Gallivan, Cavina-Pratesi, & Quinlan, 2008; Culham, Cavina-Pratesi, & Singhal, 2006; Konen & Kastner, 2008), but in my eyes the key issues are related to imaging studies that show *superior* parietal activation in the absence of covert or overt motor responses. Behavioral studies on the dissociations between illusion and action as well as the effects of delay on sensorimotor responses are also important but cannot be addressed here.

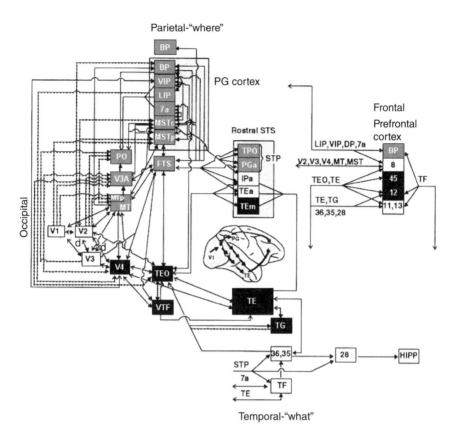

▶ **Figure 14.1**   An anatomically detailed variant of the primate two–visual systems schematic. The back of the brain is to the left of the figure. Lighter gray boxes represent distinct cortical areas of the dorsal stream (labeled by this group as *where)*; darker gray boxes represent areas of the ventral stream *(what)*. Areas of integration in the superior temporal sulcus (STS) and prefrontal cortex are also depicted.

"Pathways for motion analysis: Cortical connections of the medial superior temporal and fundus of the superior temporal visual areas in the macaque," D. Boussaoud, L.G. Ungerleider, and R. Desimone, *Journal of Comparative Neurology* Vol. 296, 1990, pgs. 462-495. Copyright 1990. Adapted by permission of John Wiley & Sons, Inc.

A second critique of two–visual systems accounts is that any idea involving only two visual streams must be grossly oversimplified and is at best a crude heuristic. It is difficult to argue with the former statement, but the latter (the crudeness of the heuristic) can be addressed by empirical evidence. In fact, in spite of all of the caveats associated with generalizing from damaged to neurologically intact brains, the evidence suggests that the heuristic is anything but crude. Furthermore, the staunchest critics of two–visual systems models must acknowledge that these models have inspired several interesting, challenging, and productive lines of experimentation, whatever the precise veracity of the original ideas that drove them.

Much of the most compelling evidence cited in support of the Milner and Goodale formulation comes from patients with optic ataxia and from one well-studied patient, D.F., who exhibited visual form agnosia. In effect, numerous experiments with D.F. suggested that her perceptual systems were severely compromised by carbon monoxide poisoning, such that she could no longer read (alexia), recognize familiar faces (prosopagnosia), or identify common objects (visual agnosia). Her variant of this latter disorder extended to making discriminations among simple rectangles of equal areas but different shapes, the so-called *visual form agnosia* (Benson & Greenberg, 1969). In 1991, we (Goodale, Milner, Jakobson, & Carey) described how, despite serious difficulties with size judgments and with judgments of orientation of a slot that could be rotated in the picture plane, D.F. demonstrated movements that were still completely sensitive to these visual attributes. When working with the rectangles that were equal in area but different in aspect ratio, although D.F. could not tell them apart perceptually, her maximum grip aperture was perfectly scaled to the size of the object while still on the move to grasp it. Similarly, when we required D.F. to use a handheld card to show us the orientation of a slot in a picture plane that we rotated from trial to trial, she performed extremely poorly. However, if instead we asked her to post her card in the slot as she would a letter in a postbox,[3] she rotated the card to match the orientation well before the card made contact with the slot (see figure 14.2). These examples show how D.F. could use visual

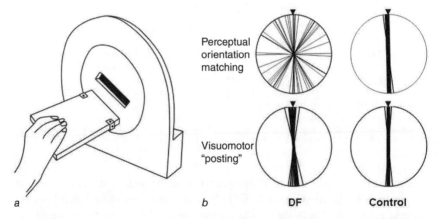

Perceptual orientation matching

Visuomotor "posting"

a   b   DF   Control

▶ **Figure 14.2** The perception–action dissociation in D.F., a visual agnosic patient. (*a*) The stimulus, which was a handheld card, and a sample visuomotor posting trial. For perceptual orientation matching, participants rotated the handheld card to match the slot's orientation. (*b*) D.F.'s performance versus a control performance on the two tasks, with correct performance normalized to the vertical (indicated by the arrow).

Adapted, by permission, from A.D. Milner and M.A. Goodale, 1998, "Visual brain in action," *Psyche* 4(12). Available: http://psyche.cs.monash.edu.au/v4/psyche-4-12-milner.html.

---

[3]Mailbox for the North American reader.

attributes such as orientation and size to control her hand actions and yet, when asked to show us what she perceived, could not function normally.

Some critics of the two–visual systems account of Milner and Goodale have suggested that the model is overly reliant on data from the single case of D.F. (e.g., Ungerleider & Haxby, 1994). Of course, if D.F. is a valid instance of a patient with a compromised ventral stream,[4] then evidence for the double dissociation with deficits and spared abilities of patients with compromised dorsal streams is logically possible. In a nutshell, double dissociations show that task A isn't failed in a single case patient because it is more difficult than task B (which patient A can do), because a different patient passes task A and fails task B (see Dunn & Kirsner, 2003).

Double Dissociations in Perception and Action

The first claim for a double dissociation between impairments after lesions to the dorsal and ventral streams appeared in 1994. Goodale and colleagues (Goodale, et al., 1994) contrasted the ability of D.F. (compromised ventral stream, intact dorsal stream) to reach and grasp irregularly shaped pebbles (see figure 14.3 for examples) with that of patient R.V. (originally described in Jakobson, Archibald, Carey & Goodale, 1991) experienced optic ataxia as part of Balint-Holmes syndrome. Optic ataxia is a disorder of reaching to visual targets that cannot be explained by low-level visual deficits. It is thought to be a consequence of damage in the superior parietal lobe (De Renzi, 1982; Husain & Stein, 1988; Ratcliff & Davies Jones, 1972; Rondot, De Recondo, & Ribadeau Dumas, 1977; although see Karnath & Perenin, 2005). The parietal lobe regions damaged in patients with optic ataxia include several important dorsal stream areas implicated in the control of eye and hand movements. R.V. had a compromised dorsal stream but a largely intact ventral stream.

Goodale and colleagues (Goodale et al., 1994) found that D.F. was extremely poor at making same–different judgments (under conditions of free viewing) about irregularly-shaped "pebble" stimuli (see figure 14.3), while R.V. was virtually flawless at this task. In other words, R.V.'s visuoperceptual performance was relatively intact, while D.F.'s was not. The opposite pattern was obtained when the participants were required to grasp the pebble stimuli between their index fingers and thumbs. Figure 14.3 is a schematic representation of the performance of R.V. and D.F. in terms of selected grasp points (as depicted by grasp lines that show the orientation of the index finger and thumb before contact). As can be seen, D.F.'s grasp

---

[4]The James, Culham, Humphrey, Milner, and Goodale (2003) fMRI study of D.F. suggests that some portions of her ventral stream are intact, more than a decade after her accident. The most extreme structural damage is to the lateral occipital cortex (area LO), which recent functional image studies (e.g., Kourtzi, Erb, Grodd, & Bülthoff, 2003) have implicated as being crucial for perceptual encoding of shape.

points tended to intersect the pebble's center of mass,[5] a finding that suggests that her dorsal stream was perfectly capable of generating effective grasps using visual information that could not be used for perceptual judgements (Goodale et al., 1994).

The second type of double dissociation between optic ataxia and visual agnosia that supports the two–visual streams model depends on a theoreti-

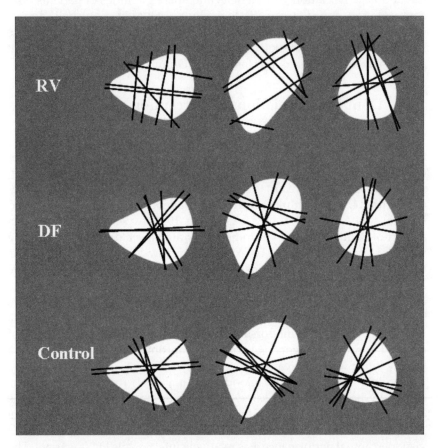

▶ **Figure 14.3** Grasp lines preceding object contact by D.F., who demonstrates visual agnosia; R.V., who demonstrates optic ataxia; and a matched control. Grasp lines of the control and D.F. tend to intersect near the center of mass of each object. While R.V. had no difficulty making same–different judgments about these objects, she clearly did not pick them up normally. On the contrary, D.F.'s grasps were indistinguishable from the control's, in spite of her difficulty in telling any two pebbles apart.

Reprinted from *Current Biology*, Vol. 4, M.A. Goodale et al., "Separate neural pathways for the visual analysis of object shape in perception and prehension," pgs. 604-610. Copyright 1994, with permission of Elsevier.

---

[5]Monika Harvey, David Milner, and I have argued elsewhere that using the principal axis to guide grasping (i.e., grasping the perpendicular axis) would produce roughly the same results, at least with these types of stimuli (Carey, Harvey, & Milner, 1996).

cal property of the dorsal stream: Its default modus operandi is to work in real time with visual information for the guidance of eye, head, and hand movements. In D.F., for example, sensitivity to both target size (her grip scaling was eliminated; Goodale, Jakobson, & Keillor, 1994) and location (her pointing accuracy dropped appreciably; Milner, Dijkerman, & Carey, 1998) was dramatically reduced when we required her to move after a delay. Paradoxically, these same delays may improve sensorimotor responses for patients with optic ataxia.

Milner and colleagues (Milner, Paulignan, Dijkerman, Michel, & Jean-nerod, 1999) investigated the effects of delay on sensorimotor responses of patients who misreach due to optic ataxia. In one study, patient A.T., who experienced bilateral parietal lobe damage 12 years previously (Jeannerod, Decety, & Michel, 1994) was required to point to peripheral targets imme-diately or 5 s after they were extinguished. Five control subjects performed somewhat worse in the delayed condition; A.T. performed substantially better. In a second study, patient I.G. (who also demonstrated optic ataxia) was tested on her ability to scale the size of her grip to different targets in immediate conditions versus a delay of 5 s, which required a pantomimed grasp (as used by Goodale and colleagues with D.F.) or a delayed real grasp. Like A.T., I.G. demonstrated an improvement after delay. The authors also found that I.G. was better when she pantomimed grasps than when she had to wait 5 s and then grasp (delayed real grasping). During delayed real grasping, presumably some dorsal stream impairments attenuated the good skills that could be driven by ventral stream mechanisms. Addi-tional evidence for this interpretation is that I.G. tended to scale her grip to the originally presented target when, in delayed real grasping trials, the target was replaced with an object of a different size. Control participants never did this (Milner, Dijkerman, McIntosh, Rossetti, & Pisella, 2003). The authors concluded that A.T. and I.G. could rely on a representation of target position or size mediated by the ventral stream to guide their actions after the compromised dorsal system response was not utilized. D.F., the previ-ously described patient with visual agnosia, had no such representation to fall back on to guide her motor responses. Therefore, her motor skills were substantially compromised by even relatively short delays (Goodale, Jakobson, & Keillor, 1994). This line of research was reviewed by Milner and colleagues in 2003 (Milner, Dijkerman, McIntosh, Pisella, & Rossetti, 2003).

Later Controversies: Diagnosing Optic Ataxia

The use of double dissociation between perception and action in optic ataxia and visual agnosia to support two–visual systems models is not without controversy. First, diagnosis in neuropsychology is not based exclusively on a particular neurochemistry, neuropathology, genetic marker, or other incontrovertible piece of hard medical evidence. The diagnosis of visual agnosia, and more specifically visual form agnosia, can depend on interpretation of the magnitude of recognition dysfunction juxtaposed with the degree of associated low-level visual disturbance. How poor does a patient have to be at recognizing Snodgrass and Vanderwart line drawings (a standard set of drawings whose psychometric properties are well described; Snodgrass & Vanderwart, 1980) before the diagnosis is made? If patients fail low-level visual subtests of standardized instruments such as the Visual Object and Space Perception Battery (VOSPB; Warrington & James, 1991) or the Birmingham Object Recognition Battery (BORB; Riddoch & Humphreys, 1993), could we reasonably expect them to be capable of normal object recognition? If not, visual agnosia should not be diagnosed.

For optic ataxia, how exaggerated does misreaching have to be (particularly in peripheral vision) before we can be confident in a diagnosis? Many of the studies examining this disorder, with only a few recent exceptions, include no control subjects matched in age or visual status. When control subjects are included, the control sample is small (and there are some serious statistical issues as a consequence; see Crawford & Garthwaite, 2005) and the selection mechanism is unspecified—often the controls are highly functioning individuals from a university community who might be not be comparable with patients with stroke, even when matched for age and sex. In some cases hand- or field-specific deficits (which of course must be consistent with lesion laterality) may allow patients to serve as control participants for themselves. However, these studies usually only describe the relatively intact performance in the unaffected arm or field—they don't typically measure it.

A second caveat for experimental work on patients with optic ataxia is that the most florid form, in which misreaching is observed even for foveated targets, occurs as part of Balint-Holmes syndrome, a complex disorder with at least a triad of symptoms. These other symptoms, including attentional and gaze difficulties, could be indirectly responsible for the misreaching, or the ataxia could be an independent symptom that depends on a different component of the large bilateral occipitoparietal lesions. Accurate eye tracking in the elderly is difficult, and when it has been done, details on calibration (which requires accurate eye movement and good control of fixation), recalibration frequency, system accuracy, and drift correction are suspiciously absent from the method sections of the reports.

The third caveat regarding optic ataxia is a critical but typically omitted demonstration: The misreaching deficits in patients who have been diagnosed with optic ataxia by definition are restricted to deficits in moving to visual targets. As I have argued elsewhere (Carey, 2004), auditory and proprioceptive guidance of movement are rarely assessed in these patients in any formal way. For example, magnetic misreaching (a very rare disorder in which patients slavishly reach to the fixation point rather than an extrafoveal target; Carey, Coleman, & Della Sala, 1997; see also Buxbaum & Coslett, 1997, 1998; Jackson, Newport, Mort, & Husain, 2005; van Donkelaar & Adams, 2005) has been labelled as a variant of optic ataxia by Buxbaum and Coslett as well as Jackson and colleagues, but we have evidence that, in our patient at least, poor guidance of limb movement is not restricted to the visual modality. Blanghero and colleagues (2007) have made similar observations in two patients previously described in the literature as demonstrating optic ataxia.

The fourth caveat relates to the distinction between foveal and nonfoveal variants of optic ataxia, which is becoming blurred or even ignored (perhaps because the former are so rare, it is becoming convenient to discuss the extrafoveal variant as the prima facie case). Misreaching in the full-blown foveal variant is so fascinating because the errors happen in spite of accurate gaze, which also in a sense serves as a crude control of visual status: The patient sees the target well enough to fixate on it. The same cannot always be said when targets are presented well into the visual periphery, which is one of the reasons why I worry about the visual status of control participants. Of course, conducting clinical experiments with the more common extrafoveal cases means ensuring fixation compliance, with all of the problems related to monitoring eye position briefly outlined earlier.

How do these concerns constrain the usefulness of any particular patient for evaluating cortical models of perception–action dissociation? I have little doubt that, in spite of her diffuse brain damage, D.F.'s recognition problems are restricted to the visual domain (for example, I tested her haptic recognition abilities in the 1990s and they were effectively normal). In spite of several attempts, other patients with a similar agnosia and perception–action profile have been difficult to find. A patient who had experienced meningoencephalitis in childhood and subsequently demonstrated relatively intact visuomotor skills in conjunction with poor visuoperceptual abilities has been described (Le et al., 2002). Nevertheless, he differs from D.F. in several important respects, including visuoperceptual matching skills and a lifetime of development that was not afforded to D.F., who acquired her disabilities in adulthood. Similarly, a few patients with agnosia have shown, similarly to D.F., dependence on binocular vision for grasping, although these people do not share many features of D.F.'s unusual profile. Recently Yang, Wu, and Shen (2006) described an anoxic patient who may have demonstrated a similar perception–action profile, but that report focussed on implicit processes related to shape and not sensorimotor skills per se. Goodale, Wolf, and others (Goodale et al., 2008; Wolf et al., 2008) have recently described a patient with visuoperceptual problems even more severe than those of D.F., who has intact grasping. Very recently, Karnath, Rüter, Mandler, and Himmelbach (2009) have found a patient with a ventral stream lesion who shows a very similar perception-action profile to D.F. using Efron square matching and grasping, as well as orientation posting and matching.

The difficulty in finding other patients with visual agnosia and such a pure dissociation has not hindered research inspired by the Milner and Goodale variant of the two–visual systems theory. Much of the recent work in support of their model has come from studies of neurologically intact samples. Work on dissociations in perception and action has proven to be fruitful as well as contentious (see Bruno, 2001; Carey, 2001; chapter 13 of this volume for reviews of dissociations in perceptual and action systems in response to visual illusions; although see Biegstraaten, de Grave, Smeets, & Brenner, 2007, for a contrary view). In parallel, claims about the rather short-term memory of sensorimotor systems (Goodale, et al., 1994) mediated by dorsal stream mechanisms have remained rather unchallenged.

One patient study (Himmelbach & Karnath, 2005) attempted to evaluate whether the effects of delay in patients represent a step function (the strongest support for a switch in processing mode from a sensorimotor representation to a more enduring, less metric perceptual representation) or a continuous drop (or improvement) in performance. These authors found some evidence for improvement with delay in two patients with optic ataxia, although this effect was relatively continuous and therefore did not suggest a step change indicative of a switch from impaired dorsal representation to intact perceptual representation. However, the two cases described in this study are not without controversy. First, no details beyond mean age were provided on the elderly control participants. Given the acuteness of the patients, a nonataxic control group with similar visual status or neglect might have been appropriate. Second, one of the patients (U.S.) had profound right-sided neglect, but we were not told of her error rates in right and left sides of space. In addition, monitoring fixation in these patients must have been extremely difficult (how was the infrared eye tracker calibrated in patients with potential difficulties in eye movement and hemispatial neglect?). Third, these cases were tested in a very acute phase of the patients' illness (6 and 8 d poststroke). In neuropsychological syndromes such as hemispatial neglect, patients with left-brain damage can show large right neglect (e.g., De Renzi, 1982) that often resolves very quickly and is made of very little by researchers. Perhaps optic ataxia, like neglect after left-brain lesions, is easier to diagnose in acute patients (although Himmelbach & Karnath do not say so explicitly). If this is the case, a more specific control group is probably more appropriate.

Optic ataxia and delay have also been linked in experiments by Schndler and coworkers (2004) and Rice and colleagues (2008). In the first study, Schindler and coworkers found that two patients with optic ataxia were impaired in adjusting their reach trajectories when two obstacles were moved in the work space from trial to trial. In the follow-up study, Rice and colleagues (2008) showed that introducing a delay between stimulus presentation and response abolished this failure. In other words, the patients showed trajectories that were appropriate for the obstacle locations in the same manner as control participants did in immediate and delayed conditions. These effects represent a third example of how optic ataxic patients behave in ways consistent with the Milner and Goodale account.

Recently, colleagues of David Milner have changed their tune somewhat by criticizing the use of patients with optic ataxia as the appropriate counter to patient D.F. (Pisella, Binkofski, Lasek, Toni, & Rossetti, 2006). One of their claims is that the deficits studied in peripheral vision in the optic ataxia cases are not strictly comparable to D.F., who performs with full foveal vision in conditions where perception and action responses are contrasted with one another. The critique is not strictly true of course: D.F. shows similar perception–action dissociations when forced to work with stimuli in peripheral vision. We have shown that D.F. reaches to target positions in peripheral vision with accuracy similar to that of controls (although interposing short delays before the response seriously impairs this skill; Milner, Dijkerman, & Carey, 1998). Figure 14.4 (from Milner & Goodale, 2008) shows data contrasting the performance of D.F. with that of A.T. (data from Milner et al., 1999). And there are examples of patients with optic ataxia operating in central vision who show the perception–action distinction, such as V.K., who we described in 1991 (Jakobson, Archibald, Carey, & Goodale, 1991).

A final study worthy of note questions the assumptions that the superior parietal lobule is the crucial site of the lesion that produces optic ataxia in humans (Karnath & Perenin, 2005). The authors of this study used a lesion overlap method (Rorden & Brett, 2001) with a large sample of patients screened for optic ataxia and found that the crucial regions of overlap did

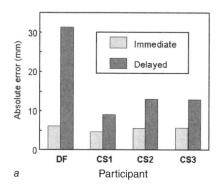
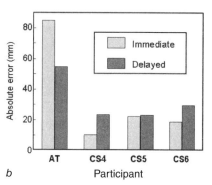

▶ **Figure 14.4**   Reaching into the periphery in (a) D.F., a patient with agnosia (from Milner, Dijkerman, & Carey, 1998), and (b) A.T., a patient with optic ataxia (from Milner et al., 1999). Note that worse performance is higher on the y-axis (absolute error = unsigned error of end point from actual target position). The scales have been modified to show the patterns from the two separate studies.

Adapted from *Neuropsychologia*, Vol. 46, A.D. Milner and M.A. Goodale, 2008, "Two visual systems re-viewed," pgs. 774-785. Copyright 2008, with permission of Elsevier.

not center on the superior parietal lobule, as suggested by early studies (e.g., Ratcliff & Davies-Jones, 1972) and the Milner and Goodale account. Instead, they found that lesion overlap centered on a region around the border of the inferior parietal lobe with occipital cortex. The precise anatomy of optic ataxia is not crucial for the Milner and Goodale model in a functional heuristic sense, but there are suggestions in the literature from neuroimaging and patient work that this region may be utilized in nonperceptual operations. This controversy warrants additional research.

Summary and Future Directions

In spite of these unresolved issues, the identification of several patients with extrafoveal optic ataxia, such as R.V., A.T., and I.G., and the first round of experiments inspired by the two–visual systems model of Milner and Goodale have reintroduced this category of dysfunction to contemporary neuroscience. For example, neurophysiological models of eye–hand transformations, inspired by data from single-unit studies in nonhuman primates (e.g., Andersen, Snyder, Batista, Bueno, & Cohen, 1998; Chang, Dickinson, & Snyder, 2008), have inspired recent experiments on the nature of eye–hand coordination deficits in neurologically intact participants as well as in patients with optic ataxia. These latter studies may never have occurred if the two–visual systems debate on dorsal and ventral streams had not reintroduced this interesting type of patient to the mainstream literature.

For example, studies by Crawford, Khan, and colleagues (e.g., Khan et al., 2007) have supported the idea that hand movements may be coded in eye-centered coordinate schemes. Some of these models may be limited because they do not necessarily acknowledge a specific role of foveation in eye–hand coordination (and retinal coordinates will do in many of these hierarchical accounts; Carey, Ietswaart, & Della Sala, 2002). Nevertheless, the eye-centered accounts have inspired additional studies of patients and neurologically intact participants from a sensorimotor control perspective (c.f., Dijkerman et al., 2006; Scherberger, Goodale, & Andersen, 2003; Verhagen, Dijkerman, Grol, & Toni, 2008). These studies will inevitably suggest greater specifications for simple two-stream accounts. Indeed, the two–visual systems models may fade from the neuropsychological literature as the specifics become elaborated. Of course, the indebtedness of those studies of the future to two–visual systems theory will remain. Ideas about a monolithic multi-feature representation of the visual world (see Goodale, 1983) have gradually been laid to rest, thanks in no small part to the literature referred to in this chapter.

In conclusion, the patient work related to the two–visual systems account of Milner and Goodale has grown dramatically in the past 15 years or so since the model first came to the attention of neuroscientists. Although contentious elements remain and some of the details have required minor rethinks (c.f., Milner & Goodale, 2008), for the most part the model has stood the test of time. What is of little debate is the amount of directed research that it has driven or at least inspired. The growing recognition of sensorimotor processes and their rightful place in cognitive neuroscience has been a long time coming.

PART III

LEARNING, DEVELOPMENT, AND APPLICATION

In this final part of the volume, we present four chapters that build on the knowledge base established in the first two parts and extend it to different theoretical and empirical contexts. Although it should be clear from many of the earlier chapters that the visual control of goal-directed movement involves many flexible and dynamic processes, the majority of the chapters in the first two parts deal with motor control. They do not explicitly address issues associated with motor learning and perceptual–motor development. In chapter 15, Tremblay reviews the most recent work associated with the specificity of learning hypothesis forwarded by his former mentor Luc Proteau more than 20 years ago (Proteau, Marteniuk, Girouard, & Dugas, 1987). Tremblay outlines not only how the use of visual information changes with practice but also how factors such as selective attention, multisensory integration, and mental imagery influence skill acquisition. His insights into individual differences in motor control and learning build nicely on research first introduced in chapter 7.

In chapter 16, we see how the perceptual–motor processes that support precision movement develop through infancy and childhood. Van Wermeskerken, van der Kamp, and Savelsbergh place their review of the literature in a unique theoretical context that combines the ecological approach to perception introduced by J.J. Gibson (1979/1986) with recent theorizing about the special roles played by the dorsal and ventral visual streams in perception and action (Milner & Goodale, 1995; see chapters 13 and 14). Thus, the chapter contributes to our understanding of both perceptual–motor development and the specific neural systems underpinning that development.

Although chapters 15 and 16 give us some insights that are important for skill instruction, chapter 17 provides the most explicit information in the volume on how visual and other information can be structured to support motor learning. Observational learning has an extremely long history in the literature on motor skill acquisition (Bandura, 1971). In chapter 17, Maslovat, Hayes, Horn, and Hodges present some of this older work in a theoretical context together with their own recent work on the variables affecting observational learning. Specifically, their review highlights the role of the mirror neuron system in skill acquisition through observation. Hence, the chapter continues on from previous chapters (e.g., chapters 3 and 4) that explore the intimate link between visuomotor behavior and the neural systems that support such behavior.

The final chapter in this volume translates our knowledge from the laboratory to the workplace. After providing a historical overview on the development of human factors psychology, Lyons explains how many of the principles outlined earlier in the volume can be applied to creating an efficient and safe work environment that optimizes the work potential of the human performer. Beyond the obvious practical implications associated with chapter 18, it is interesting to see how much of the classic work on vision and motor control was designed to solve real-world technical problems (e.g., Fitts, 1947, 1954). With its historical slant, the chapter brings us full circle by making an explicit link between theories and the practical problems they aim to solve (e.g., Woodworth, 1899).

CHAPTER 15

Visual Information in the Acquisition of Goal-Directed Action

LUC TREMBLAY

In the last few decades, a modest number of empirical investigations have been designed to identify factors influencing the use of visual information as a function of practice. During the same time, we have also observed significant debates about the use of visual information during movement execution—that is, open-loop versus closed-loop motor control models (e.g., Plamondon & Alimi, 1997, versus Elliott, Carson, Goodman, & Chua, 1991; see Elliott, Helsen, & Chua, 2001, for a review). Comparatively less attention has been devoted to whether the utilization of visual information decreases or increases as a function of practice. This is probably because the question of the use of visual information during a single trial is still not fully resolved.

After providing background information about the importance of visual feedback throughout practice, this chapter explores issues related to the use of multisensory information, attentional processes, individual differences, mental practice, and the amount of practice related to skill acquisition. These issues are used to build an argument in favor of promoting research on motor learning in order to stimulate motor control research and vice versa. For instance, some motor control models propose that visual information is important during the execution of even very rapid movements (e.g., Elliott et al., 1991). Because performers are continually trying to improve their performance over a series of movement attempts, understanding how the use of this information changes over these attempts (i.e., practice) is fundamental to the processes of limb control that occur within a single discrete movement (e.g., Elliott, Hansen, Mendoza, & Tremblay, 2004). Conversely, determining how sensory information is employed during a single movement (i.e., motor control research) can help optimize protocols for motor skill acquisition. Thus, this chapter also demonstrates the potentially symbiotic nature of motor control and motor learning research.

Background

More than 20 years ago, Luc Proteau and colleagues reported a somewhat counterintuitive data set (Proteau, Marteniuk, Girouard, & Dugas,
1987). Participants were divided into four experimental groups and were
instructed to point with their nondominant limb toward one of five possible targets. Each group performed 200 or 2,000 acquisition trials either in
a full-vision condition or in a condition where only the target was visible.
After the acquisition phases, all groups were transferred to the target-only
condition. As expected, performance in the transfer phase was better for
the groups that completed the acquisition phase in the target-only condition compared with those groups that had full vision. More interesting was
that the participants who practiced with full vision for 200 trials performed
better in the transfer phase than the participants who benefited from 2,000
full-vision practice trials. The results were compelling enough to forward
a theoretical construct that predicts the use of visual information as a function of practice.

The specificity of practice hypothesis (Proteau, 1992) has been postulated
in two parts: (1) Learning is specific to the sources of afferent information
available during acquisition, and (2) specificity increases with practice.
Proteau (1992) predicted that withdrawing—or even adding (see Proteau,
Marteniuk, & Lévesque, 1992)—sensory information after a series of acquisition trials would be detrimental to performance and that such a decrease
in performance would be larger after more acquisition trials. Although
follow-up research challenged this view for various motor skills, Proteau
and I replied to these studies and provided counterevidence that the utilization of sensory information does not decrease as a function of practice
(for research on ball catching, see Whiting, Savelsbergh, & Pijpers, 1995,
versus Tremblay & Proteau, 2001; for research on precision or beam walking,
see Robertson, Collins, Elliott, & Starkes, 1994, versus Proteau, Tremblay,
& DeJaeger, 1998;[1] and for research on powerlift squatting, see Bennett &
Davids, 1995, versus Tremblay & Proteau, 1998).

In the case of the powerlift squat (Tremblay & Proteau, 1998), we realized
that one of the fundamental premises of Proteau's (1992) hypothesis had
to be revised. Specifically, the concept that withdrawing any of the sources
of sensory information would be detrimental to performance was not supported in multiple instances (e.g., Bennett & Davids, 1995; Robertson et al.,
1994; Whiting et al., 1995). In the study of Tremblay and Proteau (1998), we
instructed participants to squat and stabilize their thighs at a horizontal
orientation under conditions of (1) normal vision, (2) normal vision aided
by a laser beam attached to the leg, or (3) lights off. After performing 20 or
100 trials with accurate KR obtained through a goniometer, all participants

---

[1]See also Robertson, Tremblay, Anson, and Elliott (2002).

performed 20 trials without KR in the lights-off condition. As expected, participants acquiring the task in the lights-off condition did not exhibit any performance loss in the transfer test. Conversely, withdrawing the laser and turning off the lights led to a significant decrement in performance. However, the participants who practiced with normal ambient vision did not exhibit any significant losses in accuracy when the lights and KR were withdrawn. These results were convincing enough to review the specificity of practice hypothesis and suggest that "one predominantly processes the source of afferent information, which is easier to use or more likely to improve performance in detriment to processing other sources of afferent information" (Tremblay & Proteau, 1998, pp. 288-289). This idea was recently revisited by Mackrous and Proteau (2007).

Mackrous and Proteau (2007) tested whether "the CNS quickly determines the source(s) of afferent input most likely to ensure spatial accuracy and processes it (them) for that purpose, perhaps at the exclusion of other sources of afferent information" (p. 182). During task acquisition, participants performed a video-based aiming task toward one of five possible targets with or without vision of the cursor. In addition to withdrawing visual information of the cursor in a first transfer test, the researchers administered a second transfer test in which they displaced the starting location of the hand (15 cm to the right or left)—but not the position of the targets relative to the hand—to assess the contribution of proprioceptive information. The results showed that perturbing the starting position of the hand had a larger effect on limb trajectories than withdrawing vision of the cursor had, although both had a significant effect. Mackrous and Proteau (2007) suggested that these results challenge the idea that one source of information is predominantly processed over the others (c.f., Tremblay & Proteau, 1998). Notably, this study provides evidence that manipulating sources other than vision can yield significant information about the utilization of visual feedback.

Utilization of Multisensory Information

One part of the problem when investigating the use of visual information as a function of practice is the coexistence of other sensorimotor systems. In this regard, some of the seminal research performed by Jack Adams and colleagues (Adams, Goetz, & Marshall, 1972; Adams, Gopher, & Lintern, 1977) is at the forefront because these researchers manipulated more than one source of afferent information during a goal-directed movement. Specifically, Adams and colleagues manipulated visual and proprioceptive information and noticed that withdrawal of visual information alone was less detrimental to end-point accuracy than was manipulating both vision and proprioception. Although these results are trivial at face value, they cast some doubt on a fundamental assumption of sensory manipulations—that the importance of a particular source of information can be assessed by examining the effects of its withdrawal (see chapter 7).

Although researchers have assumed that performance decrements following sensory manipulations merely reflect the manipulated afference, it is also possible that withdrawing vision affects how the remaining sources of information are used. Indeed, as suggested by Weiss (1941) and supported by Welch (1978), withdrawing a source of afferent information (e.g., shutting off the lights to delete visual cues) yields more important alterations to the sensorimotor systems than modifying or recombining signals for that same source (e.g., using an optical prism to transform visual cues). That is, it is not possible to use absent information, but it is possible to use biased information (see also Welch, 1978). The withdrawal of visual information may not reflect the importance of visual information when available but rather the ability of the remaining systems to satisfy the task requirements without the manipulated source. Another possibility is that withdrawing visual information alters how the remaining sources of afferent information are used. This latter option is well supported by the literature on cue combination, which suggests that for perceptual tasks sensory cues are optimally integrated into a single representation (see Ernst & Bülthoff, 2004, for a review). Thus, the preferred—and perhaps easiest—sensory manipulation, which is to withdraw visual information, may not yield the most externally valid results. Furthermore, withdrawal of vision seldom goes unnoticed by the participant, which also yields shifts of attention.

Attention and Performance

When an experimenter withdraws vision, it is virtually impossible for participants to not notice and therefore not alter their attentional focus (e.g., pay more attention to proprioceptive cues). Because shifts in attention significantly affect performance even in the absence of sensory manipulations (see Wulf & Prinz, 2001, for a review), it is reasonable to assume that attention does shift to other sensory cues (e.g., proprioception) when vision is withdrawn. The shift in sensory attention resulting from sensory withdrawal or any other noticeable manipulation could explain some of the observed performance decrements. The influence of attention on the use of sensory information is seldom discussed in fundamental motor control theories or research on the use of visual information as a function of practice; however, there is direct evidence that specificity of practice is altered by attention instructions given to participants.

In one study (Coull, Tremblay, & Elliott, 2001, experiment 2), we manipulated the focus of attention when participants were performing a continuous tracking task. Participants were asked to follow a sinusoidal target by applying force on a handheld dynamometer. They received visual feedback, auditory feedback, or both during the acquisition phase (i.e., matching a target line with visual feedback of the force produced and producing a target tone). Of particular interest are the three groups that received both auditory and visual feedback during the acquisition phase. One of these groups received no instructions, another group was asked to pay attention and learn to use the visual cues, and the last group was asked to pay attention and learn to use the auditory cues. In the final transfer tests, all three groups performed similarly when only vision was present. However, when vision was removed, the group that did not receive attentional instructions during acquisition performed significantly worse than the groups asked to pay attention to vision or audition. Thus, focus of attention on a particular sensory modality can influence the effect of vision withdrawal on motor performance. It is beyond the scope of this chapter to explain why focus of attention on a particular source of afferent information alters the effect of sensory manipulations, but the result in itself suggests using sensory manipulations that do not alter the focus of attention.

All in all, the existing literature on the withdrawal of visual information may contain multiple assumptions that must be kept in mind when interpreting results. One of these assumptions is that shifts of attention arising from sensory manipulations do not influence how the available sensory cues are used to control directed action. Considering recent technological advancements, it is perhaps advisable to employ unnoticeable manipulations (e.g., visual transformations; see Weiss, 1941) in future research rather than to continue to work under the existing assumption and performing noticeable visual withdrawal. Using a representation of the limb (e.g., a cursor on a monitor) and unnoticeably biasing its displacement is one possible option. Also, it is possible to use small physical perturbations that cannot be perceived but can be corrected. Avoiding shifts of attention is additionally relevant considering that the influence of attention on sensory cues does not alter perception the same way from person to person.

Individual Differences in Utilization of Sensory Information

Another factor to consider when assessing the use of visual information during the acquisition of goal-directed movements is that people integrate the sources of afferent information differently. One test for assessing the relative contributions of visual, proprioceptive, and vestibular cues for the perception of spatial orientation is the rod-and-frame test designed by Witkin and colleagues (e.g., Witkin & Asch, 1948). In the original version of the rod-and-frame test, participants were brought into a dark room and looked at a visual display containing a single rod that could be accompanied by a surrounding square frame. The participant's task was to orient the rod vertically or horizontally (i.e., parallel with the wall or ceiling). In some of the experimental conditions, the frame was oriented at various angles relative to gravity (e.g., –28°, 0°, and 28°), which influenced the perception of verticality and horizontality in the direction of the frame. Witkin and colleagues (1977) showed that females were more influenced by the surrounding frame than males were.[2] In other words, it appears that females make use of visual references to a greater extent than males do even if such visual cues conflict with other sensory information (e.g., vestibular information). These gender differences are not confined to perceptual tasks but also extend to goal-directed actions.

Laszlo, Bairstow, Ward, and Bancroft (1980) asked female and male participants to perform a ball-throwing task with the goal of reaching the middle of a series of flaps located at the end of a table (i.e., ward games). When visual distractions were presented just above the series of target flaps, females performed significantly worse whereas males were not reliably influenced. Thus, females were influenced more than males by irrelevant visual cues when performing goal-directed motor behaviors.

Recent research has also demonstrated that biasing visual information during the execution of a goal-directed movement can yield gender differences. Visual information available early during a limb trajectory has greater potential to influence movement end point than visual information available late during the movement (e.g., Hansen, Cullen, & Elliott, 2005). Hansen, Elliott, and Tremblay (2007) showed that this was not necessarily similar for males and females since females took more advantage of visual information early in the movement. Using prismatic displacement at movement onset and during movement, we observed that manipulating visual information influenced females' upper-limb trajectories to a greater extent. Thus, if females and males use vision differently during movement execution, it is not difficult to imagine that practice influences the use of sensory information differently for females and males. Many researchers shy away from investigating gender differences, perhaps because simple and apparently irrelevant factors (e.g., how diligently the task was performed) can be used to explain these differences. As a result, the literature on gender differences in the use of visual information for motor skill acquisition is scarce at best.

Although there is no direct evidence that specificity of practice differs between males and females, gender differences are often neglected, if not avoided. However, current strategies by funding agencies encourage researchers to include gender as a factor. Past experience (e.g., pharmaceutical research) has shown that not considering gender can yield significant

---

[2]Asking participants to pay attention to sensory cues during the rod-and-frame test significantly changes performance in females but not in males (Reinking, Goldstein, & Houston, 1974). We also replicated this flexibility in the female use of sensory information with a spatial orientation task with altered body orientations (Tremblay, Elliott, & Starkes, 2004).

problems and represents a guiding principle of considering individual differences such as gender when forwarding neurobehavioral models. After all, the link between perceptual processes and hormones has been laid out (e.g., the perception of spatial orientation and testosterone levels; see Kimura, 1996, 2000), and it is not a big step to extend this link to goal-directed action, or even imagined movements.

Modulating the Utilization of Sensory Information Does Not Require Physical Practice

The formation of an internal representation of limb movements is perhaps one of the most evolutionary useful capacities that humans have developed. Without moving a limb, we can estimate our degree of accuracy at performing a skill. If failing the task is life threatening, we have a risk-free opportunity to try solving the task with a series of coordinated muscle contractions before physically trying the solution, although the imagined solution is not always successful.

We can imagine movements that will be unsuccessful even if the expected sensory consequences generated before movement initiation are those of a movement intended to be successful. Indeed, a person can make a mental attempt at a task in which success is anticipated even though the result of that imagined movement is different from the expected outcome. An example is when a gymnast attempts to imagine a perfect double somersault but actually imagines failing the skill. Thus, imagining movements (i.e., mental practice or visual imagery) may involve additional processes related to afferent information, which represents a much more complex notion than simply playing the predicted series of afferent signals.

In 2004, Rick Grush published a target article in *The Behavioral and Brain Sciences* titled, "The Emulation Theory of Representation: Motor Control, Imagery, and Perception." One theoretical concept forwarded by Grush was the idea of an emulator that replaces the missing sensory consequences during mental practice. Specifically, when people are imagining movements, the prepared motor response and associated expected sensory consequences are used to emulate the sensory signals normally generated by limb movements. Such emulated afferent signals differ from the expected afferent signals, and as a result it is possible that humans are capable of detecting discrepancies between expected and emulated signals and therefore imagine amendments to the planned trajectory. Considering that some athletes experience difficulty imagining successful movements despite genuine attempts to succeed, the emulation theory is relevant to ideas on the importance of sensory information in skill acquisition.

The emulation theory allowed us to explain how current views of the specificity of practice hypothesis are supported in a visual imagery study.

Following up on Proteau and colleagues (1998), which is one of the strongest lines of support for the specificity of learning hypothesis, we sought to determine whether people could develop a reliance on visual information for precision walking when 90% of the practice was performed using visual imagery (Krigolson, Van Gyn, Tremblay, & Heath, 2006). Participants performed 10 or 100 attempts to walk along a 12 m line under conditions of full vision, no vision, or full vision and visual imagery trials combined in a 1:9 ratio. After the acquisition phase, all participants performed 10 trials without vision or KR.

The participants who performed 100 trials revealed an expected advantage for practicing with eyes closed. However, no significant differences were observed between the full-vision and visual imagery groups. Our results prompted us to suggest that a person can develop a dependence on visual feedback even if the movement is imagined. Taken into the context of Grush's (2004) theory, it appears that humans can optimize their use of emulated visual feedback during visual imagery as they normally do during physical practice. Thus, the effect of vision withdrawal on performance after visual imagery is no different than it is after physical practice. Of course, these studies have employed amounts of practice that may not necessarily be ecologically valid, which is another factor to consider.

Utilization of Sensory Information as a Function of Practice

The last—but definitely not least—factor to consider when assessing the use of visual information as a function of practice is the actual amount of practice and, more importantly, its distribution over time. The two studies directly related to specificity of practice that involved the largest number of trials were Proteau and colleagues (1987) and Khan, Franks, and Goodman (1998). Both studies involved practicing a goal-directed movement with normal or full vision or with target-only vision as well as performing a transfer test in the target-only condition after different amounts of practice. Proteau and colleagues used 200 and 2,000 trials spread over 1 wk or less, whereas Khan and colleagues used 100, 1,300, and 2,100 trials spread over 2 wk or less. Both studies lent significant support to the specificity of practice hypothesis: Vision withdrawal was more detrimental to performance after 100 trials than after 1,300 for Khan and colleagues (1998), and it was more detrimental after 200 trials than after 2,000 for Proteau and colleagues (1987). However, Khan and colleagues also noted a larger difference between the full-vision and target-only groups in the transfer test after 1,300 trials compared with 2,100 trials. Though it could be argued that this effect was caused by repeated transfer tests (i.e., the same participants performed all transfer tests), which was not an issue with the study by Proteau and colleagues (1987), the mere distribution of practice over many weeks could also explain this reversal in specificity.

One major argument to be made is that although Proteau and colleagues (1987) and Khan and colleagues (1998) employed what could be considered very large amounts of practice, none of the work on the specificity of practice hypothesis has used ecologically valid distributions of practice—not in the sense of the number of trials but in the sense of their distributions over time (i.e., 1 wk or 2 wk). Empirical support for this assertion includes an fMRI study published by Karni and coworkers (1995). Participants were asked to perform a sequential finger–thumb opposition task for 10 to 20 min/d for 5 wk. Also, participants were asked to perform their assigned sequence as well as a control sequence in the fMRI scanner once a week. As would be expected from the power law of practice (Schmidt & Lee, 2005; see Crossman, 1959; Snoddy, 1926), the largest improvements in performance for the practiced task were observed after 1 wk.[3] However, when performing the task in the fMRI scanner, the representation of the movement in the primary motor cortex was specific to the practiced sequence (versus control sequence) only after 3 wk or more. Thus, although the utilization of visual feedback may increase as a function of practice, brain plasticity associated with the acquisition of a goal-directed skill takes more than a few weeks of acquisition. By extension, the optimization of goal-directed movements may take more than 3 wk and could be accompanied by less detrimental effects of vision withdrawal, which is what Khan and colleagues (1998) may have observed on their third transfer test.

It is possible that visual information is more efficiently processed as practice progresses but that learners also improve their ability to interchangeably use combinations of sources of afferent information after a few weeks of practice. Such increases in sensory flexibility with prolonged practice make sense, considering how easy it is to disrupt visual feedback.

Conclusions and Future Directions

The hypothesis that the utilization of sensory information does not decrease as a function of practice has received overwhelming support in the last two decades. Parallel development in other research areas has also helped identify the potential weaknesses and assumptions associated with studies on the use of vision with practice.

First, findings concerning the convergence of multisensory signals on multimodal cells such as superior colliculi (Meredith & Stein, 1986; see Stein & Stanford, 2008, for a review) provide a strong rationale for manipulating sources other than vision. Such a statement is valid even when determining

---

[3]Snoddy (1926) manipulated the time interval between acquisition sessions and noticed a significant effect of intervals between sets of trials and rate of change in performance (see figure 15.1 on page 291).

the use of visual information is the sole purpose of the study. Showing that manipulation of vision influences performance to a greater extent after more practice can be supported if a proprioceptive manipulation influences performance to a lesser extent during the same time frame.

Second, the sensory manipulations employed in most empirical studies are noticeable by the participants and therefore could alter their focus of attention. In turn, instructing people to pay attention to sources of sensory information alters how afference is utilized to control goal-directed movements (e.g., Coull et al., 2001). Thus, another recommendation is to employ less conscious or noticeable manipulations to determine how sensory information is used as a function of practice.

Third, future research should systematically include gender as a factor in investigations of the utilization of sensory information. Because there are individual sensory differences even at the structural level (e.g., vestibular level; see Sato, Sando, & Takahashi, 1992), it is difficult to imagine that such physiological differences have no effect whatsoever on perceptual and motor functions. Furthermore, the relationship between hormones and perception (see Kimura, 1996, 2000) substantiates the need to better understand individual differences in neurobehavioral research pertaining to the utilization of vision during motor skill acquisition.

Fourth, physical practice does not appear to be absolutely necessary to understand the use of sensory information as a function of practice (e.g., Krigolson et al., 2006). Visual imagery not only provides a practical solution to physiological limits in training but also represents a theoretical challenge (e.g., Jeannerod, 2006) that in turn could be used to assess the utilization of sensory information during goal-directed behaviors.

Fifth, there is a clear need to include longer acquisition protocols (i.e., distribute acquisition trials over more than 2 wk). The seminal work of Snoddy (1926) included a comparison between massed and two types of distributed practice (see figure 15.1). The results demonstrated that distributing practice over 20 d yielded larger performance improvements in acquisition than did massing all practice trials in 1 d. Even the two longest protocols assessing the use of information as a function of practice (i.e., Khan et al., 1998; Proteau et al., 1987) are significantly shy of the amount of practice required to elicit significant brain plasticity (e.g., Karni et al., 1995) and thus still may not have shed the most externally valid results.[4]

Altogether, the most employed methodology to understand the utilization of visual information as a function of practice—visual information withdrawal—is the most trivial and is perhaps a counterproductive alternative. The factors influencing the effect of vision withdrawal on motor performance (multisensory integration, individual differences, attention)

---

[4]It has been suggested that specific alternation between rapid eye movement (REM) sleep and non-REM sleep is a sine qua non condition for learning (see Maquet, 2001, for a review). As such, distributing practice over many days may be necessary for ecologically valid tests of motor learning.

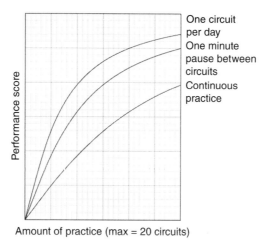

One circuit per day
One minute pause between circuits
Continuous practice

Performance score

Amount of practice (max = 20 circuits)

▶ **Figure 15.1** Performance as a function of practice for three practice distribution schedules. Adapted from G.S. Snoddy, 1926, "Learning and stability: A psychophysical analysis of a case of motor learning with clinical applications," *Journal of Applied Psychology* 10: 1-36. Used with permission.

represent motor control issues that can be used in the design of novel and prolific motor learning studies. Reciprocally, the effects of mental practice and distributed acquisition sessions on the use of sensory information as a function of practice are a promising avenue for closed-loop models in motor control research. Thus, it could be argued that motor control and motor learning studies can bring about symbiotic research that is more promising than separate investigations of these fields.

The strongest line of evidence for open-loop control may come from deafferented patients. Yet, the complete absence of sensory information is virtually impossible in living organisms. The seminal work of Lashley (1917) reported investigations on a patient with "partial anesthesia of both legs" (p. 170). However, even the most respected textbooks mention the term *deafferented* when referring to Lashley's seminal paper (e.g., Schmidt & Lee, 2005, p. 166). The main problem here is the insidious use of the term *open loop*, which requires (among many possibilities) complete dorsal rhizotomy, section of the optic nerves, section of all extraocular muscle afferent fibers, section of the vestibular nerves, and section of the auditory nerves.[5] Such a subject would not have any means to determine the target or goal for the movement. Thus, there is no question as to whether sensory information is used throughout practice; the only question is whether it is being used during movement execution. Perhaps demonstrating how the utilization of online afferent information varies with practice would close the debate on open-loop versus closed-loop models.

---

[5]From that point, it would still be necessary to demonstrate the absence of afferent fibers in the ventral roots of the spinal cord.

CHAPTER 16

Early Development
of the Use
# of Visual Information
for Action and
Perception

MARGOT VAN WERMESKERKEN, JOHN VAN DER KAMP, AND GEERT J.P. SAVELSBERGH

At the age of 3 mo, infants can already intercept slowly moving objects (van Hof, van der Kamp, & Savelsbergh, 2002, 2006, 2008; von Hofsten, 1980, 1983; von Hofsten & Lindhagen, 1979). Obviously, these infants are not yet proficient reachers, but their reaching quickly becomes more sophisticated between ages 6 mo and 12 mo. For example, 6 mo old infants reach and look toward the future interception position of a moving object rather than reach and look to its present position. This is particularly evident when the object suddenly stops moving or changes direction. In these cases, 6 mo old infants reach toward the original future location of the object (von Hofsten, Vishton, Spelke, Feng, & Rosander, 1998). Findings such as these provide clear evidence that, from 6 mo on, infants are able to anticipate the spatiotemporal properties of moving objects. Intriguingly, however, habituation experiments with visual events similar to those in this reaching study show that it is not until the age of 8 mo that infants perceive the future position of a moving object when they are not reaching for it (Spelke, Katz, Purcell, Ehrlich, & Breinlinger, 1994).

These findings suggest that the development of action and the development of perception are not necessarily intrinsically linked. Each may follow its own temporal trajectory. The relationship between action and perceptual development has been the subject of several theories (e.g.,

Atkinson, 2000; Bertenthal, 1996; Netelenbos, 2000; Piaget, 1952). It has been assumed, for instance, that the development of action precedes the development of perception (e.g., Piaget, 1952; see also Held, 1965). Though the findings discussed earlier do not exclude such a view, further empirical findings do question this claim. After all, research has indicated that infants have rather refined perceptual abilities at birth or shortly thereafter (Atkinson, 2000; Gopnik & Meltzoff, 1996; Kellman & Arterberry, 1998; Rochat, 2001).

Thus, a reconsideration of the relationship between the development of action and the development of perception is needed. The working hypothesis of this chapter is that the development of action and development of perception are not necessarily related, at least as far as the exploitation of visual information is concerned. We consider neither action nor perception as privileged in development. The theoretical framework of the present chapter is formed by the work of Gibson (1979/1986) and Milner and Goodale (1995, 2008). Gibson, the founder of the ecological approach to perception and action, argued that perception results from the direct pickup of visual information—that is, to perceive is to detect meaningful information that specifies the to-be-perceived or to-be-acted-upon environmental property. From this perspective, development is a process of convergence to more useful information.

Following a great deal of neuropsychological work, Milner and Goodale (1995, 2008) suggested that there are two independent but interacting visual systems: one for visual control of movements and one for visual perception of the environment (i.e., obtaining knowledge about the environment). According to Milner and Goodale, these two visual systems are functionally and anatomically separate. Therefore, it is appropriate to distinguish between the use of visual information for action and the use of visual information for perception, as well as to distinguish between the timescales at which the systems operate. In this chapter, we explore the consequences of this theoretical framework for the relationship between the development of action and the development of perception.

In the next sections, we elucidate the perspectives of Gibson and then Milner and Goodale in more detail, resulting in the proposition that the development of action and perception may not be necessarily related. Unfortunately, empirical work that directly tests this contention is scarce and often circumstantial. However, we will review literature on the early development of action and perception that suggests that the early development of eye and arm movements for moving objects and the visual perception of motion direction and velocity of moving stimuli follow distinct trajectories. We then review the development of the control of eye and arm movements in situations in which the object is temporarily out of sight in order to explore how the interaction between action and perception processes may develop in the first year of life.

Ecological Approach to Perception

Gibson (1979/1986) introduced the ecological approach in psychology. His approach broke with the traditional view that the ambiguous retinal image forms the starting point for visual perception (Reed, 1996). This approach held that visual perception is the formation of an internal representation of the world by transforming, encoding, or decoding the sensory stimuli that impinge on the retina. Gibson rejected the idea that perception is such a process of enrichment. Rather than beginning with the retinal image, Gibson took the optic array as the starting point for visual perception. The optic array comprises a pattern of light coming from all directions of the environment to a single point of observation. It is structured and consists of optical patterns that are specific and as such are lawfully related to objects, events, and places. Consider, for instance, an infant looking at an approaching ball (figure 16.1). As the distance between the infant's head and the approaching ball diminishes, the optic array encompasses an expansion pattern that specifies the time remaining until the object reaches the infant, or tau, which is expressed as $T(\phi)$ and is the inverse of the relative rate of optical expansion of the angle subtended by the ball (Lee, 1976). In other words, there is a one-to-one mapping between optical information and environmental properties, making enrichment processes redundant. The detected information is meaningful in itself. Gibson referred to this process of picking up information as *visual perception.*

The empirical agenda of the ecological approach is to identify the visual informational variables that specify objects, events, and places for perception

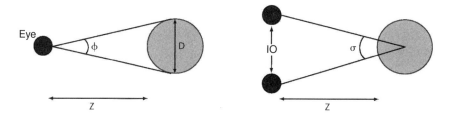

▶ **Figure 16.1**   A ball with diameter (D) approaching at distance (Z) from the perceiver's eyes. *(a)* Representation of monocular viewing. The angle subtended between the eye and the ball is the optic angle (ϕ), which is a function of the ball's diameter (D) and distance (Z). The available monocular variables are the optic angle (ϕ); its derivative $(\dot{\phi})$, which is the rate of change of the optic angle (ϕ); and $T(\phi)$, which is the inverse of the rate of change of optic angle (ϕ). Whereas the variables (ϕ) and $(\dot{\phi})$ are affected by object size, $T(\phi)$ is not. *(b)* Representation of binocular viewing. The angle subtended between the eyes and the ball is (σ), which is a function of the interocular separation (I) and the distance (Z). The available binocular variables are the optic angle (σ); its derivative $(\dot{\sigma})$, which is the rate of change of the optic angle (σ); and $T(\sigma)$, which is the inverse of the relative rate of change of the optic angle (σ). None of these variables is affected by object size.

and for the guidance of action (Gibson & Pick, 2000). Again, the infant looking at a moving ball can serve as an example. Suppose the infant tries to grasp or hit the approaching ball. The infant needs visual information that specifies, for example, when to start reaching for the ball. Figure 16.1a illustrates the situation. The optical angle (ϕ), the angle subtended by the edges of the ball and the infant's eye, increases with the approach of the ball. The infant might use this variable and initiate the catching movement whenever the optical angle reaches a critical value. In the case where the diameter of the ball (D) is constant, optical angle (ϕ) specifies the distance between the ball and the eye.

However, for objects with different or unknown diameters, the information that this variable provides is ambiguous. In that case, it would be better to use the inverse of the relative rate of change of the optical angle, or tau ($T[\phi]$; figure 16.1). Tau specifies the time until the ball reaches the eye, provided the ball approaches with constant velocity. Since tau is independent of ball diameter, it provides information about time or distance across a broader range of objects and events. An infant who exploits this variable would be better adapted to the task compared with an infant who relies on the optic angle (ϕ). By coupling the more useful optical variables to movement variables, actions are guided more efficiently. Hence, movement and information are directly coupled with each other, and inferential processes are superfluous.

One important task for the newborn, then, is to attune to the more useful optical variables to obtain knowledge about the environment and to guide actions (van der Kamp, Oudejans, & Savelsbergh, 2003). This process of attunement was demonstrated by van Hof and colleagues (2006), who presented 2 to 8 mo old infants with moving balls of varying sizes under monocular and binocular viewing conditions. Because the use of any binocular information (e.g., σ or $T(\sigma)$; see figure 16.1b) is independent of ball diameter, reliance on this type of information yields better performance across a larger range of objects than reliance on monocular information only (e.g., ϕ) yields; the timing of a catching action is independent of ball size under binocular but not monocular viewing (van der Kamp, Savelsbergh, & Smeets, 1997).

It was therefore hypothesized that infants capable of exploiting binocular visual information should tune their actions independent of ball size under binocular viewing. By contrast, infants relying only on monocular information should show timing patterns affected by ball size under both binocular and monocular viewing. By means of a cross-sectional and longitudinal experimental design, van Hof and colleagues (2006) demonstrated that with increasing age, infants came to rely more on binocular information. More specifically, from the age of 5 mo onward, the initiation of the reaching movements became increasingly independent of ball size under binocular viewing but not under monocular viewing. In contrast, among the 3 to 4 mo old infants, the timing of the reaching movements was affected by the size of the approaching ball irrespective of the viewing condition, indicating that these infants used monocular information. Similar findings of attunement to more useful information with increasing age were also provided by Kayed and van der Meer (2000, 2007) for defensive blinking and by van Hof and colleagues (2008; Savelsbergh, Caljouw, van Hof, & van der Kamp, 2007; van Hof, 2005) for intercepting moving balls.

Evidence for the process of convergence can also be found in studies of infant visual perception (e.g., Johnson, 2004; Johnson et al., 2003; Sitskoorn & Smitsman, 1995). These studies are typically concerned with whether infants perceive possible and impossible events in accordance with certain laws (e.g., law of inertia, law of continuity) by means of preferential looking or habituation methods (Sitskoorn & Smitsman, 1995; Spelke et al., 1994; Wattam-Bell, 1996a, 1996b). They indicate that with age, infants exploit visual information that specifies properties of objects or events across a larger range of experimental conditions.

Thus far, we have only superficially touched upon the distinction between the use of visual information for online control of movements and the use of visual information for perception. This distinction between action and perception is not imposed by the ecological approach (Michaels, 2000). However, neuropsychological evidence, to be discussed shortly, suggests that such a distinction between the two processes exists. In the next section, we elaborate on the distinction between the use of visual information for action and the use of visual information for perception. We then explore the consequences of this distinction for development.

Two Visual Systems

Goodale and Milner (1992, 2004; Milner & Goodale, 1995, 2008) claim that there are two structurally and behaviorally distinct visual systems. One is involved in action or the visual control of movements, whereas the other is concerned with the visual perception of objects, events, and places. The dorsal stream, which projects from V1 to the posterior and superior parietal cortex, is thought to support action. The ventral stream, on the other hand, supports perception and projects from V1 to the inferior temporal cortex. This distinction of the use of visual information in action and perception is derived from observations of patients with neuropsychological deficits (see chapter 14). Patients with visual agnosia (i.e., with damage to the ventral stream) are unable to accurately perceive object shape, size, and orientation but nevertheless are able to appropriately guide actions to these objects.

One of the most frequently studied patients is D.F., whose ventral system was damaged by carbon monoxide poisoning. D.F. shows good performance (i.e., at a level comparable to participants without neurological deficits) on a posting task in which a handheld card is inserted into a slot set to various orientations (Goodale et al., 1994; Goodale, Milner, Jakobson, & Carey, 1991). By contrast, D.F.'s performance deteriorates dramatically when she has to match the orientation of the card to the slot without inserting it in the slot. Conversely, patients with optic ataxia (i.e., with damage to the dorsal stream) are able to recognize objects and use information about size, shape, and orientation to describe them. However, these patients are not capable of using this information to control actions. They perform poorly in the posting task but are able to perceptually distinguish among the slot orientations (Perenin & Vighetto, 1983, 1988; see Milner & Goodale, 1995).

A similar phenomenon is observed in children with Williams syndrome (WS), a rare genetic condition that is associated with deficits of the dorsal stream (Atkinson, 2000; Atkinson et al., 1997). In line with observations of patients with optic ataxia, children with WS encounter difficulties when performing the posting task but not when matching the orientation of the card to that of the slot. In addition, these children fail to smoothly perform a movement; instead, they perform a sequence of small actions that are continuously controlled visually (Atkinson et al., 1997, 2003, 2006; Elliott, Welsh, Lyons, Hansen, & Wu, 2006). Taken together, these patient studies show that there are perception and action tasks that involve distinct visual processes related to ventral and dorsal stream functioning.

Before we further elucidate the differences between the use of visual information for action and the use of visual information for perception, we should emphasize that Milner and Goodale's view of visual perception and the visual guidance of action stands in sharp contrast to the ecological approach (Michaels, 2000; van der Kamp & Savelsbergh, 2000, 2002). For example, Milner and Goodale defined visual perception as a process that "allows one to assign meaning and significance to external objects and events" (Milner & Goodale, 1995, p. 2) and as the "creation of an internal model or percept of the external world . . . a model that can be used in the recognition of objects and understanding their interactions" (Goodale & Humphrey, 1998, pp. 206-207). According to Milner and Goodale, the two visual systems differ in the way visual stimuli are transformed or encoded. Perception and action require different transformations of the same visual stimulus; the stimulus is encoded into allocentric or egocentric frames of references, respectively.

In contrast, proponents of the ecological approach refute the necessity for these enrichment processes. They explain the difference between action and perception in terms of distinct sources of visual information that are picked up and used (Michaels, 2000; van der Kamp, 1999; van der Kamp, Rivas, van Doorn, & Savelsbergh, 2008; van der Kamp, Savelsbergh, & Rosengren, 2001). In this view, action and perception differ in their reliance on egocentric (body-centered, viewer-dependent) information and allocentric (world-centered, viewer-independent) sources of information. The visual control of goal-directed action primarily relies on egocentric sources of information. By contrast, visual perception is chiefly based on allocentric sources of information that specify objects, events, and places relative to each other. These latter sources of information are thought to result in perceptual illusions (see chapter 13). The Ebbinghaus illusion, for instance, consists of a circle surrounded by smaller or larger circles (see figure 16.2). When the outer circles are smaller than the inner circle, the inner circle is perceived to be larger than it is. Conversely, the inner circle is perceived to be smaller when it is surrounded by larger circles. However, if the inner circle is grasped, hand aperture is scaled to the real size of the circle and not to the perceived size. Thus, visual perception takes the visual context into account, but the visual control of action remains largely unaffected (Aglioti, Goodale, & DeSouza, 1993; van Doorn, van der Kamp, & Savelsbergh, 2007).

Besides relying on different sources of visual information, action and perception are also distinguished by the timescale at which they operate. Action entails the pickup of information to instantaneously control the ongoing movement. The information is used online (i.e., immediately) and decays quickly thereafter—it is short lived. In contrast, visual perception does not involve a time constraint—visual information used to obtain knowledge about the environment can be exploited over longer time intervals.

These differences in timescale can be shown by introducing a temporal delay between information pickup and action execution. Due to the quick decay of the information, a delay results in perturbation of the online

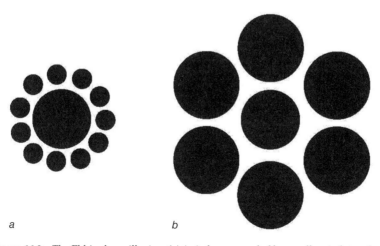

a   b

▶ **Figure 16.2**   The Ebbinghaus illusion. *(a)* A circle surrounded by smaller circles makes the inner circle appear larger. *(b)* A circle surrounded by larger circles makes the inner circle appear smaller.

movement control processes. It appears that under these circumstances, movement control becomes more reliant on allocentric sources of information, resulting in specific changes in the kinematics of the movement (e.g., Hu, Eagleson, & Goodale, 1999). For example, a delay causes a perceptual illusion (i.e., allocentric information) to affect movement execution (e.g., Mendoza, Hansen, Glazebrook, Keetch, & Elliott, 2005; Westwood, Chapman, & Roy, 2000; Westwood & Goodale, 2003; Westwood, McEachern, & Roy, 2001). These findings indicate that not only the use of visual information for action and perception entails different timescales but also the two processes complement each other. If one process is compromised, the contribution of the other may increase.

In sum, there is good evidence that the use of visual information for action and perception is dissociated. Action and perception rely on different sources of information and operate at different timescales. However, even though these processes are separate, they work together and may serve complementary functions. Consequently, it is not appropriate to make the distinction between action and perception based on the exploitation of egocentric versus allocentric sources of information absolute. Indeed, whether to make the distinction at all is currently under debate (Mendoza et al., 2005; Milner & Goodale, 2008; see also Rossetti & Pisella, 2002). Handlovsky, Hansen, Lee, and Elliott (2004), for instance, found that the Ebbinghaus illusion (see figure 16.2) affects online movement control. In their study, the presence and absence of illusory stimuli (i.e., allocentric information) before and during movement execution were manipulated independently. Participants were presented with a circle that was (1) not surrounded by circles, (2) surrounded by smaller circles (see figure 16.2a), or (3) surrounded by larger circles (see figure 16.2b). During aiming movements toward the inner circle, the display remained the same or changed by eliminating the surrounding circles (in the cases that stimulus 2 or 3 was displayed) or by adding small or large surrounding circles (in the case that stimulus 1 was presented). When a surround of small circles was added, the time the participants needed to perform their aiming movement decreased significantly. This reduction was attributed to a decrease in time between peak velocity and termination of the movement, a portion of the movement that is associated with online control (Handlovsky et al., 2004; see Mendoza et al., 2005). The other manipulations, however, did not result in significant differences in movement time. Nevertheless, the findings suggest that the online visual control of movement does not exclusively rely on egocentric information; allocentric information may be exploited as well. It is possible to argue, therefore, that distinguishing between action and perception based on egocentric and allocentric information is inappropriate (e.g., Mendoza et al., 2005; Smeets & Brenner, 1995). However, considering other sources of evidence, we think that the distinction is still tenable (and valuable) if it is kept in mind that the distinction is not absolute.

Development of the Use of Visual Information for Action and Perception in Infancy

In the previous section, we discussed the distinction between using visual information for action and using it for perception. We argued that there are two independent but interacting visual systems, one concerning the visual control of goal-directed action and the other dealing with obtaining knowledge about the environment. The distinction between the uses of visual information in adults raises the issue of the early development of these two processes, as well as their interaction.

In the remaining sections of this chapter, we explore these developmental issues. First, we focus on the findings of earlier studies that suggest separate developmental trajectories for action and perception. We do this by assessing the involvement of egocentric and allocentric information in infants' action and perception processes. Second, we evaluate whether action and perception operate at different timescales (online versus off-line) in early development. More precisely, we discuss studies that suggest an interaction between the two processes early in infancy.

Early Development of Action

For adults, it has been demonstrated that the visual control of movements is primarily guided by egocentric information, whereas allocentric information seems of lesser importance. We explore whether this is also true during the first year of life, examining whether goal-directed actions that manifest during early development (i.e., eye movements and reaching) are more reliant on egocentric information than on allocentric information.

Eye Movements   Research on tracking visual stimuli indicates that infants use egocentric information to control eye movements. Von Hofsten and Rosander (1996, 1997; Rosander & von Hofsten, 2000, 2002) have examined infants' ability to track moving objects under various conditions, including manipulations of egocentric and allocentric sources of information. These researchers investigated 1 to 3 mo old infants who were tracking a target that oscillated in front of them. The target was so big that it covered the entire field of view so that there was no background information (von Hofsten & Rosander, 1996). The authors found that infants as young as 1 mo of age are able to track the moving target and that tracking performance improves substantially with age. The lag with which infants tracked the target was smaller for older versus younger infants. The authors argued that this decrease in temporal lag was due to an improved ability to couple eye movements with head movements both spatially and temporally. The findings suggest the use of egocentric sources of information. Specifically, the movements of head and eyes are controlled based on information that specifies the movement of the target relative to the infant. This conclusion was based on the fact that, because of the size of the target, there was no background that could provide additional information about the position of the target. In effect, allocentric information was eliminated.

The same results were found for tracking smaller objects that moved relative to a homogeneous background, which also fails to provide additional allocentric information about the target position (Rosander & von Hofsten, 2002; von Hofsten & Rosander, 1997). Tracking performances in 1 to 5 mo old infants were similar. However, when the small object moved in front of a patterned background (i.e., allocentric information), tracking was facilitated only in infants aged 3 mo and older (Rosander & von Hofsten, 2000). Von Hofsten and Rosander argued that the background provided additional information (i.e., allocentric information) that served as a reference frame to guide eye movements at the turning points. Consequently, it might be concluded that, until 3 mo, infants rely solely on egocentric information to control eye and head movements when tracking a moving object. Infants at that age do not appear to benefit from additional allocentric sources of information; however, allocentric information seems to improve tracking performance beyond that age.

Further evidence suggesting that young infants rely on egocentric sources of information to control eye movements is provided by Gilmore and Johnson (1997, 1998). In their studies, they presented 4 to 6 mo old infants with a visual stimulus on a central monitor located in front of the infants followed by a sequence of two brief visual stimuli that flashed first 30° to the left of the center of fixation and then 30° to the right of the center of fixation (see figure 16.3a). The flashes occurred before the infants shifted gaze. The infants had to integrate the positions of both flashes to accurately fixate them. The authors argued that if an infant relies on information relative to the eye position (what they denote a *retinocentric reference frame*),[1] then the infant would not be able to fixate both stimuli sequentially; the second saccade would fall short (see figure 16.3b). More specifically, picking up information specifying the location of both target stimuli relative to the current eye position prevents the information from being veridical across eye movements. That is, when an eye movement (e.g., gaze shift) is made to the first target, the exploited information of the second target location remains specific to the former eye position but not to the new eye position. By contrast, picking up information combining the retinal and eye position (i.e., a *head-centered reference frame*) would result in fixating both target stimuli, since this information remains veridical across eye movements as long as the head does not move.

It was found that 6 mo old infants were capable of making accurate eye movements to both stimuli, suggesting that they detected information about the locations of the flashed stimuli relative to their head position.

---

[1]The term *reference frame*, also used by Milner and Goodale (1995), is equivalent to *sources of information* (i.e., retinocentric sources of information).

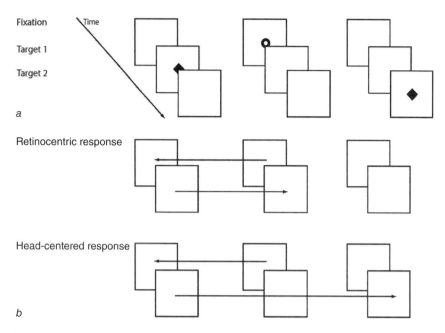

▶ **Figure 16.3**   A pictorial summary of the main conditions of Gilmore and Johnson's (1997) experiment. *(a)* Display sequence of the visual stimuli. After fixation of the first stimulus, two stimuli were flashed on the right or the left monitor, one after the other. *(b)* Response types in accordance with the exploited egocentric information (i.e., retinocentric or head centered).

Infants who were 4 and 5 mo old, however, did not succeed in guiding eye movements to the second target; they made errors that were consistent with the use of retinocentric sources of information. Importantly, all infants relied primarily on egocentric sources of information to control eye movements; the exploited information specified a relationship between the infant and the visual stimuli. However, Gilmore and Johnson (1997, 1998) did not specifically aim at disentangling egocentric and allocentric sources of information. Consequently, similar results would have been obtained when the older infants had used allocentric information, because with a stable head position (relative to the environment), head-centered egocentric and background allocentric sources of information covary. Nevertheless, the youngest infants did clearly rely on retinocentered egocentric information.

These findings strongly suggest that during early development, infants' eye movements primarily rely on egocentric information. There is no evidence that infants before the age of 3 mo exploit allocentric sources of information. Yet, beyond this age allocentric information may add to the accuracy of eye movements. The evidence, however, is partly circumstantial because direct tests, for instance by manipulating egocentric and allocentric information, are lacking.

Reaching   In a similar vein, infants were found to primarily exploit egocentric information when reaching for moving objects. As mentioned earlier, by 3 mo of age, infants are already capable of intercepting moving objects. Of course, this does not by itself imply that infants use egocentric information. After all, they might gain knowledge about where to move the hand in space relative to a location in the environment rather than relative to the self. For example, a ball that moves on a set trajectory (as is usually the case in infant studies) can be intercepted at a fixed location relative to some feature in the environment. However, von Hofsten (1980, 1983; von Hofsten & Lindhagen, 1979) argued that infants reaching toward objects that approach on a fixed trajectory from different directions (from the left and right of the baby) with different velocities (3.4-30 cm/s) are guided by egocentric information. He argues that "the infant reaches in reference to a coordinate system fixed to the moving object instead of to the static background" (von Hofsten, 1983, pp. 83-84). In other words, infants extrapolate the future position of the moving ball and control their reaching accordingly (von Hofsten, 1980, 1983; von Hofsten et al., 1998). Infants' reaching behavior is not characterized by stereotyped reaching toward a fixed position relative to other objects in the environment; rather, it seems to be adapted to the approach characteristics relative to the self. This indicates use of egocentric information when controlling reaching movements.

The use of egocentric information while reaching for a moving object is also consistent with the findings of van Hof (2005; see also van Hof et al., 2008). She revealed that 3 to 9 mo old infants who reach for moving objects approaching frontally at different speeds (10-200 cm/s) detect and use visual information specifying the temporal relationship between the infant and the object (i.e., egocentric information). Moreover, older infants exploited more useful egocentric information to guide their reaching movements than the younger infants; 3 to 5 mo old infants timed their reaching based on the optical angle (ϕ). Recall that this variable is defined as the angle subtended by the edges of the ball and the infant's eye (see figure 16.1 on page 295). Thus, the optic angle is an egocentric (head-centered) source of information. Reliance on this variable yields initiation of the reach when the object is at a fixed distance from the observation point. The older infants, in contrast, used the absolute rate of change of the optical angle $(\dot{\phi})$ or tau $(T[\phi])$. As a result, these infants timed their reaching movements based on time rather than distance. This strategy is more sophisticated. It yields better performance because a distance strategy causes the infant to initiate the reaching too late in the case of high ball velocities. Either way, these findings suggest that infants use egocentric information when controlling reaching movements toward moving objects.

The results are consistent with the use of egocentric information, but they are not definite because none of the studies involved the manipulation of allocentric information. Fortunately, there is a series of studies that provide insight into the reliance on allocentric sources of information (Clifton, Muir, Ashmead, & Clarkson, 1993; Clifton, Rochat, Robin, & Berthier, 1994; McCarty & Ashmead, 1999; McCarty, Clifton, Ashmead, Lee, & Goubet, 2001; Robin, Berthier, & Clifton, 1996). Robin and colleagues (1996), for instance, presented 5 and 7.5 mo old infants with moving and stationary objects in two illumination conditions (light and dark). In the dark condition, a glowing object was presented in an otherwise dark environment. Consequently, the infants could pick up only egocentric information; all sources of allocentric information were eliminated.

In accordance with earlier research of Clifton and colleagues (Clifton et al., 1993, 1994), the study found that the infants' reaching behavior toward stationary objects was comparable for both illumination conditions. The authors argued that sight of the hand does not affect the reaching, an observation that is compatible with findings concerning reaching in adults (e.g., Elliott, 1990). Importantly, the observation that reaches remained unperturbed also indicates that infants at this age do not rely on allocentric sources of information when controlling their arm movements. In addition, the authors reported that when presented with moving objects, infants showed fewer reaches in the dark condition than in the light condition (Robin et al., 1996), but once they attempted to reach for the ball, they performed at a level comparable to that of the light condition. The latter finding suggests that elimination of allocentric information may make it more difficult for infants to perceive what the environment offers for action (i.e., affordance perception; Gibson, 1979/1986). Yet, the use of vision to control the movement was not affected by the presence or absence of allocentric information.

In sum, the evidence on the use of egocentric and allocentric information in movement control during early development is largely circumstantial. That said, these studies indicate that during early development, the control of eye and arm movements is primarily guided by egocentric information. Furthermore, the studies suggest that only at later ages does allocentric information come into play, with egocentric information still being the most pertinent source in movement control.

Early Development of Visual Perception

Having considered the empirical evidence for the use of egocentric (and allocentric) information in the early development of movement control, we now describe the use of visual information in the early development of perception. In adults, visual perception is thought to rely on allocentric rather than egocentric information (Milner & Goodale, 1995). In this section, we assess whether this is also true for the early development of visual perception. To allow for comparison with the findings on action in the previous section, we restrict ourselves to perception of speed and direction of motion of moving stimuli.

Infant perception is commonly investigated using habituation or preferential looking methods (e.g., Dannemiller & Freedland, 1989, 1991; Kaufmann, Stucki, & Kaufmann-Hayoz, 1985; Mason, Braddick, & Wattam-Bell, 2003; Wattam-Bell, 1991, 1992, 1996a, 1996b). In preference-looking experiments, an infant is presented with two visual stimuli simultaneously. By measuring the infant's looking time for each stimulus, it is determined whether the infant has a preference for one of the stimuli. In that case, it is assumed that the infant visually discriminates the stimuli. In habituation experiments, an infant is repeatedly shown the same stimulus. Habituation occurs when the infant loses interest in the stimulus, indicated by a significant decrease in looking time. If a new stimulus elicits longer looking times, dishabituation is said to occur. Once again, the inference is that the infant visually discriminates the two stimuli. (Note that these methods do not entail the assessment of how infants control eye and head movements when they look at the visual stimuli. The researcher's interest is only in the duration of looking as an indicator of what infants perceive.)

To date, the contributions of allocentric and egocentric information sources in the early development of the perception of motion direction and velocity have received scant attention. Identification of their contributions would entail independent manipulation of the two. Given the difficulties involved in manipulating egocentric sources (e.g., moving the baby in synchrony with the moving object), the manipulation of allocentric information may be more fruitful. It is predicted that eliminating allocentric sources of information (e.g., by presenting the stimulus in an entirely darkened environment or on a screen that encompasses the infant's entire field of view) would have profoundly adverse effects on the perception of motion direction and motion velocity early in development.

Perception of Motion Velocity   Infants who are 1 mo perceive motion velocity when presented with a stimulus that moves relative to a static environment (e.g., the boundaries of a monitor), although this ability is restricted to a narrow range of velocities that expands with age (Dannemiller & Freedland, 1989, 1991; Kaufmann et al., 1985; Volkmann & Dobson, 1976; Wattam-Bell, 1992). Infants who were 6 wk old detected differences in velocity of 9°/s (Aslin & Shea, 1990), whereas infants who were 20 wk old were able to perceive much smaller differences in velocities of 2.3°/s to 1.2°/s (Bertenthal & Bradburry, 1992; Dannemiller & Freedland, 1989). Unfortunately, these studies do not provide insight into the contributions of allocentric and egocentric information. These sources of information always covaried because they were not independently manipulated. Hence, further research is needed to discover whether infants primarily rely on allocentric sources of information for the perception of motion velocity.

Perception of Motion Direction   Infants' perception of motion direction has been studied in more detail. Wattam-Bell (1992, 1994, 1996a, 1996b) examined 1 to 4 mo infants' ability to perceptually discriminate stimulus displays. Infants' looking behavior for displays with a static stimulus pattern and displays with a coherently moving uniform stimulus pattern were compared, or infants' looking behavior for displays with a coherently moving uniform stimulus pattern was contrasted with looking behavior for displays with segregated stimulus patterns moving in opposite directions (see figure 16.4).

These studies revealed that 1 mo old infants discriminated between the static and moving stimulus patterns. However, it was not until the age of 7 to 8 wk that infants discriminated between the uniform and segregated stimulus patterns. In other words, although 1 mo old infants could perceive motion per se, it took at least 2 wk more before they were able to perceive the direction of motion (Atkinson & Braddick, 2003; Wattam-Bell, 1992, 1994, 1996a, 1996b; see also Dannemiller & Freedland, 1989, 1991). Banton, Dobkins, and Bertenthal (2001), who used similar segregated stimulus patterns but with motion directions that ranged between 0° and 180°, found that the ability to detect differences in motion direction improved with age. For the 6 wk old infants, no threshold could be obtained. Consistent with the findings of Wattam-Bell, even the opposite motions (i.e., 180°) were not discriminated by these infants. By 12 wk, however, infants discriminated a difference in motion direction of 22°, whereas the 18 wk old infants were able to discriminate differences of 17°.

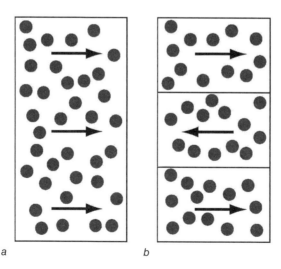

a   b

▶ **Figure 16.4** Typical display used in studies employing random-dot stimuli to investigate the perception of motion direction in infants. *(a)* Uniform display: All dots move uniform and coherently (as shown by the arrows). *(b)* Segregated display: In the upper and lower box of the display, the dots move uniformly, whereas the dots in the middle box move in the opposite direction (as illustrated by the arrows in the boxes).

In addition to presenting egocentric information (i.e., motion direction of the stimulus pattern relative to the stationary infant), these studies also presented allocentric information about motion direction. This information was directly available from the segregated stimulus patterns within a display. These studies therefore cannot elucidate infants' reliance on egocentric versus allocentric information. However, Wattam-Bell (1996a, 1996c) conducted several habituation experiments that do speak to the issue. He used coherent and uniform motion displays in which allocentric information was not always present. In the first study (Wattam-Bell, 1996a, experiment 3), infants aged between 3 and 8 wk were habituated to a display that either contained uniform rightward motion or uniform leftward motion. In the subsequent test phase, infants were presented with a display that contained both uniform motion directions. Wattam-Bell (1996a) reported that the infants did not discriminate between the original and the new motion direction. Rather than providing allocentric information within a display (as in the segregated displays shown in figure 16.4), this experiment allowed infants to extract allocentric information about motion direction only by comparing two displays. It might have been these differences in the sources of allocentric information that prevented the 6 to 8 wk old infants from discriminating motion direction when looking at two displays that contained opposite but uniform stimulus patterns (Wattam-Bell, 1996a). In contrast, infants of the same age discriminated motion direction when they looked at segregated stimulus patterns (Wattam-Bell, 1996a, 1996b).

More convincing evidence that these young infants rely on allocentric sources of information comes from an experiment in which infants were habituated to upward and downward motion (Wattam-Bell, 1996c, in Atkinson, 2000, and in Braddick, Atkinson, & Wattam-Bell, 2003). In the subsequent test phase, the infants were presented with only the opposite motion direction. Moreover, care was taken to eliminate all sources of allocentric information. No motion boundaries or alternative sources of background information were available (Atkinson, 2000, pp. 80-81; see also Braddick et al., 2003). In other words, the only information available on motion direction during the habituation and test phases of this experiment was relative to the infant (i.e., egocentric). Wattam-Bell found that infants did not dishabituate before the age of 12 wk. Therefore, the ability to perceive absolute motion direction using only egocentric information does not appear to emerge before the age of 12 wk. By contrast, perceptions of motion direction occur between 6 and 12 wk when allocentric sources of information are available.

To conclude, although the evidence is scarce and incomplete, it seems that allocentric sources of information are much more important than egocentric sources in the development of visual perception. Infants younger than 3 mo seem completely reliant on allocentric information for the perception of motion direction. By contrast, egocentric information contributes only after 3 mo of age.

Interaction Between Action and Perception Processes in Early Infancy

Up to this point, we have considered the early development of visual information usage in movement control and perception of the environment separately. The present review suggests that egocentric sources of information play a major role in the early development of action, whereas allocentric sources of information appear central in the early development of perception. This suggests that action and perception follow separate developmental trajectories. Yet, adult studies have shown that the two separate processes work together and may serve complementary functions. Recall that a temporal delay between the detection of information and the execution of action can have profound influences on movement kinematics (Hu et al., 1999). The temporal delay perturbs the dorsal online movement control processes, which results in the engagement of ventral perception processes in movement control. This ventral contribution is demonstrated by the presence of an illusion bias in the movement kinematics (e.g., Westwood et al., 2000, 2001). The present section assesses the development of this interaction during infancy. If the use of visual information in action and perception separates shortly after birth and follows different trajectories (Atkinson, 2000; Bertenthal, 1996; Rochat, 2001; van der Kamp & Savelsbergh, 2000, 2002; von Hofsten et al., 1998), what does this mean for the interaction between the two processes? Is the interaction already present at birth, or does it emerge later, and does it need further development? To explore these issues, we discuss studies in which infants tracked or reached for objects. These are actions that, under normal circumstances, are guided by egocentric information. In these studies, however, a temporal delay was introduced by either darkening the room and target or by placing a screen between the moving object and the infant.

Effects of Temporal Delay on Infants' Reaching and Tracking   Clifton and coworkers demonstrated that 4 mo old infants presented with a stationary sounding object in the dark are able to touch and grasp the object (Clifton et al., 1993; Clifton, Perris, & Bullinger, 1991; see also Bower & Wishart, 1972). This is at approximately the same age as the first successful reaching for objects in the light and could be interpreted as a well-developed interaction. Specifically, the ventral perception system is capable of taking over the control of reaching.

However, at least two observations qualify this claim. First, during these experiments the lights were turned off shortly after the reach was initiated. The reason for this procedure was that otherwise the infants did not reach (Clifton et al., 1991; see also Hood & Willats, 1986). In other words, it seems that 4 mo old infants do not reach, or reach less frequently, for objects when a temporal delay is introduced. Second, even the reaching movements that were initiated when the room was darkened were less accurate and had kinematic characteristics that were substantially different from reaching for objects in the light (Clifton et al., 1993; Clifton et al., 1991). The reaches in the dark had higher velocities and were of shorter duration compared with reaches in the light (McCarty & Ashmead, 1999). Temporal delays in adults, however, commonly result in lower velocities and longer durations (Hu et al., 1999). The reason for the opposite effects between infants and adults is unclear. It might be related to the auditory information available from the sounding objects in the infant studies. The findings are not unambiguous, but they do suggest that young infants are less likely to reach when a temporal delay is introduced.

Research that used moving objects is less ambiguous. These studies introduced a temporal delay between the pickup of information and movement execution by using a brief blackout (i.e., total darkening of the environment and moving target) or occlusion (i.e., placing a screen between the infant and the path of motion of the object). These studies revealed that infants before 4 mo of age do not track, and infants before 5 mo of age do not reach for objects that move temporally out of sight. It is only beyond these ages that infants perform predictive tracking and reaching movements under these circumstances (Jonsson & von Hofsten, 2003; Munakata, Jonsson, Spelke, & von Hofsten, 1996; Rosander & von Hofsten, 2004; van der Meer, van der Weel, & Lee, 1994; von Hofsten, Kochukhova, & Rosander, 2007). Recall that predictive tracking and reaching without temporal delays emerges at 1 and 3 or 4 mo of age, respectively. Clearly, infants initially are not capable of dealing with the perturbations to the online control process caused by a temporal delay. It seems to take at least 1 mo more before they start to compensate for these perturbations. It is likely that this ability reflects the first interaction between action and perception processes.

The way that 4 mo infants perform predictive tracking differs for situations in which the object is or is not temporally out of sight—that is, infants' tracking over an occluder is saccadic rather than smooth (Rosander & von Hofsten, 2004; von Hofsten, 2004; von Hofsten et al., 2007), and the head lags the moving target to a larger extent during the occlusion and blackout conditions than in a full-vision condition (Jonsson & von Hofsten, 2003). Furthermore, until 5 mo of age, infants do not reach when the trajectory of a moving object is partially occluded (van der Meer et al., 1994). Beyond that age, infants increasingly reach for the occluded ball, though the amount of reaching is less frequent compared with full-vision conditions (Jonsson & von Hofsten, 2003). Van der Meer and colleagues (1994) also reported that 5 to 8 mo old infants initiated their reach at a fixed location (i.e., relative to the screen), whereas older infants started their reach at a certain time before the ball reappeared. More kinematic data are not available from these studies.

Taken together, the findings indicate that, as in adults, the introduction of a temporal delay between information pickup and movement execution perturbs infants' control of tracking and reaching. In the youngest infants, predictive tracking and reaching broke down, suggesting that no other processes (including those involved in perception) could compensate for the perturbation of the action system. It follows that the action and perception processes do not work together in the beginning. Nonetheless, from 4 mo (in the case of tracking) to 5 mo (in the case of reaching), infants seem able to guide their actions when the object is briefly out of sight. Because the kinematic characteristics of these actions are distinct from situations in which the object is not occluded from sight, it might be that ventral perceptual processes contribute. Support for the latter contention would be provided if it could be shown that predictive tracking and reaching for objects that are temporarily out of sight involve allocentric information. We explore this issue in the next section by comparing the findings from blackout and occlusion studies.

Comparison Between Blackout and Occlusion Studies The information sources that are available to control predictive tracking and reaching in the blackout and occlusion studies differ. In the blackout studies, where both the environment and target are completely darkened, all visual information is eliminated. By contrast, in the occlusion studies, where a screen is placed between the moving object and the infant, only the egocentric sources are eliminated; several allocentric sources remain. For instance, the borders of the occluding screen provide information about where the moving object disappears and reappears. If infants' successful predictive tracking and reaching for objects that are temporarily out of sight is supported by ventral perceptual processes, it would be expected that infants would perform better in the occlusion situations than in the blackout situations because the former provides allocentric sources of information. Indeed, tracking performance is more proficient in occlusion situations versus blackout situations (Jonsson & von Hofsten, 2003; Munakata et al., 1996). Infants frequently stopped tracking the moment the object disappeared and then shifted their gaze to the other edge of the screen to where the object would reappear. Sometimes, infants were observed to shift their gaze to the far edge of the screen where the object would reappear, return to the edge of the screen where the object disappeared, and make a final gaze shift back to the location of reappearance (Rosander & von Hofsten, 2004; von Hofsten et al., 2007). It thus seems that infants exploit information from the screen to predict where the object will reappear and use that information to guide their eye movements. In the blackout situation, this information was not available, resulting in less predictive tracking. Tracking movements in the blackout situation were slower, which resulted in lags larger than those observed in occlusion situations (Jonsson & von Hofsten, 2003; Munakata et al., 1996).

It is somewhat surprising that reaching performance deteriorates more in occlusion versus blackout situations (Jonsson & von Hofsten, 2003). This finding is not what would be expected. Instead of inhibiting predictive reaching, allocentric information sources in the occlusion situations should have facilitated it. Two explanations come to mind. First, it might be that our hypothesis that the ability of 5 mo old infants to successfully reach for moving objects that are temporarily out of sight points to the contribution of ventral perceptual processes simply is incorrect. Alternatively, the screen might absorb the infants' visual attention after the object disappears behind it (Jonsson & von Hofsten, 2003; Rosander & von Hofsten, 2004; von Hofsten, 2004; von Hofsten et al., 2007).

In conclusion, the evidence suggests that interaction between action and perception processes develops within the first year of life. It is not until about 1 mo of age, after infants can successfully track and reach for objects, that they can deal with a temporal delay between the detection of visual information and the execution of action. With respect to tracking, certain circumstantial evidence suggests the involvement of allocentric information sources in overcoming the temporal delay. However, much more experimental work is needed to substantiate this claim.

Conclusions and Future Directions

In this chapter, we explored whether the early development of visual information usage for perception and of visual information usage for action follow separate developmental trajectories. Following the neuro-psychological work of Milner and Goodale (1995) and Gibson's ecological approach to perception and action (Gibson, 1979/1986), we argued that the use of visual information for perception and the use of visual information in movement control differ in the type of information that is exploited for the processes as well as in the timescale at which the two processes operate. Movement control processes primarily but not exclusively involve the instantaneous use of egocentric sources of information, whereas visual perception is much more reliant on allocentric sources of information that are available over longer amounts of time. Importantly, the two processes must interact to achieve successful performance. If, for example, the action processes are perturbed, the contribution of the perception processes in performance is likely to increase.

A selective review of the development of visual information usage in action and perception suggests different developmental trajectories. On the one hand, the control of tracking and reaching movements for objects moving in different directions and with different speeds primarily relies on egocentric information between 1 mo (in the case of tracking) and 3 mo (in the case of reaching) after birth. It appears that allocentric information does not contribute before 3 mo of age, at least as far as it concerns tracking. The role of allocentric information in reaching is less clear, although reaching in the dark for glowing objects suggests that until 7 mo of age, allocentric information plays a minor role at best. On the other hand, the perception of motion direction, which emerges about 6 wk after birth, chiefly relies on allocentric information. There is tentative evidence that egocentric information sources do not get involved before 3 mo of age. In other words, on a developmental timescale there may be a differential involvement of egocentric and allocentric information sources. If true, this would lend support to the idea that the separation between the use of visual information in action and the use of visual information in perception already exists shortly after birth. However, caution is warranted since much of the evidence that we presented is circumstantial and needs further testing

The same is true for the empirical evidence related to the development of the interaction between the two processes. Research suggests that until the age of 4 mo (in the case of tracking) to 5 mo (in the case of reaching), a temporal delay between the detection of the information and movement onset leads to a breakdown of action. It is only beyond these ages that infants learn to deal with this type of perturbation. One hypothesis is that this is due to the visual perception system becoming engaged in the control of action. Hence, the first indications of interaction between action and perception processes would occur between 4 and 5 mo of age, depending on the task. At this stage of research, this interpretation is rather speculative, and alternative explanations cannot be ruled out.

Clearly, the first round of research should be directed at substantiating the claims we have made here. However, if we speculate that they are at least partly true, then a second round of research will have to deal much more explicitly with the relationship between the development of action and the development of perception. As mentioned early in the chapter, several theories posit that the development of action precedes the development of perception, but there are equally strong claims to the contrary (e.g., Atkinson, 2000; Kellman & Arterberry, 1998; Piaget, 1952). We have argued that neither action nor perception is privileged in development but that each follows its own developmental trajectory. This does not mean that action and perception develop in total isolation. On the contrary, we are convinced that they mutually influence each other. Van Hof and colleagues (2008), for example, showed in 3 to 9 mo old infants that improvements in the perception of whether a moving object can be caught are related to the infant's proficiency in controlling the catching movements, suggesting that the development of perception is constrained by the development of action. It is for future research to unravel exactly how and when the development of action and the development of perception influence each other.

CHAPTER 17

Motor Learning Through Observation

DANA MASLOVAT, SPENCER HAYES, ROBERT R. HORN, AND NICOLA J. HODGES

Motor skill acquisition typically involves the transfer of information between instructor and learner. A common method of transfer is demonstration. *Observational learning* is the term for the process by which observers watch the behavior of a model and adapt their movement as a result, typically as assessed in a delayed retention test (see Hodges, Williams, Hayes, & Breslin, 2007; Horn & Williams, 2004; McCullagh & Weiss, 2001; Newell, Morris, & Scully, 1985; Vogt & Thomaschke, 2007; Williams, Davids, & Williams, 1999, for reviews). Relevant to this review is the difference between observational learning and observational practice (Vogt & Thomaschke, 2007). Observational learning relates to a situation where a demonstration and physical practice are interleaved (i.e., observe, practice, observe). Observational practice relates to a situation that merely requires the learner to observe and does not involve physical practice.

It has long been thought that observational learning is a more efficient method of learning than verbal instructions (McCullagh & Weiss, 2001). It is considered a powerful means to transmit patterns of behavior to a learner (Bandura, 1986). The results of a meta-analysis of the literature on observational learning reflected a significant advantage of modeling over practice-only (i.e., discovery) conditions (Ashford, Bennett, & Davids, 2006). Compared with discovery learning, observational learning has been shown to provide both immediate performance benefits and long-term learning benefits in a range of behavioral measures. These include improvements in movement form and outcome, recall and recognition, decision making, and self-confidence, as well as reduced fear and anxiety (see Hodges et al., 2007, and McCullagh & Weiss, 2001, for more detailed reviews). Although it is clear that observational learning can be an effective teaching tool, understanding the mechanisms underlying this process provides valuable information to optimize the use of demonstrations.

This chapter summarizes the theories, methods, and techniques that have influenced research in the field of adult observational learning. We hope this information will help researchers determine the information and processes guiding this perceptual–motor learning process. We start with some definitions followed by a review of the theoretical approaches that have guided research into observational learning, practice, and imitation. This includes an examination of traditional behaviorally based theories as well as current behavioral approaches and theories that have been guided by neurophysiology and brain imaging research. In the remaining sections we look at measures and manipulations that have been used to explore variables related to the observational learning process. The effectiveness of observation for learning appears to depend on a complex interaction among the observer, model, and task, and thus these characteristics are discussed in relation to the various methods that have been used to assess model effectiveness (e.g., movement kinematics, eye movement recording, brain imaging, point-light models).

Cognitive Mediated Learning

An initial theoretical explanation for how information is transferred to the observer through modeling was offered by Bandura (1971) in his social learning theory, later revised to social cognitive theory (1986). Building upon Sheffield's (1961) concept that behavior is stored in symbolic form, Bandura proposed that a representation serves as the mediator between observation and action. Therefore, the quality of the symbolic representation (i.e., the learner's internal standard) was believed to be critical for modeling effectiveness (see Carroll & Bandura, 1982, 1990). Although this theoretical approach has led to numerous experiments exploring task, model, and observer characteristics that maximize learning, it has generally failed to prompt researchers to examine what information is perceived and how it guides subsequent actions. Moreover, the underspecification of the nature of the cognitive representation has afforded researchers few testable hypotheses (Heyes, 2002). Bandura's theory is also primarily based on social learning principles rather than motor learning, and it is possible that the mechanisms for these two functions are quite different (see Horn, Williams, & Scott, 2002).

In Bandura's formulation, the cognitive representation that guides imitation is acquired before the observer attempts to perform the skill. This was originally termed *no-trial learning* (Bandura, 1965). More recent discussions of when observational learning takes place in the perception–action process have resulted in the terms *late* and *early mediation* (Vogt, 2002; Vogt & Thomaschke, 2007). In late mediation, the motor representation (and hence the motor system) is only formed (or engaged) during movement reproduction and physical practice. In early mediation, the motor system is believed to be involved during observation and no physical practice or translation is needed for motor learning to occur. Although superficially it is tempting to equate Bandura's no-trial learning with early mediation, Bandura did not discuss the involvement of the motor system during observation and argued that the observed information was translated through cognitive processes (see also Heyes, 2002). In view of these latter factors, and that the motor demands in Bandura and colleagues' tasks were low, we equate his ideas more with late-mediation accounts of observational learning.

The positive effects of observation in the absence of physical practice do not necessarily imply that the motor system is engaged during observation. Considerable evidence suggests that demonstrations help to convey an explicit, cognitive strategy that could result in immediate performance improvements. For example, throwing a dart with an unusual underarm throw to hit a target on the floor (Al-Abood, Davids, & Bennett, 2001), moving a ball quickly to attain a target in the shoot-the-moon task (Martens, Burwitz, & Zuckerman, 1976), and learning to anticipate the trajectory of a stimulus (Kohl & Shea, 1992) are strategies which can be picked up through observation. It is likely that many motor skills have similar explicit strategies that can be acquired merely by observational practice (sometimes to the performer's detriment; see Hodges & Franks, 2002b).

The degree of verbalizable knowledge about the strategy used during performance might indicate the degree of motor involvement during observation, with less-verbalizable knowledge indicative of early mediation. For example, Mattar and Gribble (2005) provided an example of early mediation during observational practice. Observers acquired a novel motor action that required dynamic adaptations to motor perturbations even though they performed an attention-distracting arithmetic task during observation. Because the participants still learned the action, the authors argued that learning occurred at an unconscious level through the utilization of the motor system. Furthermore, a second group of participants who performed a nonrelated motor action during observation showed compromised performance. The authors concluded that the motor system was involved at the observation stage and that a cognitive strategy was not responsible for learning. Similarly, Heyes and Foster (2002) found that the degree of positive transfer in a keyboard sequence task depended on the effector. This finding would suggest some priming of the effector during observation and hence supports early mediation views of learning (see also Porro, Facchin, Fusi, Dri, & Fadiga, 2007).

We hypothesize that in motor tasks where the rule or strategy governing performance is difficult to ascertain, the motor system is likely to be more engaged during observation, a finding that is somewhat supported by neurophysiological evidence, as discussed later (Buccino et al., 2004). Indeed, there is evidence from sequence learning tasks that explicit instructions concerning the regularity of the sequence can interfere with performance and perhaps change the mode of control (and hence involvement of the motor system) in a similar manner to the strategies discussed here (see Berry & Broadbent, 1988; Green & Flowers, 1991; Magill & Clark, 1997).

A number of authors have extended Bandura and colleagues' early work (e.g., Carroll & Bandura, 1990) showing that cognitive processes such as detection and correction of error are aided by demonstrations, supporting the idea that a cognitive representation for the motor skill is acquired through observation. For example, observational practice was as effective as physical practice when error recognition was assessed during a serial keypress task (Black & Wright, 2000; Black, Wright, Magnuson, & Brueckner, 2005). Although Shea, Wright, Wulf, and Whitacre (2000) found advantages during retention for a physical practice group versus an observation-only group, both groups performed similarly on a transfer task where adaptability of the acquired cognitive strategy was required. Factors such as practice schedule (Wright, Li, & Coady, 1997; however, see Lee & White, 1990) and augmented feedback (Badets, Blandin, Wright, & Shea, 2006), which have been shown to influence physical practice, have also been shown to affect the observation process. Because these effects are believed to be mediated by processes related to recall, effort, and elaboration, it is argued that demonstrations engage the observer in cognitive and neurological processes similar to those adopted during physical practice (Badets & Blandin, 2004, 2005; Blandin & Proteau, 2000; Meegan, Aslin, & Jacobs, 2000).

In summary, there is significant evidence that observational practice and learning typically engage the cognitive system of the observer and that this higher-level processing of the perceptual information might facilitate transfer to new yet similar task situations (e.g., Shea et al., 2000). Observational practice is rarely equal to physical practice, and as suggested by a number of authors, motor practice appears necessary to calibrate the motor system (Shea et al., 2000) and aid in the development of a motor representation of the action (Vogt & Thomaschke, 2007).

Visuomotor Coupling and Direct Learning

One of the mechanisms that has been proposed to mediate observational practice and learning is mental imagery. Jeannerod (1994) proposed that observational practice involves neural mechanisms similar to those involved in mental imagery, with the only difference being the presence or absence of an external stimulus (for reviews, see also Annett, 1996; Jeannerod, 2001; Jeannerod & Frak, 1999; Vogt, 1996). For example, first-person actions (as would be self-generated in imagery) and third-person actions (as would be observed in demonstrations) share similar neural pathways (e.g., Anquetil & Jeannerod, 2007). Motor imagery also results in increased activity in cortical motor areas, suggesting that covert action simulation as a result of imagery or observation engages processes similar to those engaged by the actual action (e.g., Decety, Sjoholm, Ryding, Stenberg, & Ingvar, 1990; Grafton, Arbib, Fadiga, & Rizzolatti, 1996; Tomasino, Werner, Weiss, & Fink, 2007). People have also shown difficulty imaging actions they cannot perform, a phenomenon again suggesting the commonality of the observation for action and imagery processes (see Mulder, Zijlstra, Zijlstra, & Hochstenbach, 2007).

Despite evidence showing the similarity of these processes, Ram, Riggs, Skaling, Landers, and McCullagh (2007) found that observational learning was better for acquiring form and outcome in weightlifting and balance tasks compared with imagery conditions. In these experiments, participants were not able to form an accurate image of the action in the absence of demonstrations, thus hindering any covert action simulation and development of an appropriate cognitive representation. From a theoretical perspective, imagery might be involved in both early and late mediation, facilitating covert action simulation during observation and movement recall and reproduction processes during physical practice, respectively.

Studies on imitation in newborns showed that facial and hand gestures performed by adults could elicit similar actions in the newborn (Meltzoff & Moore, 1977). The active intermodal matching (AIM) theory resulted from this work and similar studies, which proposed an innate supramodal system in infants that had a common pathway for observation and execution of motor acts (Meltzoff & Moore, 1997). Similar theories have been proposed for adults, including common-coding theory (Prinz, 1997), whereby perceived events and planned actions share a common representational domain, and direct matching, where it is proposed that perception automatically activates the observed response (Meltzoff, 1993; Meltzoff & Moore, 1983, 1989, 2002). Several lines of evidence support these viewpoints. These are reviewed below in reference to neurophysiological data and then behavioral measures.

The discovery of similar patterns of cortical activation during both observation and physical production of a movement provides the best support for the capability of direct matching between action and perception (see Brass & Heyes, 2005; Rizzolatti, Fogassi, & Gallese, 2001; Rumiati & Bekkering, 2003; Vogt & Thomaschke, 2007; Wilson & Knoblich, 2005). As a result of advances in methodologies for measuring brain activity, a neurophysiological network that is involved in imitation, the mirror neuron system (MNS), has been discovered (see Rizzolatti & Craighero, 2004, for review). Mirror neurons were first discovered in the macaque monkey in area F5 of the premotor cortex and in the rostral section of the inferior parietal lobule, and strong evidence has been provided that similar structures are present in humans (di Pellegrino, Fadiga, Fogassi, Gallese, & Rizzolatti, 1992; Fogassi et al., 2005; Gallese, Fadiga, Fogassi, & Rizzolatti, 1996; Rizzolatti, Fadiga, Gallese, & Fogassi, 1996). The most common explanation of why these areas are activated during observation is that observation automatically evokes a motor representation of the action, forming the basis of action imitation, understanding, and anticipation (for reviews, see Elsner & Hommel, 2001; Fadiga & Craighero, 2003, 2004; Iacoboni, 2005; Prinz, 2006; Rizzolatti & Craighero, 2004; Rizzolatti et al., 2001; Wilson & Knoblich, 2005).

It does not appear that this cortical system directly transforms perceived motion information into action commands. Activation of mirror neurons in monkeys did not occur when an action was mimicked without an object (Gallese et al., 1996). Umilta and colleagues (2001) showed mirror neuron activity during observation of a reaching movement when the object was hidden yet the monkey knew it was present. Kohler and colleagues (2002) showed mirror neuron activity in monkeys for a recognizable action sound (e.g., ripping paper, breaking a peanut). As a result of this work and similar findings in humans, Rumiati and colleagues (2005) proposed a dual-route theory of imitation. A direct route or mechanism enables novel actions to be transformed into motor output, and a semantic mechanism allows reproduction of known actions through stored memories. It has been shown that meaningful actions (i.e., pantomime of hammering or writing) and meaningless actions (i.e., nonsensical hand movements) activate different cortical areas (Decety et al., 1997; Grezes, Costes, & Decety, 1998). Meaningful actions engage the left frontal and temporal regions (areas associated with the MNS), whereas meaningless actions mainly engage the right occipitoparietal pathway. By examining strategy selection during action imitation, Tessari, Bosanac, and Rumiati (2006) showed that once a meaningless action was acquired, it was then processed in a manner similar to meaningful actions. Similar dissociations in cortical areas have been shown as a result of practice expertise, as discussed later (e.g., Calvo-Merino, Glaser, Grezes, Passingham, & Haggard, 2005). One of the implications of this dual-route theory is that the more meaningful an action is perceived to be, the more likely it is to engage the MNS. Therefore, demonstrating an action within its appropriate context and keeping it goal directed should be a requirement for observational practice and learning.

Behavioral evidence suggests that the translation between action and perception is relatively direct and bidirectional. Hecht, Vogt, and Prinz (2001) controlled motor and visual experience and showed that participants who only received physical practice of a relative timing movement improved visual judgments on a related task, which they called *action–perception transfer*. Similar results have been shown for the production and discrimination of a gait pattern displayed via point of lights at the joints (Casile & Giese, 2006) and for the perception of limb position when the observer is moving (Reed & Farah, 1995). The bidirectional nature of translation between perception and action is strong support for the idea that both processes share a common neurological pathway. From an observational learning perspective, these findings raise interesting questions about the utility of demonstrations in some situations in view of the dependency of perception on action experience. These issues are discussed further when we consider observer and model interactions.

Evidence for direct matching also comes from studies showing that visual perception affects the execution of a related but irrelevant action. For example, Kilner, Paulignan, and Blackmore (2003) studied participants making sinusoidal arm movements during observation of either a human or robotic arm making similar or dissimilar movements. Participants' movements were negatively affected by observation of dissimilar human movements only, suggesting that perception of incongruent biological motion interfered with action generation. Similar interference effects have been shown for participants observing one point of light moving along a biologically realistic trajectory incongruent to the participant. No interference effects were observed when the trajectory was artificial (Bouquet, Gaurier, Shipley, Toussaint, & Blandin, 2007). Observation of task-irrelevant actions can also facilitate action in what is called *visuomotor priming* (e.g., Brass, Bekkering, & Prinz, 2001; Brass, Bekkering, Wohlschlager, & Prinz, 2000). Motor–visual priming has also been demonstrated in which preparation of the movement affects future processing of visual information. When participants were asked to prepare a grasping movement before a visual prime, the grasping responses were faster if the visual prime was compatible with the end state of the prepared movement (Craighero, Bello, Fadiga, & Rizzolatti, 2002; Miall et al., 2006; Vogt, Taylor, & Hopkins, 2003).

The eye movements that participants show in response to observed manipulative actions have also been presented as evidence for the direct matching hypothesis. Direct matching manifests itself if observers show evidence that they are implementing covert action plans in real time with the actor (Flanagan & Johansson, 2003; Rotman, Troje, Johansson, & Flanagan, 2006). Flanagan and Johansson (2003) found that the eye movements of participants observing actors who were performing a block-stacking task were similar to, and in phase with, the eye movements they produced when they performed the task themselves. In both instances, attention was directed proactively to the upcoming point of contact. When observers cannot see the actor's hand, their behavior is no longer coupled to the gaze of the actor but is instead reactive (Falck-Ytter, Gredebäck, & von Hofsten, 2006). The common-coding framework has been developed further into the theory of event coding (Hommel, Musseler, Aschersleben, & Prinz, 2001), also referred to as *ideomotor theory* (Prinz, 2002, 2005) based on early ideas of James (1890). These theories suggest that voluntary actions are initiated by anticipatory ideas or representations. Actions are automatically activated by anticipation of their effects. Similarly, actions are automatically activated by visual events that correspond to these effects. Therefore, observation can be an alternative mechanism to action initiation.

Despite evidence suggesting that perception and action are closely linked during observation, as with the neurophysiological literature, it is unlikely that matching is as direct as implied by the term itself (see Decety & Grezes, 1999, for a review). Meltzoff (2002) has acknowledged that direct matching in newborns becomes less direct with age and involves more understanding of the intentions of the model (e.g., Gergely, Bekkering, & Kiraly, 2002). Young children will often imitate the outcome or intended goal of the movement, such as reaching to touch their ear, but not the means, such as reaching across the body (Bekkering, Wohlschlager, & Gattis, 2000; Wohlschlager, Gattis, & Bekkering, 2003). On the basis of this work, Wohlschlager and colleagues (2003) developed the theory of goal-directed imitation (GOADI). Action reproduction and imitation are based on emulatory processes that result in achievement of the outcome by the most efficient means. The imitation process is based on a decomposition of the observed action and its ordering into a hierarchy of goals and subgoals. At the top of the hierarchy is the outcome of the action, which is given more importance than the process by which the outcome is achieved when these differ.

In support of these ideas, it has been shown that observation of both process (i.e., grasping and moving without an action goal) and outcome (i.e., placing) results in similar cortical activation of the DLPFC, which is thought to be involved in action goal representation (Chaminade, Meltzoff, & Decety, 2002). The authors interpreted this result as evidence that the goal of the action is constructed even if it is not present during observation— that is, making the action meaningful (see also Kohler et al., 2002; Umilta et al., 2001). The GOADI approach is consistent with the dual-route theory described earlier since meaningful actions should involve a concrete action goal. Observation of meaningful, goal-related behaviors would result in more activation of the MNS and thus allow for easier imitation. However, there is evidence showing that MNS activity increases when attention is directed toward the means rather than the outcome of the action (Hesse & Fink, 2007) and that distal goals do not always take precedence in imitation, particularly when action features are highlighted (see Bird, Brindley, Leighton, & Heyes, 2008).

Thus, the advance of technology has provided extensive evidence for a neurophysiological mechanism by which perception can be translated into action. The discovery of the MNS has led to a number of theories detailing how observation can lead to the acquisition and improved performance of a motor skill. Additionally, considerable behavioral evidence speaks to commonalities of perception and action. It is evident, however, that matching perception to action is not as direct as first imagined but rather involves understanding and experience with the task, especially if observation is used to guide the learning process. It is still unclear whether this necessitates two routes to action (a qualitative difference as a function of task) or just differential activation in similar areas (a quantitative difference).

Visual Perception Perspective

It is unlikely that imitation is governed explicitly by a direct perception-to-action matching mechanism such that an exact copy of the observed action is imitated. An observational learning perspective that seems to be based primarily on this assumption is the visual perception perspective (VPP) proposed by Scully and Newell (1985). Although there have been issues concerning the link between perception and movement reproduction, this perspective has played an important role in observational learning research, prompting the question as to what visual information is used by the observer during the observation learning process.

VPP is based on motion and perception research (e.g., Johansson, 1971) and Newell's (1985) model of motor learning. Common to these approaches is the idea that the acquisition of coordination (i.e., the relationship between joints and effectors) defines the initial stage of learning with respect to both observing and performing. In VPP, people are believed to be directly attuned to coordination information through the perception of biological motion (Johansson, 1971, 1973, 1975). Johansson showed that movements presented in point-light form were automatically identified (within about 100 ms) through the motions of individual elements relative to each other (i.e., relative motion). VPP links the concept of relative motion to motor control and coordination (Kugler, Kelso, & Turvey, 1980, 1982; Newell, 1985). The immediate problem for a learner is coordinating the many degrees of freedom of the motor system. Because actions are identified (and described) by the relative motions of the body and limbs, this information was believed to be essential and directly extracted and imitated during observational learning.

Although there is evidence that relative motion is an important constraining source of information for perception, other sources of information appear to be just as or even more important for observational learning when motor learning is required. As detailed in the GOADI account of learning, the means (relative motion) do not always dominate observational learning. Attempts to make relative motion salient through point-light models have failed to produce beneficial effects (e.g., Al-Abood et al., 2001; Horn, Williams, Scott, & Hodges, 2005; Scully & Carnegie, 1998), and in some cases these point-light models have been detrimental relative to video models (e.g., Hayes, Hodges, Scott, Horn, & Williams, 2007; Romack, 1995).

To directly examine the importance of relative motion information for action reproduction, Hodges, Hayes, Breslin, and Williams (2005) removed this information in a kicking task. One observation group viewed only the toe marker (i.e., no relative motion information), a second group observed two points of light pertaining to the foot (toe and ankle), and a third group viewed three points of light pertaining to the lower leg (toe, ankle, and knee). No other contextual cues were presented to show that a kicking action was required, although participants realized what joints the markers represented. The toe-marker group approximated the model's coordination profile as well as, and in some instances (e.g., hip–knee coordination) better than, the foot or leg groups. When the three groups transferred and observed a full-body relative motion model, there was no significant improvement in the coordination profiles, indicating that end-point information was the constraining source of information for action reproduction. In the final phase of the experiment, participants were required to imitate the action conveyed by the model in order to propel a ball over a height barrier to land on a target. The requirement to achieve an external goal led to the closest approximation of the model's intralimb coordination pattern.

Based on these data, there are two findings that call into question the importance of relative motion for successful observational learning. First, it seems that end-point information was sufficient to successfully imitate a full-body movement. This suggests that at least part of the imitation process is based on action understanding, where the person is able to fill in the gaps. Relative motion is not imitated in a direct fashion (see also Umilta et al., 2001). Second, the variable that brought about the closest approximation of the model's intralimb coordination pattern was the requirement to propel a ball. A change in a person's coordination profile to more closely approximate a model should not be taken as evidence that relative motion was used during learning.

These findings have been partially replicated in experiments involving overarm cricket bowling and lawn bowling actions for which the action has been presented in whole-body video and point-light display (PLD) formats, as well as partial PLD format (see Hayes, Hodges, Huys, & Williams, 2007, and Hayes et al., 2007, for details of underarm bowling task and methods; see Breslin, Hodges, & Williams, in press, and Breslin, Hodges, Williams, Kremer, & Curran, 2005, 2006, for details of the cricket bowling action and manipulations). Rather than end-point information alone, it appears that end-effector information (i.e., the bowling arm, rather than just motions of the wrist) is an important source of information during observational learning of whole-body actions. From these experiments, Breslin and colleagues suggested that during goal-directed imitation, people adopt a local processing strategy (see Mataric & Pomplun, 1998; Mather, Radford, & West, 1992) in which attention is directed toward the motion of a distal effector. This suggestion would be congruent with the GOADI theory of movement imitation. This does not mean that relative motions are not perceived; rather, it means that this information, particularly at a between-limb level, is not necessarily prioritized during observational learning (see Pinto & Shiffrar, 1999).

There is also evidence that the end point of the action does not even have to be in direct contact with the body for it to be useful in bringing about the desired coordination pattern. Participants who observed and received feedback pertaining to only the trajectory of the ball in a kicking task showed better retention than participants who observed only the model (Hodges, Hayes, Eaves, Horn, & Williams, 2006). In line with this finding is evidence that actions are planned and executed based on anticipation of their end effects (see Ford, Hodges, & Williams, 2005; Ford, Hodges, Huys, & Williams, 2006; Koch, Keller, & Prinz, 2004), and hence this type of strategy encouraged through outcome-based demonstrations might be fruitful for teaching movement skills. As noted in neuroimaging studies (e.g., Umilta et al., 2001), there is no reason for the observer to actually see the action to engage the MNS. As long as an action is implied and there is some correspondence between the action and the object, motor skill acquisition can take place through observation of an object's trajectory.

A few researchers have attempted to more directly examine the information used in observational learning using eye tracking techniques. Because the point of gaze does not guarantee the extraction of visual information from that location, visual search evidence is also an indirect supposition of both the information used and the guiding, underlying processes. Mataric and Pomplun (1998) found that when participants watched arm, hand, and finger movements, they consistently fixated on the end point, arguing that an internal kinematic model of the action helped the observer fill in the gaps. Horn and colleagues (2002) did not find consistent end-point tracking during observational learning of a kicking motion. However, tracking of the foot did generally decrease as a function of practice and observation for the video group, perhaps suggesting that this information is prioritized early in learning. In a later study, this narrowing of search was seen only among participants who did not show improvements in movement form (Horn et al., 2005).

In summary, we have reviewed key theoretical approaches that affect research in observational learning (see table 17.1). We have differentiated these approaches based on their emphasis on cognitive processes mediating observation and action. To date, the social learning model of Bandura has had the greatest influence on the field of observational learning. However, methodological and theoretical advances in neurophysiology are starting to influence the way mainstream behavioral and neuroscience researchers think about observational learning. In particular, the sophisticated resonance that can take place during observation (as evidenced by MNS activation) allows a mechanism for information transfer in the absence of memory stores and cognitive representations of the act. This does not mean that some sort of image or representation of the act does not guide movement reproduction during physical practice; rather, it means that motor learning can take place during observation (i.e., early mediation) such that the details of the act do not need to be contained within any representation of the act. If observation and action share common neurological pathways, observation would supposedly assist the learner in a manner similar to that of physical

TABLE 17.1

PRIMARY RESEARCH QUESTIONS AND THEIR ASSOCIATED METHODS, AND REFERENCES IN OBSERVATIONAL LEARNING RESEARCH

Research area	Primary research questions	Method used to test the question	Research examples
What is the representation guiding action?	Is a motor representation of the movement evoked during its observation, or is it formed during movement production (i.e., early mediation versus late mediation)?	Performance of a distracting cognitive task and an unrelated motor task during observation of a force-field perturbation task Sequence learning of serial RT Test for effector dependence in observational practice of finger-sequence serial RT	Mattar & Gribble (2005) Howard et al. (1992); Heyes & Foster (2002); Bird & Heyes (2005)
	Do observation and action share common neural pathways (i.e., is there common coding)?	Imaging tests (e.g., fMRI) of common neural activation during observation and reproduction of movements	di Pellegrino et al. (1992); Gallese et al. (1996); Rizzolatti et al. (1996)
	Does perception of the event activate the observed response (i.e., direct matching), or is the response mediated by a memory representation (i.e., semantic, dual route)?	Tests of cortical activation during observation of meaningful and meaningless actions Tests of cortical activation during imitation of actions performed with and without an object Tests of similar eye movements in observers and actors	Rumiati et al. (2005); Decety et al. (1997); Grezes et al. (1998) Gallese et al. (1996) Flanagan & Johansson, (2003); Rotman et al. (2006)
	Does movement and action experience mediate (and facilitate) perception of the same movement?	Discrimination of perceptual events (e.g., gait) with and without motor practice Tests of motor–visual priming on RT to a visual stimulus Comparison of motor experts and novices	Hecht et al. (2001); Casile & Giese (2006) Craighero et al. (2002); Miall et al. (2006); Vogt et al. (2003) Calvo-Merino et al. (2005, 2006); Buccino et al. (2004)
	Does motor imagery facilitate imitation?	Tests of activation in cortical motor areas during imagery	Decety et al. (1990); Grafton et al. (1996); Tomasino et al. (2007)
What information is perceived and imitated?	Do observers perceive and use relative motion in the imitation of skills?	Changes in observer's relative motion toward that of model Tests of imitation in the absence of relative motion	Al-Abood et al. (2001); Horn et al. (2005); Hodges et al. (2005); Breslin et al. (2005)
	Do observers emulate the goal of the performer rather than the means (i.e., is there goal-directed imitation)?	Gesture imitation in children Observer's visual search prioritizing the end effector in finger, hand, and arm movements	Bekkering et al. (2000); Bird et al., (2007); Wohlschlager et al. (2003); Mataric & Pomplun (1998)

practice. However, because overt action is inhibited during observation, the learner would not receive any feedback during observation, thus limiting the information required to adjust future skill attempts.

Our section on the VPP provided data on the type of information used during observational learning. Although there does not seem to be a definitive information source guiding observational learning, there is evidence that the learner is goal oriented, which promotes a distal focus on the end effector. Most theorists acknowledge that the observational learning process likely depends on a number of factors, such as the task, model, and observer characteristics, and as such the route to learning is quite complex. The GOADI theory (Wohlschlager et al., 2003), in which imitation depends on the goals and intentions of the learner, is one theory where this task dependency is an inherent feature of the model. As well, the dual-route model of imitation proposed by Rumiati and colleagues (2005) offers a neurophysiological explanation for discrepancies in observational learning research based on the type of action and characteristics of the model and observer. Next we review how these characteristics affect observational learning and consider the empirical evidence in view of the theories discussed thus far.

Task Characteristics

We will examine the role of task characteristics in affecting the observational learning process first in terms of behavioral data then in view of neurophysiological evidence. The previously mentioned meta-analysis outlining the benefits of observational learning (Ashford et al., 2006) revealed different effects of modeling depending on the type of motor skill. Observation was most beneficial for serial or sequencing tasks (involving several subtasks), with reduced effects for continuous tasks and smallest effects for discrete tasks. According to these findings, tasks that emphasize memory and cognition are more susceptible to positive observational learning effects than are tasks that emphasize motor learning. Ashford and colleagues (2006) also noted that positive effects of observational learning were typically obtained from studies involving a small range of relatively simple skills that had limited interactions among the components. There has been considerable discrepancy in research findings related to observational learning when multilimb coordination movements have been examined. For example, Whiting, Bijlard, and den Brinker (1987) showed benefits from observing a model performing on a ski-simulator task, yet they failed to replicate this result in a later study. In what they referred to as *discovery learning*, they even found that not watching a model was more beneficial for performance compared with watching the model (Vereijken & Whiting, 1990). In the latter study, the authors attributed the poor performance during observation to goal confusion (Gentile, 1972; Whiting

& den Brinker, 1982), where attention becomes divided between the task demands and the movements of the model (see Hodges & Franks, 2002b, for further discussion on this topic).

In tasks requiring the acquisition of a difficult, continuous, bimanual coordination pattern, where the limbs are offset by 90° relative phase, demonstrations have also been found to be relatively ineffective at conveying the desired movement (Hodges, Chua, & Franks, 2003; Hodges & Franks, 2000, 2001, 2002a). The most effective method of acquisition in these experiments was providing the learner with augmented feedback that displayed the trajectory of one limb as a function of the other so that correct performance resulted in a circular pattern (see also Lee, Swinnen, & Verschueren, 1995). This strategy arguably helped make the task more meaningful in that participants now had a goal to achieve (i.e., make a circle) rather than just an abstract movement to copy. Experiments are currently underway to determine whether perception of the means (i.e., a model performing a difficult coordination pattern) changes as a function of practice such that understanding develops as a result of motor experience—that is, action-to-perception transfer (e.g., Edwards, et al., 2008; Maslovat, Hodges, Krigolson, & Handy, 2009). However, there has been evidence that observational practice of a model performing a single-limb, between-joint (rather than between-limb) coordination task facilitates later performance of that skill (Buchanan, Ryu, Zihlman, & Wright, 2008). It appears that these differences are due to task-related factors, rather than factors related to the skill of the model and the amount and type of feedback (Maslovat et al., 2009). Further, observers are relatively proficient at performing the motion pattern of a model within a limb (such as the arm during an overarm cricket bowl), yet they are less proficient at modeling the required relative motions of the two arms (Breslin et al., 2006; in press).

Another determinant of modeling effectiveness pertains to how the goals of the task are achieved and measured. Learning effects associated with observation have generally been stronger for measures of movement form versus movement outcome, although these results are task dependent (Ashford et al., 2006). For example, when the task environment does not have an explicit outcome goal, as in learning a ballet technique (e.g., Scully & Carnegie, 1998), the model's movement pattern is the primary goal and observing for imitation purposes is elevated in importance. This was shown in two studies by Horn and colleagues (2002, 2005). When the task had competing goals, such as imitating the model's movement (soccer kick) and attaining the outcome (landing the ball on a target), learners prioritized the external-outcome goal at the expense of imitating the model's movement. We have illustrated the results from these two studies in figure 17.1, where the hip–knee coordination patterns of two expert models have been compared with those of typical participants as angle–angle plots. Only general strategic features of the action were imitated, such as the number of

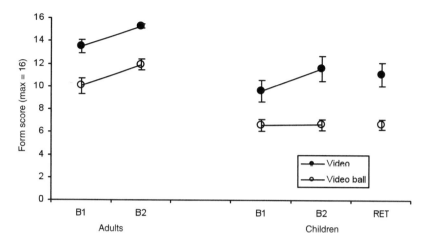

▶ **Figure 17.1** Hip–knee angle–angle plots illustrating the kinematics from two expert models in comparison with movements in retention (after 15 observation trials) from typical participants in the studies by Horn and colleagues (2002) and Horn and colleagues (2005).

Adapted from R.R. Horn and A.M. Williams, 2004, Observational learning: Is it time we took another look? In *Skill acquisition in sport: Research, theory and practice*, edited by A.M. Williams and N.J. Hodges (Oxford, UK: Routledge), 175-206.

approach steps to the ball, and not the general relative motion pattern. In support of conclusions from the meta-analysis by Ashford and colleagues, seeing a model did not lead to improvements in outcome, and improvements in movement form were observed only when feedback about task success was withheld. In a subsequent experiment, a direct manipulation of task goal feedback was made. Adult and child observers were asked to imitate a lawn bowling action either with or without a ball (Hayes, Hodges, Scott, Horn, & Williams, 2007). They were scored based on similarity to the model in terms of the step and lunge pattern. As illustrated in figure 17.2, the lunge was more correctly imitated when there was no additional outcome goal (no ball) and hence feedback about performance. The children who bowled with a ball made no improvements in form scores compared with the no-ball group.

When the external goal within a motor task can be solved in different ways, there might be no outcome performance advantage in adopting the technique demonstrated by the model. For example, comparisons of a demonstration and control group during the acquisition of an underarm dart throw by Al-Abood and coworkers (2001) showed that the control group adopted a different action than the model and the demonstration groups adopted (e.g., standard overarm dart throw), but there was no difference in outcome performance across the groups. This result is a prediction from VPP, whereby coordination (form) is facilitated by demonstrations but features related to scaling of the movement, such as timing and accuracy,

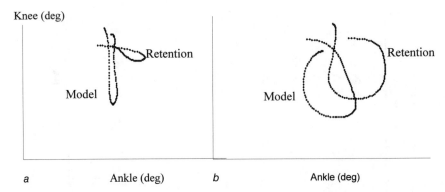

▶ **Figure 17.2**   A comparison of form scores during observational learning of an underarm lawn bowling technique across two blocks of practice (B1 and B2) and in a retention test for four groups of adults and children bowling (*a*) with and (*b*) without a ball.

Adapted, by permission, from S.J. Hayes et al., 2007, "The efficacy of demonstrations in teaching children an unfamiliar movement skill: The effects of object-orientation and point-light demonstrations," *Journal of Sports Sciences* 25: 559-575. http://informaworld.com

are facilitated by physical practice (yet see Blandin, Lhuisset, & Proteau, 1999; Hayes, et al., 2006).

In contrast, when the task outcome goal is directly linked to a specific coordination pattern, having access to a model is more helpful. In a three-ball juggling task, Hayes, Ashford, and Bennett (2008) found that observational learning conditions were better for performance and learning than a control condition where only basic verbal instructions were provided. In this case, the juggling movement was not acquired in the control condition. A visual demonstration encouraged the adoption of the desired movement and hence the ability to juggle. It is not clear what the important information within the demonstration was, however. If participants only saw the trajectory of the balls without the trajectory of the hands, would this be sufficient to encourage learning, or is the interaction between the two necessary? Furthermore, because observation conditions were not examined independently of physical practice, it is not possible to make conclusions about early and late mediation and hence whether the demonstrations alone were sufficient to bring about learning.

In summary, evidence suggests that the effectiveness of demonstrations for motor learning depends on a number of task-related factors, including whether the task is goal or outcome oriented compared with tasks where the movement is the goal of the action, whether the primary measure of performance is outcome or form based, and whether the task comprises discrete components that require sequencing together versus a task requiring interacting components and continuous movements. Because of the goal-dependent nature of these findings, it would appear that the GOADI theory of movement imitation is a good candidate explanation for these discrepant findings. As detailed next, task dependencies might also have a cortical explanation related to judgments of meaningfulness and goal directedness.

In an attempt to understand the link between perception and understanding, researchers have examined what types of activities elicit human MNS activation during observation. Activation has been shown for both transitive (i.e., tool- or object-oriented) and intransitive (i.e., meaningless or non-object-oriented) actions across various effectors, including hand, mouth, and foot (e.g., Buccino et al., 2001; Fadiga, Fogassi, Pavesi, & Rizzolatti, 1995; Grezes, Armony, Rowe, & Passingham, 2003). Cortical activation is decreased for observed movements that are robotic rather than biological (Tai, Scherfler, Brooks, Sawamoto, & Castiello, 2004), virtual rather than real (Perani et al., 2001), and biologically impossible rather than possible (Stevens, Fonlupt, Shiffrar, & Decety, 2000). These results have led to the hypothesis that MNS activity is seen only during observations of actions that the observer can physically produce. These results are congruent with dual-route theories outlined earlier since the goals and means of the movement cannot be constructed for actions the observer cannot perform and hence the actions would be considered meaningless. These findings raise the question as to the usefulness of demonstrations in encouraging movements that are not part of the observer's repertoire (an important goal in early learning). It might be that this initial route for the learning of novel tasks is primarily cognitive, occurring via late mediation. Difficult or unusual movements are strategized and represented explicitly. At a representational level, the action system would have little or no involvement until physical practice takes place. This action experience that emerges as a result of practice now informs perception.

However, there is evidence to show that impossible and meaningless movements should perhaps be considered on a continuum or on an individual or task basis. When seemingly impossible human movements can be made to look possible (by exaggerating certain movements), the goal and general meaning of the action can be constructed, leading to activation of the MNS (Candidi, Urgesi, Ionta, & Aglioti, 2007). In a related study, Gazzola, Rizzolatti, Wicker, and Keysers (2007) hypothesized that the lack of activation in previous studies involving robotic actions (e.g., Tai et al., 2004) may have been a result of repetitive presentation of the same video stimuli. By using different robotic movements within an observation block rather than the same movement each time, Gazzola and colleagues (2007) were able to elicit MNS activation (see also Press, Gillmeister, & Heyes, 2007, who showed that practice moderates activation of the MNS for robotic movements). A similar desensitization effect was observed by Hamilton and Grafton (2006), who showed that repeated observation of identical movies resulted in decreased MNS activation (i.e., habituation). This latter finding supports the use of learning rather than expert models in facilitating observational practice (see also Mattar & Gribble, 2005). Similar arguments exist concerning MNS involvement during early or late learning, as detailed later. These findings show that the MNS is tasked with making sense of actions, not just resonating with actions that already make sense.

Indeed, understanding of the action appears to be more important than being able to actually perform the movement. For example, observation of a biologically impossible movement showed different interference effects (in terms of movement error) if the participants were told the movement was performed by a human versus a computer (Stanley, Gowen, & Miall, 2007). It has also been shown that the MNS codes the same observed action differently depending on the complexity (Molnar-Szakacs, Kaplan, Greenfield, & Iacoboni, 2006) and perceived intention of the movement (i.e., grasping a cup to drink versus grasping a cup to clear a table; see Iacoboni et al., 2005).

Collectively, these results provide strong support for the involvement of the MNS in action understanding rather than simply action recognition. The perception and understanding of the task by the observer affects MNS activity and thus potentially the effectiveness of observational learning, as discussed later. Although there is evidence that MNS involvement is greater when the task is meaningful to the observer, this does not imply that only easy tasks within the performer's repertoire activate the MNS.

Model Skill Level

Much of the initial work involving observational learning focused on the model's characteristics and their influence on the learner's performance. Bandura (1977) predicted that observers would pay more attention to models that are more skilled, higher status, and the same sex as the learner. A highly skilled model should create a more accurate cognitive representation and thus result in increased learning, at least from a late-mediation view of observational learning. Early examination of model type showed that model skill level was not important when participants were required to learn a skill of low cognitive demand, such as rolling a ball to a target, versus a skill of high cognitive demand, such as having to employ a strategy to get the ball to the target (Martens et al., 1976).

Landers and Landers (1973) manipulated skill level (high versus low) and status (teacher versus peer) of the model during observational learning of the Bachman ladder-climbing task. Participants who observed the skilled teacher performed the best at the task, whereas participants who observed the peer model performed better when the model was of low rather than high skill level. The fact that an expert model was more effective in encouraging learning supports late-mediation views of learning, in which the quality of the acquired cognitive representation of the desired movement dictates accuracy of movement replication. However, the fact that a low-skill peer model was better than a high-skill model seems to support early mediation accounts of observational learning. Increased similarity between the observer and model might result in greater covert action simulation, especially if there is variability across trials, as would be expected with a learning model (Hamilton & Grafton, 2006; yet see Desy & Theoret, 2007, for alternative findings regarding model similarity).

When peer models were used to convey a swimming stroke, skilled models were more effective than novice models for observational learning (d'Arripe-Longueville, Gernigon, Huet, Cadopi, & Winnykamen, 2002). The authors attributed this result to increased motivation by the observer to emulate the skilled model and thus work harder in practice. Other authors have failed to show differences between models of differing skill levels (learning versus expert) on a computer video-game task (Pollock & Lee, 1992) or a weightlifting task (Lee & White, 1990; McCullagh & Meyer, 1997). These equivocal results have been attributed to task differences, such as the difficulty of the task, and the lack of control over model status (e.g., Weir & Leavitt, 1990).

Learning models allow the observer to determine the information that is most related to task success, since only specific actions result in desirable outcomes. This information would not be as salient in observation of repetitive, correct performance (Pollock & Lee, 1992). Furthermore, actions would be modified as a result of errors, resulting in the observer being more engaged in the cognitive problem-solving processes (Adams, 1986). In support of this latter argument, Adams (1986) found that improvements in learning a timing task were observed only if the model's feedback was also available to the observer, arguably engaging the learner in the process of error correction (see also Herbert & Landin, 1994; Hodges et al., 2003; McCullagh & Caird, 1990). The possible benefits of a learning model have been further underscored by neurophysiological evidence (EEG) showing that motor-related areas in the brain that are activated when observers view a person making errors are similar to the areas that are activated when errors are self-generated (van Schie, Mars, Coles, & Bekkering, 2004). It seems the observer needs to see the conflict between the desired and actual movement in order to engage the motor (or MNS) system to learn through observational practice alone (e.g., Mattar & Gribble, 2005).

Model Status and Similarity

Skill level of the model can affect both cognitive effort and the degree of covert motor simulation during observation (i.e., both late and early mediation). How the model is perceived could also affect these observational learning processes. Effects of model status could be due to attention differences (as hypothesized by Bandura, 1977), differences in information presented by the model, or the perception of different information due to the learner being more motivated and concentrating harder on imitation (Gould & Roberts, 1981). Evidence against the first hypothesis was provided by McCullagh

(1986), who found that regardless of whether participants were cued to the status of the model before or after observation, participants who viewed a high-status model performed better on the Bachman ladder-climbing task than participants who viewed a low-status model.

Model similarity has been shown to be an important variable mediating the effectiveness of observational learning. Same-sex models are more beneficial than opposite-sex models for observational learning (e.g., Griffin & Meaney, 2000). One way to control for model similarity is to use learners as their own model. However, simply watching oneself on videotape has not proved to be an effective strategy (Newell, 1981; see Rothstein & Arnold, 1976, for a review). This may be because learners do not need to see all their performances. It may be more effective to select good trials and remove those containing undesirable performance (see Dowrick, 1999, for a review). In addition, augmenting video observation with verbal (and visual) cues helps focus the learner's attention on the salient features of the presentation (e.g., Janelle, Champenoy, Coombes, & Mousseau, 2003). Further testing is necessary to determine whether these effects are motivationally mediated or a result of early mediation such that the more similar the model is to the observer, the more likely the motor system is engaged during observation.

Model–Observer Interactions and Observer Experience

If action understanding is a key requirement for activation of the MNS during observation, a question that has arisen is whether watching an unfamiliar movement (one that is not in the observer's motor repertoire) will result in MNS activity. If the observer does not have the necessary experience with a task to understand the actions or goals of a movement, will a demonstration activate MNS circuitry? Observation of someone playing a piano produced greater motor cortical activation in pianists than in musically naive participants, although no differences were found during observation of control stimuli involving finger and thumb movements (Haslinger et al., 2005). When skilled dancers observed similar movement patterns from two dance styles that were either familiar or unfamiliar, MNS activity was observed only for movements that were within the observer's motor repertoire (Calvo-Merino et al., 2005; Calvo-Merino, Grezes, Glaser, Passingham, & Haggard, 2006).

The differential MNS activity for learned versus unlearned movements suggests that this activation develops during the learning process. Although there is considerable evidence that the cortical connections mediating motor activation through observation are formed through experience (see Brass & Heyes, 2005, and Kelly & Garavan, 2005, for reviews), few studies have examined how MNS activation changes as a function of practice. Examination of the change in MNS activation during the learning process may help clarify how observational learning occurs. One exception was a study in which expert dancers practiced a new dance sequence for 5 wk, with observation and fMRI recordings of the practiced movement and a nonpracticed movement interspersed within each week of the acquisition phase (Cross, Hamilton, & Grafton, 2006). Increased activity in MNS areas occurred during the learning process for the practiced movement. It would also be worthwhile to examine whether changes in MNS activation occur with observational practice (i.e., without physical practice). If motor practice is necessary for MNS activation, it would seem that the information obtained through observation is more cognitive or strategic in nature.

One limitation of some studies examining expertise differences in MNS activation (i.e., Calvo-Merino et al., 2005, 2006) is that the observers were instructed to evaluate the movement based on symmetry or perception of effort rather than with the goal of imitating the movement. Instructions have been shown to affect cortical activity; more activity occurs in the brain structures associated with action planning when imitative instructions versus evaluative instructions are given (Decety et al., 1997; Zentgraf et al., 2005). In contrast to the findings of Calvo-Merino and colleagues, motor activation has been shown for observation of unfamiliar movements when imitation was required. Buccino and colleagues (2004) had nonguitarists imitate unfamiliar guitar chords. They showed MNS activation during observation, preparation, and imitation. Increased MNS activity has also been seen in the early stages of imitative learning, a result again attributed to instructions requiring reproduction of the task (Vogt et al., 2007).

These effects of the learner's intention are similar to the intention superiority effect seen in behavioral studies. When observers were told that they would have to reproduce an observed motor skill (e.g., a key-press, timing task), they performed significantly better during retention than observers who were told they would only have to recognize or describe the task (Badets, Bladin, Bouquet, & Shea, 2006; Badets, Blandin, & Shea, 2006). The differences were mainly in terms of relative timing rather than absolute timing, suggesting that intention moderated what information was attended and observed, perhaps encouraging early mediation.

In summary, the effectiveness of modeling depends on an interaction of several factors, including the characteristics of the model, the observer, and the task being learned. We have summarized the general research areas and methods along with some examples in table 17.2. Although practitioners are often hoping for a golden rule to use with modeling, such a rule may not be possible due to the complexity of the interaction. Not all tasks and skills respond equally to observational learning, particularly when the goals and means of the movement are different. Thus, important considerations when evaluating the success of observational learning include the task requirements (i.e., outcome versus process) and how they will be evaluated. There is clear evidence that the type of model affects the observer's motivation and attention, which in turn affects the learning process. Although research

TABLE 17.2

OBSERVATIONAL LEARNING VARIABLES AND THEIR ASSOCIATED RESEARCH QUESTIONS, METHODS, AND REFERENCES

Research area	Primary research questions	Method used to test the question	Research examples
Task characteristics	Does the effectiveness of observational learning depend on how the goal of the task is achieved (i.e., external goals versus performance of the movement pattern)?	Examination of coordination tasks in which the movement pattern is the goal Manipulation of feedback and task goals	Buchanan et al. (2008); Hodges et al. (2003); Hodges & Franks (2002a, 2002b); Scully & Carnegie (1998) Hayes et al. (2007); Horn et al. (2002, 2005)
	How do understanding and implied meaning of the observed task affect activation of cortical motor areas?	Examination of cortical activation during observation of robotic movements Examination of cortical activation during observation of impossible movements	Gazzola et al. (2007); Press et al. (2007); Tai et al. (2004) Candidi et al. (2007); Stevens et al. (2000)
Model characteristics	Does the observer need to see errors in performance?	Manipulation of model skill level	d'Arripe-Longueville et al. (2002); Landers & Landers (1973); Lee & White (1990); Martens et al. (1976); McCullagh & Meyer (1997); Pollock & Lee (1992)
	Can the type of model affect cognitive effort and degree of motor simulation?	Manipulation of model status and similarity to observer	Griffin & Meaney (2000); McCullagh (1986)
Observer characteristics	Does observer intention affect observational learning?	Manipulation of instructions	Badets, Blandin, Bouquet, et al. (2006); Badets, Blandin, & Shea (2006); Decety et al. (1997); Zentgraf et al. (2005)
	Does the performer need experience with the observed task to activate cortical motor areas?	Comparison of motor experts and novices Examination of within-participant cortical activation changes during skill practice	Buccino et al. (2004); Calvo-Merino et al. (2005, 2006); Haslinger et al. (2005) Cross et al. (2006); Vogt et al. (2007)

in this area has not provided a consensus regarding optimal model characteristics, it helps if the learner can adequately determine the proper performance of the skill and if feedback is available regarding both the model's performance and the observer's own performance (during observational learning), facilitating error detection and correction.

Finally, the observer's mind-set affects observational learning. Intention to reproduce the observed movement affects later performance, which can be influenced by the instructions. Although the interaction of task, model, and observer characteristics makes it difficult to establish guidelines for modeling, it is hoped that neurophysiological techniques will advance our understanding of these interactions, at least in terms of motor involvement during observation, so that more specific behavioral recommendations can be made.

Conclusions and Future Directions

In this review, we have outlined the major theories that influence thinking and empirical research about observational learning. We have focused on the implications of these theories for behavioral research and ways of modifying the learning process. In discussing how various characteristics play a role in the observational learning process, we have highlighted factors to consider when designing effective procedures for observational learning, as well as drawn attention to areas of debate in this field. It is difficult to draw general conclusions across studies because of the experimental inconsistency regarding instructions, provision of feedback, and conveyance of the goals of the action. In addition, studies have varied as to whether goals are means or outcome oriented and hence have varied in how performance is assessed in terms of these measures.

Continued research on demonstrations may help clarify the mechanisms by which observation benefits learning, thus providing clearer guidelines for practitioners. Further exploration comparing observational learning, observational practice, and physical practice at different times in the learning process may clarify the roles of watching versus performing motor skills, particularly if motor skills are examined that place differing emphasis on movement form (dynamics) and outcome attainment (see Weeks & Anderson, 2000). For example, if observational practice provides the learner with primarily strategy-related information, then demonstrations would perhaps be most valuable early in the learning process to speed up acquisition (unless there are benefits from task exploration and discovery learning for later retention and transfer; see Vereijken, 1991).

Future studies will need to consider how demonstrations facilitate learning in terms of early and late mediation and whether one route is better than another with respect to rate of acquisition, retention, and later transfer. In terms of behavioral evidence, effector specificity has been the strongest evidence of motor system involvement during observation (see Heyes & Foster, 2002; Vogt & Thomaschke, 2007). It will be helpful to consider other types of behavioral evidence for and against early mediation, such as performance on related perceptual discrimination tasks and errors in action that could not be attributed to explicit strategy use. This might be achieved through examination of learning models or expert models who make occasional errors that are not consistent with explicit strategy use. Measurement or manipulation of visual gaze or kinematics during the observation phase would also help to indicate the degree of direct motor involvement during observation.

It is also likely that people will acquire the same skill via observation with different degrees of motor system involvement during observation. Although this question has been examined through comparisons of expert and novice performers and as a function of learning, there has not been a systematic attempt to examine the consequences of these different ways of learning and to examine behavioral changes when the motor system is more involved in perception. Potential benefits of observational practice or learning in relation to physical practice also have not been explored. At least with respect to late mediation, there might be more generality in the type of representations acquired through observation, which could be beneficial for transfer.

Of primary importance to the practitioner is how the information gathered can be used to increase the effectiveness of demonstrations during observational learning. One implication is that the instructions given to the observer may change the involvement of the MNS, since observing with the intent to imitate appears to activate more MNS structures than observing with the intent to evaluate. In addition, modeled actions must be possible to perform and must be understood by the observer. Understanding appears to be an important determinant of MNS activation, perhaps due to the observer being able to imagine the movement or make the movement more meaningful with respect to task goals (see Milton, Small, & Solodkin, 2008).

We have summarized pertinent research involving the examination of observational learning from diverse areas, including traditional behavioral measures, perturbation or occlusion research, eye tracking studies, and neurophysiological techniques. All provide a unique contribution to understanding what information is important during observational learning and how this information is translated from perception into action. Behavioral measures provide the basics of how the types of task and model characteristics affect learning, but they are limited in their appraisal of what is attended to and how translation occurs. Occlusion (e.g., point-light displays) and eye tracking studies help provide the *what* and neurological studies help provide the *how* of observational learning; so far these areas provide only limited information that can be applied to practical observational learning. As we continue to gain understanding of the mechanisms by which observation benefits performance, we also hope to gain insight into how to accelerate this process and maximize the use of demonstrations in the learning environment.

Although we appreciate that practitioners would like simple guidelines for maximizing learning, the development of skill acquisition is not a simple process, and thus this expectation may be unreasonable. The hope is that future work will involve a coalition of the research in these varied areas to provide a useful framework to guide observational learning. In addition, new technologies and methodologies will provide new avenues of research that further contribute to our understanding of imitative processes. Regardless, it should be evident from this chapter that observation assists the learning process and demonstrations are a useful tool for skill acquisition. However, rather than assuming that any demonstration will naturally lead to maximal performance, careful consideration of skill type, model type, characteristics of the observer, and instructions will lead to guidelines regarding the type and amount of observation to optimize learning.

CHAPTER 18

Optimizing Performance Through Work Space Design

JAMES L. LYONS

Almost 10 years before Paul Fitts published his landmark work formalizing the speed–accuracy trade-off for aiming movements, he was developing the genesis of this model with work targeted at the commendable goal of stopping airplanes from falling from the sky (Fitts & Jones, 1947; Fitts, Jones, & Milton, 1950). These studies into pilot error were some of the first to develop and apply theoretical models of motor control to the maximization of performance and the reduction of error in applied human–environment interactions. In this chapter, we explore how work spaces, as well as objects and displays within work spaces, can influence motor performance. We begin with an overview of applied motor behavior research, with an emphasis on human performance psychology, and examine how that research gave rise to the modern discipline of human factors. From there, we review topics pertaining to performance vis-à-vis human–environment interactions. Subtopics in this section include the role and function of the human sensory systems and the processes of perception and cognition. At the end of each section, we discuss how our understanding of these issues can either help or hinder our daily interactions with a working environment.

A Little History

Throughout history, humans have sought ways to make work easier, more cost and resource efficient, and safer. The term *ergonomics* (derived from the Greek "science of work") has been used since the early 1940s to describe an eclectic body of research aimed at achieving these goals by exploring the psychology, physiology, anthropometry, and biomechanics of human interactions with work environments. At its most basic level, this research seeks to optimize the functioning of people with respect to their activities. Because the term *ergonomics* is necessarily broad, practical distinctions are now drawn between the physiological, anthropometric, and biomechanical contributions to this relationship (functional ergonomics) and those engendered by the sensory, perceptual, and cognitive limitations of the human performer or operator (cognitive ergonomics, or human factors). This chapter focuses on human factors and the perceptual–motor aspects of human–environment interactions.[1]

The scientific discipline of human factors is a neophyte compared with well-established research areas that are supported by several hundred years of published literature. Nevertheless, it has a long and distinguished academic lineage. Given the integrative nature of the field, it is impossible to determine precisely when human factors research began; however, a good starting point is Ernst Weber's and Gustav Fechner's pioneering work exploring human perceptual sensitivity (e.g., Fechner, 1860/1966; Weber, 1846/1978). This work provided clear evidence of human sensory and perceptual limitations and led to the development of the field of psychophysics (the relationship between physical events and psychological events). Following were many landmark investigations that blazed a trail directly toward the point where human factors research stands today. A small sampling of these includes Donders' (1868/1969) application of chronometric subtractive logic procedures to mental processes (forming the central core of the information processing approach to human performance), Bryan and Harter's (1899) work with the learning of Morse code telegraphy (a seminal study for those interested in the broader field of motor skill acquisition), and Elton Mayo's (1933) 8 y series of studies on worker productivity at Western Electric's Hawthorne Illinois plant.[2]

Although the genesis of human factors research lies in studies conducted many years before the discipline started, the 20 or so years following the advent of World War II represented a true watershed for the discipline. This era brought together some of the most influential minds in human performance psychology (e.g., Frederic Bartlett, Margaret Vince, W.E. Hick, A.T. Welford, Donald Broadbent) in an attempt to answer specific questions arising from a general problem: how to better understand human operator capabilities and limitations in the face of the unprecedented technological improvements to machinery and work environments brought about by the war effort.

Studies from this time drew heavily on research dealing with issues such as depth perception, light and dark adaptation, gun sighting, target

---

[1]The term *human factors* was first used in its current context in 1957 (Edwards, 1988).

[2]Although these studies were originally intended to determine the degree to which worker productivity was affected by workplace illumination, their most enduring legacy was the revelation of the Hawthorne effect. The term, coined by Landsberger (1958), refers to a short-term performance improvement caused by the observation of workers by persons in a position of authority.

tracking, and the effects of fatigue on task performance. In England, much of this work was conducted at the Applied Psychology Research Unit at Cambridge University under the direction of Kenneth Craik (upon Craik's death in 1945, the directorship of the unit passed to Sir Fredrik Bartlett). In the United States, the driving force was provided by Alphonse Chapanis during his time (as the only psychologist) at the Aero Medical Laboratory (AML) at the Wright-Patterson Air Force Base in Ohio. In 1945, Paul Fitts joined Chapanis at AML, was appointed director of the laboratory's first psychology branch, and immediately set into motion a comprehensive, well-defined research program aimed at increasing aviation safety.

Fitts' work at AML was astonishing in terms of both volume and theoretical import (e.g., Fitts, 1947; Fitts & Crannell, 1950; Fitts & Jones, 1947; Fitts, Jones, & Milton, 1950). One excellent example of this research illustrated the new drive to feature the end user as a critical variable in the design of equipment (Fitts & Jones, 1947). Given numerous reports from pilots of problems experienced during instrument-only landings, Fitts and colleagues developed a link analysis procedure in which they recorded and analyzed the visual scan patterns of pilots across the cockpit instrument panel during runway approaches. Their idea was to identify which display instruments (e.g., air-speed indicator, directional gyroscope, altimeter) were viewed most frequently and in which order and then to compare this information to the spatial location of the instruments on the display panel.

The results showed that the greatest proportion of total gaze shifts occurred between two specific displays: the cross-pointer and the directional gyroscope. The problem was that a third instrument, the air-speed indicator, was situated directly between these two displays. Fitts and colleagues argued that this arrangement could be the reason for the reported pilot confusion (i.e., from what would now be referred to as a *visual distractor)* and that a simple repositioning of the display elements would solve the problem. This link analysis protocol, in which link values are established among elements within an environment and then used to best position those elements (i.e., such that the highest calculated link values are closest together), is still used today in the design of work environments ranging from data-entry systems to restaurants and bars.

As evidenced from these studies on scan patterns, Fitts was initially interested in how processing limitations in the human visual system had the capacity to constrain performance. In a series of studies run concomitantly with the link analysis work, Fitts investigated the accuracy of no-vision reaching movements to targets that were situated in various three-dimensional locations in space. These were some of the first attempts by Fitts to explore goal-directed aiming movements and served as the forerunners for the seminal information transfer work that was to follow (and subsequently give rise to Fitts' law).

In the first of these studies, Fitts (1947) had pilots memorize letter-coded locations of 20 targets and then use a pencil to aim at the center of a specified target while fixating visually on a red light situated directly in front of them. He found an asymmetry in accuracy performance, with straight-ahead movements being more accurate than reaches to either side. In addition, he found that smaller movements were also more accurate. Fitts and Crannell (1950) modified this procedure by changing the position of the reaching hand at movement initiation (i.e., placed at the sides of the body rather than in front of it). Again, reaches made to targets located directly in front of the participant were the most accurate. However, accuracy to other locations differed noticeably from those in the earlier study (i.e., where the start of the movement was in front of the body). Together, the results of these experiments suggested that the starting point of a given movement, the movement amplitude, and the movement end point all influence the accuracy of reaching when vision of the movement environment is not available.

Of the many applied and practical discoveries during this time, arguably the most important to the emerging field of human factors was the theoretical view of humans as information channels (i.e., the human is an active information processor, similar to a modern computer). Although Fitts was instrumental in the development of this metaphorical line of reasoning as an explanation for the results of his pilot studies, the origins of the concept lie in the engineering master's thesis of Claude Shannon. In this thesis, Shannon addressed the practical problem of how to maximize the amount of information that could be transmitted through noisy mechanical communication channels by arguing that electronic switching circuits could operate at peak efficiency when conforming to the binary principles of Boolean logic.

Ten years later, Shannon expanded on these ideas in collaboration with Warren Weaver in a two-part paper titled "A Mathematical Theory of Communication" (Shannon, 1948; Shannon & Weaver, 1949). At the heart of this paper was a mathematical definition of information that was revolutionary in that it ignored the everyday view of information as images, sounds, and so on, as well as the specific ways in which that information was eventually transmitted (e.g., sound waves, microwaves). Instead, Shannon conceptualized the rather abstract notion of information as a physical entity that describes the degree to which uncertainty and disorder (entropy) exist within a physical system (see Adler, 2002). In so doing, Shannon was able to devise a system of information processing based on the premise that the sole purpose of information is to reduce uncertainty. Furthermore, he proposed that this process is optimally accomplished in a binary fashion wherein each piece (or bit) of information reduces any remaining system uncertainty by half (i.e., a $\log_2$ function). This formalization and adaptation of binary logic principles to information processing signaled the beginning of the information age and are still the standard by which today's most complex supercomputers operate.

Three important concepts in Shannon's ideas were immediately seized upon by Fitts: (1) All environmental information must be processed against a background of noise, (2) processing channels have exceedable limits on the amount of information that can pass through them, and (3) the more complex the information (i.e., the greater the degree of uncertainty), the longer the binary reduction process will take. Using these foundational precepts as a starting point, Fitts made the conceptual leap between machines and humans. For example, whereas mechanical systems are perturbed by white thermal noise generated by electrical circuitry, humans process information against a background of variability-inducing neural noise. Whereas mechanical systems are limited by the size of the processing channel, humans are limited by the sensory, perceptual, and perceptual–motor resources available at any given time.

Fitts was not alone in pursuing this line of reasoning. Contemporaneous studies conducted by Hick (1951, 1952; see also Hyman, 1953) also assumed some degree of human processing limitation based upon the efficiency of information transfer from stimulus perception to the initiation of a response. Specifically, the Hick-Hyman law of reaction time holds that choice RT (i.e., the time taken to initiate a response to one of several equally likely alternatives) varies linearly with the logarithm of the base 2 of the potential stimulus set. The big difference between Fitts and Hick, however, was that Fitts carried the information transfer logic not only to the rate at which humans can internally process stimulus information but also to the efficiency of human movement execution. In other words, human processing capacity was constrained not only by the rate of processing of input information but also by the generation of motor output information. This conceptualization is based on the premise that interactions with any stimulus within a given environment are constrained by the amount of information provided by that stimulus.

Human–Machine System

To best understand the relationship between humans and the objects that they control, it is useful to cast the discussion in the conceptual framework of a human–machine system. For the purposes of this discussion, such a system is defined as one or more human beings and one or more physical components interacting to bring about, from given inputs, some desired output (see Proctor & Van Zandt, 1994). In this definition, a machine is simply a physical object and thus can refer to anything from a pencil to a nuclear reactor. The interactions are continuous and primarily closed loop, with the machine providing the operator with ongoing information regarding its current status and the operator in turn using this information to plan and execute actions back to the machine (see figure 18.1).

This framework assumes essentially parallel processing systems in both the human and the machine. Both have mechanisms by which information is inputted from one side of the system to the other (sensory systems of the person; control functions of the machine), means for processing that information (cognitive mediation in the human; mechanical or electrical central processors in the machine), and some way of relaying the processed output back to the other side (motor processes or action systems in the human; displays in the machine). Although conceptually simplistic, each of these components is subserved by many highly complex variables, all of which exert significant influence on the efficiency of the system. These are discussed in some detail in the sections to follow.

In addition, this system operates within the boundaries of a larger external environment. The characteristics of this broader environment influence both the individual system components noted previously and the manner in which the human and machine interact. Traditionally, this larger environment is thought to influence the human–machine system at three basic hierarchical levels: the general environment (e.g., city, community, transportation systems), the intermediate environment (e.g., home, office, factory), and the immediate environment (e.g., workstation, computer, chair).

Because this is a closed-loop, fully interactive system, the point at which we can begin the discussion is arbitrary. Furthermore, it would be possible to write several chapters on each of the stages within this human–machine framework. Given the general scope of this book, however, the focus of this chapter is the two elements of the model most directly related to the

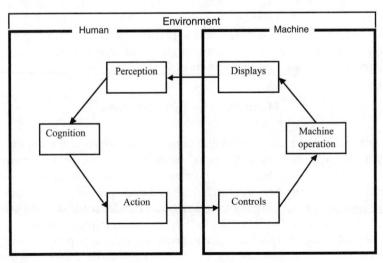

▶ **Figure 18.1**   Conceptualization of the human–machine system.
(Source: Proctor & Van Zandt, 1994, pg. 4).

sensorimotor attributes of the human operator—sensation and cognition. The contributions to action are discussed in the context of both stages in the form of several recommendations for design.

Sensory Stage

Inherent in the human–machine concept is the notion that our daily inter-actions with objects are governed by three broad classes of constraint: The environmental context under which the interaction takes place, the physi-cal properties of the object (e.g., size, shape, texture), and the perceptual–motor resources available to the actor. For this human–machine system concept to be viable, the person must receive information from elements within the external environment in some usable form. The gateways are the sensory systems that are available to us, including the visual, auditory, vestibular, haptic, and proprioceptive systems, which allow for the recep-tion of different sources of environmental information regarding system status. Although all are useful, far and away the most important sources of stimulus information in terms of system operation are the visual and audi-tory structures. Assuming they are intact (i.e., no structural impairment), these two sensory inputs serve as early warning systems, able to receive information distal to the body. Subjected to rigorous scientific study for more than 400 years, the human visual system is perhaps better understood than any of the other sensory receptor systems. Although a comprehensive review of this literature is not possible here, there are several areas that make visual perception of critical importance when considering any human–environment interaction.

Early theory in the field of psychophysics held that the most important characteristic of a stimulus, at least in terms of sensory stimulation, is salience—that is, the quality of the signal provided by the physical elements that make up the stimulus (typically defined in terms of size and intensity). Thus, it is important to bear in mind stimulus attributes such as brightness, loudness, and texture when considering the design of work space. Although this is fairly obvious, there are other factors to consider that complicate matters. Because human sensory systems operate at variable rates of speed (based upon the type, location, and firing rates of sensory receptors), it is also important to consider the nature of the information that is conveyed by a given stimulus. For example, whereas considerable information can be communicated by a visual stimulus, auditory stimuli are preferable when the message is relatively simple or some type of alerting function is required (e.g., a warning alarm).

The unique physiology of the eye suggests that stimulus location is also of vital importance at this stage.[3] Consider that visual stimuli come from

---

[3]In 1604, Johannes Kepler's *Ad Vitellionem paralipomena* likely became the first attempt at explanation of the optics of the human eye. In 1619, Christoph Scheiner's *Oculus* provided the first accurate diagrams of the human eye.

light reflected from a narrow band in the electromagnetic spectrum (400-700 nm). When this light energy enters the eye, it is absorbed by two types of photoreceptors: cones and rods. Rods, located primarily in the periphery of the retina, are sensitive to light and are able to detect motion in extremely low illumination. Thus, although they are instrumental in our capability to visually detect movement, they are not receptive to color, nor are they sensitive to detail. Cones, on the other hand, are concentrated centrally and are more densely packed. Although they are sensitive to color and are able to discern fine detail, they are not well suited to the detection of motion and they require relatively high levels of illumination. Thus, it is likely that two distinct but parallel physiological systems subserve visual perception—a focal system centered within the foveal region, characterized by high acuity and color sensitivity, for accurate stimulus identification, and an ambient system located within the periphery that is sensitive to motion and allows for stimulus localization. Designers must take these physiological attributes into account. For example, environmental interactions that must necessarily take place in poorly (or variably) illuminated settings are most efficiently designed when critical visual stimuli are located in the periphery.

Further complicating matters are the cooperative but often competitive interactions both within a single sensory system and between two or more sensory systems. A good example of the former involves voluntary control of eye movements. When viewing any moving stimulus, we have at our disposal at least three cooperative mechanisms of eye movement. The first of these are smooth pursuit movements that keep moving objects fixed on the retina (see chapter 9). The velocity of these eye movements can be voluntarily altered to track objects that are moving at variable speeds (e.g., a cursor moving on a computer screen). The second mechanism, termed *optic saccades*, is characterized by short bursts of eye movements, the velocities of which are determined by the distance between stimuli and are not subject to voluntary control (see chapter 10). The third, allowing for the perception of depth, is vergence, wherein the eyes move in opposition (i.e., as an object gets closer, the eyes rotate inward; as an object recedes, the eyes turn in parallel).

Whereas voluntary control of eye movements demonstrates the cooperative nature of a within-system sensory operation, there are also many examples where multisensory interactions compete. Perhaps the most significant occurs when the visual and auditory systems are activated simultaneously. In a classic study by Colavita (1974), participants were asked to differentially respond to visual and auditory stimuli either in isolation or during simultaneous presentation. Although this study revealed much about the nature of these two individual sensory systems, perhaps the most striking results occurred during the simultaneous presentation. Specifically, when auditory and visual information competed, participants invariably responded more quickly and accurately to the auditory stimulus. So strong was this auditory advantage that participants often failed to even notice that a visual stimulus was present. The message from this study for designers is clear: If performers are expected to act on specific sensory information, it is critical to isolate the source of that information. For example, if the primary source of task-specific information is auditory (e.g., sonar tracking), using visual stimuli to impart critical information, such as warnings or changes to system operation, may result in that visual information being ignored.

Recommendations for Design

Before any form of useful cognition can occur, elements within a working environment must communicate with the human actor. Because this is necessarily accomplished through the display of information to one or more set of sensory receptors, it is critical that designers consider the differing characteristics (including strengths and weakness) of these sensory processes. An understanding of the limitations of the sensory systems is crucial if we are to maximize the performance of the human–machine system.

Although such environmental information can be either direct or indirect, researchers of human factors are primarily concerned with direct information (i.e., information that is represented by displays).[4] There are several things to take into account from a design point of view when considering the sensory perception of action-relevant cues transmitted through these displays. In general, it is vital to ensure appropriate levels of salience for all imperative stimuli. For visual displays, there are a minimum of four qualities that will enhance their effectiveness: conspicuity, visibility, legibility, and intelligibility.

Conspicuity means the display should attract attention by being prominent, novel, and relevant. This is aided by ensuring appropriate size and brightness for visual stimuli, location and loudness for auditory stimuli, and texture gradient for tactile stimuli. Visibility means the display must be visible under all expected viewing conditions. Given the unique physiology of the visual system, designers are well advised to play to its strengths and mitigate its weaknesses. For example, be cognizant of low or variable levels of illumination while at the same time avoiding unnecessary glare. Be judicious in the use of color. Since only the central visual field is sensitive to color, any stimuli relying on color to impart information should be centrally located. A rule of thumb is to always design first in monochrome. If all of the necessary information can be displayed in this form, the use of color is redundant and potentially problematic. Legibility includes consideration of contrast ratio between imperative stimuli and any associated backgrounds (visual and auditory), as well as the size and simplicity of any lettering. It is easy to mask important information with background noise,

---

[4]Displays include any indirect method of presenting information (e.g., visual, auditory, tactile, olfactory, oral). The majority of displays are visual or auditory.

thus reducing sensitivity to imperative cues. Finally, intelligibility means any messages must be unambiguous and emphasize the most important aspects of the display.

Under some conditions, the auditory modality can offer advantages over the visual modality. Situations in which auditory displays may be preferable include simple and short messages, warnings or messages that require immediate action, an overburdened visual system, poor illumination, or a required verbal response. However, every attempt should be made to avoid situations in which sensory information is imparted across two or more sensory modalities. Because of the constraints associated with each sensory input system, important information that is delivered in one modality (i.e., visual) can be easily masked by information that is delivered through another (e.g., auditory).

Cognition

From the earliest psychophysical investigations into human perceptual sensitivity, it was thought that stimulus salience was the single most important variable subserving stimulus detection. Though this is true to a point, subsequent research has long demonstrated that other characteristics of objects and signals within a given environment are equally important, if not even more so, in terms of perception with a view toward action. This is because the act of simply becoming aware of a stimulus is only the first step in understanding the meaning of that stimulus and using that understanding to plan and execute an appropriate response toward it. These action processes are mediated by many higher-order cognitive operations that are complex, highly interactive, and often situation specific (e.g., attention, memory, experience). These processes, which make up the next stage in the human–machine model, are considered now.

For decades, researchers have been intrigued by questions regarding the mechanisms that drive the translation process in which stimulus information is transformed into action. If errors occur in any human–environment interaction, either through the selection of an inappropriate response or in the incorrect execution of a correct response, the problem almost invariably lies in this information–action translation process. The first formal research on human factors, described earlier in this chapter, tackled this problem directly. What has become evident since these early studies is that several characteristics of stimuli beyond those that operate at a sensory level will either help or hinder actions toward them. At the risk of oversimplifying the issue but in the interest of space, discussion of these attributes focuses on stimulus size and spatial location.

As discussed earlier, the work of Paul Fitts in the 1950s was groundbreaking from both an applied and a theoretical perspective. Although this research was important in many ways, Fitts' greatest legacy was the application of information theory to human motor behaviors. The outcome was Fitts' law. The intricacies of Fitts' law as they pertain to variations in aiming movements have been discussed at length elsewhere in this book, so an in-depth discussion is not required here. However, because it is so fundamental to human–object interactions that are undertaken in applied settings, it is useful to reconsider the basic tenets of the law before moving on to some examples. Fitts' law (Fitts, 1954) describes the linear and lawful nature of the speed–accuracy trade-off that exists when people engage in accuracy-constrained, target aiming situations. Specifically, MT increases as either the distance between targets increases or the size of the targets themselves decreases. It is thought that the longer MT results from the increased demands placed on human information processing systems that are occasioned by conformation to increasingly constrained task demands (i.e., smaller targets or longer distances). These constraints have been quantified in Fitts' law, which states that in any target aiming task, the index of difficulty (ID) is derived as $\log_2$ of $2A \ / \ W$, with A representing the distance between targets and B representing the width of the targets.

Anyone who has used an automated bank machine will notice the instantiation of this law in that the keys (targets) that are used most often or are most important (i.e., the *Enter* or *OK* commands) are the largest and closest. If the operator is under no temporal constraints (i.e., can move as slowly or as quickly as desired), these size and amplitude constraints are seldom problematic. If, on the other hand, the time required to acquire the target is of some great importance (e.g., hitting an emergency cutoff on a power tool), then these variables take on a much greater significance.

Another point to consider, however, is that it is possible to have identical IDs for two qualitatively different movements. These situations occur when increases in target size cancel out different movement amplitudes. For example, 10 cm movements to a 5 cm target (i.e., 2 bits) will create an ID identical to movements of 20 cm to a 10 cm target (i.e., 2 bits). Theoretically, the information processing demands in each of these situations are identical, and common convention considers these two instances as equal. Though this is seldom problematic when considering most aiming movements, it can sometimes be misleading. Consider, for example, any operator who must control a cursor on a computer screen so as to move it to a specific icon. The speed at which the operator can accurately move the cursor is still lawfully governed by how close and how large the icon is, but the nature of the size–distance relationship is fundamentally different from that of a three-dimensional aiming situation (e.g., reaching out to push a button).

Evidence for this comes from Graham and MacKenzie (1995, 1996), who demonstrated that for mouse-controlled cursor movements, the effects of changing amplitude on MT were much more pronounced than the effects of changing target size, even though those movements were constrained by an identical ID. Similar effects have been demonstrated when the generation of a movement trajectory is compromised by age or injury. For example, we (Lyons & Hansen, submitted; Passmore, Burke, & Lyons, 2007) have shown that people with spinal cord injury execute faster movements to shorter-amplitude targets (versus longer-amplitude targets of the same ID), whereas people without spinal cord injury complete movements to both target conditions in a similar amount of time.

The spatial location of stimulus events affects more than MT, however. One of the most robust findings in both theoretical and applied research, and one that has often been used as a window into many of the processes underlying motor control, has been that of stimulus–response compatibility.

Stimulus–response compatibility effects refer to variations in performance (usually measured by RT) that are a function of the ways in which stimulus–response pairings are arranged. Specifically, the time that it takes to respond to stimuli depends on the relationship between the stimulus patterns and the possible response options (Fitts & Seeger, 1953). At its simplest conceptual level, pairings that lead to faster RT are termed *compatible* and pairings that lead to slower RT are termed *incompatible*. Since the seminal work by Fitts and Seeger (1953), it has long been known that spatial location is an important determinant of stimulus–response compatibility.

Traditionally, spatial stimulus–response compatibility effects have been explained in one of three ways: an innate tendency to respond in the direction of the source of the stimulation (e.g., Simon & Small, 1967), the degree of correspondence between the spatial codes associated with the response effector and the stimulus (e.g., Anzola, Bertoloni, Buchtel, & Rizzolatti, 1977; Kornblum, Hasbroucq, & Osman, 1990), or an attentional bias favoring whichever effector occupies the same spatial location as the stimulus (e.g., Heilman & Valenstein, 1979). Early evidence (e.g., Fitts & Seeger, 1953; Wallace, 1971) directed theoretical accounts of the stimulus–response phenomenon toward a coding explanation of stimulus–response effects that was based on the same premises of information theory. These coding explanations of stimulus–response effects generally maintain that mental representations of the task environment are formed and then used to execute the required action. The efficiency and accuracy of these representations ultimately result in the latencies evidenced through chronometric measures (such as RT). Thus, the translation of stimulus information into action is determined by the degree of correspondence between stimulus codes and response codes. In other words, stimulus–response compatibility effects reflect the efficiency of translation between codes that are derived from the spatial (e.g., Fitts & Seeger, 1953) or symbolic (e.g., Hedge & Marsh, 1975) characteristics of the stimulus and codes that are formed for a response. Note that it is not physical correspondence between stimulus and response per se that induces stimulus–response compatibility effects but rather the correspondence between mental codes that are constructed to represent stimuli and response sets.

Coding hypotheses have been postulated to occur at several levels of cognitive complexity (Michaels, 1988). For example, a finding by Simon and Rudell (1967) suggests that even if the spatial position of the stimulus is irrelevant to the task, that position still exerts considerable influence by directing, or biasing, the direction of the response toward the irrelevant location (Simon effect). In such situations, it appears that if the irrelevant location of the stimulus corresponds to the response, translation of stimulus codes to response codes is affected and response to the relevant stimulus is negatively affected.

Many years of research in this area have led to the development of taxonomies of stimulus–response compatibility. One such taxonomy (Simon, Sly, & Vilapakkam, 1981) distinguishes three types of potential compatibility: symbolic compatibility resulting from verbal labels associated with stimulus and response, spatial compatibility between the position of the stimulus signals and the position of the response, and the Simon effect. A more comprehensive taxonomy was developed by Kornblum and colleagues (Kornblum et al., 1990). This taxonomy stresses that the degree of dimensional overlap within the stimulus–response arrangement (i.e., the degree to which the stimulus shares attributes with the response set) will generate varying degrees of response compatibility. Kornblum and colleagues distinguished between relevant and irrelevant task dimensions and specified four stimulus–response ensemble types, ranging from type I ensembles (no dimensional overlap) to type IV ensembles (stimulus and response sets overlap on relevant and irrelevant dimensions).

These taxonomies have proved useful in the development of several models that try to account for stimulus–response compatibility effects. One such model, a strict representational coding-based account of stimulus–response compatibility, was proposed by Heister and colleagues. In a series of experiments spanning several years, Heister and colleagues (Heister, Ehrenstein, & Schroeder-Heister, 1986, 1987; Heister & Schroeder-Heister, 1987) distinguished three potential forms of stimulus–response compatibility that differ with respect to the spatial coding of the response. They suggested that compatibility effects are observed as a function of compatibility due to the coding of response key position, response effector position (responding hands or fingers), or spatio-anatomical mapping. Furthermore, the results of these studies suggest a hierarchical order of effectiveness, with coding of response keys being the dominant factor. In situations where no spatial difference between response goals is evident, however, spatial coding of effector position becomes the dominant factor. If coding of response effector position is not possible (e.g., where there are orthogonal stimulus–response arrangements), then spatio-anatomical mapping takes precedence. This model captures a large amount of empirical data that show RT dependence on the spatial arrangement of stimuli and their associated responses.

Another model positing hierarchical control was suggested by Ladavas (1990). This model also suggests that representational coding takes place at three levels: the spatial coding of the goal, the spatial coding of the response effectors, and the coding of the anatomical status of the effector (i.e., which hand makes the response). Again, at least in situations of dimensional overlap, these hierarchical levels are listed in order of dominance, with goal coding superseding effector coding and both of these dominating anatomical status coding. In instances where dimensional overlap between stimulus and response locations is not present, anatomical status of the responding hand dominates the other two factors.

Both models suggest that relative, rather than absolute, spatial coding underlies stimulus–response compatibility effects. However, different coding mechanisms are available to direct responses when spatial coding is not possible. In addition, Umilta and Nicoletti (1985) suggest that, even within spatial coding, there appears to be a certain stimulus–response hierarchy. Specifically, horizontal coding will dominate vertical coding in situations where both are possible (Umilta & Nicoletti, 1985), with both of these coding relations dominating depth coding (Merry, Weeks, & Chua, 2003).

Although issues of spatial stimulus–response compatibility are certainly dominant in workplace design, it is worth mentioning that other forms of compatibility will affect the efficiency of information processing. These include issues related to movement compatibility, where the movement of displays and controls relative to the response of the system being displayed can help or hinder the movement (e.g., a clockwise movement of a control knob usually means an increase in the control parameter and vice versa); modality compatibility, where certain stimulus–response modality combinations are more compatible with some tasks than with others (e.g., a verbal response to a verbal command is faster than a manual response and vice versa); and conceptual compatibility, where codes and symbols correspond to conceptual associations of meaning (e.g., an airplane on a sign rather than a colored square to indicate an airport).

Upon completing the cognitive processing of all available sensory information, a decision is made. This decision is translated into neuromuscular commands and an overt action ensues. For the purposes of this discussion, *action* refers to all those processes involved in the selection, programming, and execution of a response. Actions are the manner by which the human transmits information to the machine. Generally speaking, if the cognitive mediation processes have gone well, the original stimulus information provided by environmental stimuli (i.e., those originating from the machine display) will elicit an appropriate response (i.e., one that is either desired or required to continue the human–machine cycle). Remember that this action plan is considered the optimal course for achieving a specific goal that has been defined by system constraints that have been successfully resolved during the cognitive mediation stage. Of course, if these constraints have not been successfully resolved, the action plan will lead to an interaction with the environment that is either less than optimal (e.g., too slow, too much applied force) or incorrect (e.g., pressing the wrong key on a keyboard, missing a target). Errors can occur in any of the selection, programming, and execution phases of a response.

In terms of human factors, errors can generally be grouped into those that are latent and those that are active. Latent errors are usually a series or combination of operator or design errors that are present in the system long before the frontline operator or user commits an active error. Examples of latent errors include faulty design, poor maintenance, poor communication, and so on. Of more interest, however, are active errors, those committed by frontline operators. Most active errors arise during the cognitive stage of processing and are felt immediately (e.g., pushing the wrong button, incorrectly setting a dial, leaving the door of a ferry open). Action errors can be further classified into those of omission (failing to perform a required action) or commission (performing an incorrect action). In the more general literature on motor behavior, these types of errors have been described as response selection and response execution errors (see Schmidt, 1976).

Newer Issues and Future Directions

As noted earlier in this chapter, the field of human factors originally developed to address the challenges brought about by the rapidly accelerating technological advances of World War II. It is a truism of the field that although the abilities and limitations of human operators remain relatively stable across time, progressive changes to the technologies with which they are expected to interact continue to move forward. Perhaps the most recent significant shift in this direction was the widespread acceptance of computing technology in the early 1980s. The advent of computers as a major construct of daily activity has brought a new set of issues that challenge the way we think about our place in the human–machine system. Indeed, the past 20 years have seen the development of a wholly novel field of research (human–computer interaction, or HCI) that is dedicated exclusively to understanding the unique relationship between humans and computers. We will focus here on only a few examples of the ways in which the nature of HCI differs from interactions conducted in typical three-dimensional space.

One major issue that complicates human interactions with computers and other virtual environments occurs at the display stage of the human–machine system. In most cases, system information is transmitted to the user-operator through a monitor screen that is situated both distally and in an orthogonal plane to the work space (e.g., keyboard, mouse). The frame of reference for users is fundamentally different from that in which the user operates during everyday interactions within a three-dimensional environment. Under these types of display conditions, the system necessitates a dissociation of the space in which the user is making a movement and the space in which the movement actually occurs (i.e., the hand moves the mouse and the mouse moves the cursor). This dissociation requires the frame of reference for stimulus perception and eventual action to be adapted such that the egocentric, person-centered reference frame that guides typical three-dimensional movements is modified to an allocentric, environment-centered frame that remains independent of the user's current position.

To illustrate, consider a control-room operator of a fabricating plant in the 1960s. To activate a particular machine, the operator would find the appropriate switch in an array of switches, isolate that particular switch as a target, and then formulate and execute a motor plan that would move the arm to throw the switch. These actions would all be governed by the information processing constraints of Fitts' law (switch size and movement amplitude) and stimulus–response compatibility (the composition of the switch array). In the modern version of this plant, the operator would likely view a schematic drawing of the plant machinery on a computer monitor, receive current system status information from this display, identify and isolate a symbolic representation of the target machine (presented as a screen icon), and then plan and execute a motor plan to move a mouse. These mouse movements would then result in the movement of a cursor on the screen. Under this scenario, the cursor assumes the representative role of the arm and hand. When the cursor arrives over the icon, a terminal action (pressing a mouse button) would be executed and system feedback monitored by the operator to ensure that the appropriate end result was achieved.

Although this example appears quite simplistic, careful consideration of the variables at play reveals a significantly altered human–machine dynamic. In addition to the allocentric and egocentric distinctions described previously, additional factors are at play in HCI situations that differentially affect movements. For example, the target itself is represented symbolically by an icon, which is mediated in turn by comprehension of the symbol, which requires an additional degree of learning. Furthermore, indirect movements such as mouse pointing often result in temporal lags between action and effect. These particular characteristics of the HCI typically result in two types of temporal lag that can dramatically affect performance (e.g., So, Chung, & Goonetilleke, 1999).

The first type of temporal lag, display lag, occurs as a result of both the additional stimulus processing time required for the translation of symbolic (icon) information into a meaningful referent and differences in a computer operator's field of view. The second type, control lag, refers to delays that exist between the initiation of movement and the point at which the movement representation (the cursor on the screen) records the movement.

Empirical studies of the effects of these lags suggest that MT increases with increasing lags and that these increases are proportional to the ID of the movement—that is, the greater the lag, the greater the ID (Hoffmann, 1992). Using these data, Hoffman (1992) proposed a modification to Fitts' law to predict the effects of lag on manually controlled pointer MT: $MT = a + b$ $(c + lag) \log_2(2A / W)$. Furthermore, and as noted earlier, mouse-controlled cursor movements are affected more by changes in amplitude than by changes in target size (e.g., Graham & MacKenzie, 1995, 1996).

These examples detail specific issues in HCI that arise from principles of motor behavior. As is the case with typical three-dimensional environmental interactions, however, errors in HCI occur most often at the processing stage of the human–machine system. Wickens and colleagues (Wickens, Lee, Liu, & Gordon-Becker, 2004) have developed a useful taxonomy of design principles in HCI that can reduce operator error. These principles are grouped according to perception, mental models, attention, and memory. As an example of a perceptual principle, Wickens and coworkers suggest the avoidance of absolute judgment limits (i.e., not asking the user to determine the level of a variable on the basis of a single sensory variable such as color, size, or loudness since these sensory variables can contain many levels).

Of course, as technology continues to advance, the complexity of work environments, both real and virtual, will increase. Future directions in research on human factors will have to consider issues such as the increased use of teleoperation and telemedicine (operation of machines and surgical procedures at a distance), a rapidly aging population and workforce and the associated decrements in perceptual–motor processing, the increasing prevalence and fidelity of simulators in the workplace, and, as was the case 50 years ago when it all began, extraordinarily rapid advances in military technology.

REFERENCES

PART I

Elliott, D., Helsen, W.F., & Chua, R. (2001). Woodworth's (1899) two-component model of goal-directed aiming. *Psychological Bulletin, 127,* 342-357.

Khan, M.A., Franks, I.M., Elliott, D., Lawrence, G.P., Chua, R., Bernier, P.-M., Hansen, S., & Weeks, D. (2006). Inferring online and offline processing of visual feedback in target-directed movements from kinematic data. *Neuroscience and Biobehavioral Reviews, 30,* 1106-1121.

Tipper, S.P., Lortie, C., & Baylis, G.C. (1992). Selective reaching: Evidence for action-centered attention. *Journal of Experimental Psychology: Human Perception and Performance, 18,* 891-905.

Woodworth, R.S. (1899). The accuracy of voluntary movement. *Psychological Review, Monograph Supplements 3*(13), 1-119.

CHAPTER 1

Beggs, W.D.A., & Howarth, C.I. (1970). Movement control in man in a repetitive motor task. *Nature, 221,* 752-753.

Beggs, W.D.A., & Howarth, C.I. (1972). The accuracy of aiming at a target: Some further evidence for a theory of intermittent control. *Acta Psychologica, 36,* 171-177.

Binsted, G., & Elliott, D. (1999). The Muller-Lyer illusion as a perturbation to the saccadic system. *Human Movement Science, 18,* 103-117.

Brebner, J. (1968). Continuing and reversing the direction of responding movements: Some exceptions to the so-called "psychological refractory period." *Journal of Experimental Psychology, 78,* 120-127.

Carlton, L.G. (1979). Control processes in the production of discrete aiming responses. *Journal of Human Movement Studies, 5,* 115-124.

Carlton, L.G. (1981). Visual information: The control of aiming movements. *Quarterly Journal of Experimental Psychology A: Human Experimental Psychology, 33,* 87-93.

Carlton, L.G. (1992). Visual processing time and the control of movement. In L. Proteau & D. Elliott (Eds.), *Vision and motor control* (pp. 3-31). Amsterdam: North-Holland.

Carlton, L.G. (1994). The effects of temporal-precision and time-minimization constraints on the spatial and temporal accuracy of aimed hand movements. *Journal of Motor Behavior, 26,* 43-50.

Chua, R., & Elliott, D. (1993). Visual regulation of manual aiming. *Human Movement Science, 12,* 366-401.

Crossman, E.R.F.W., & Goodeve, P.J. (1983). Feedback control of hand movement and Fitts' law. *Quarterly Journal of Experimental Psychology A: Human Experimental Psychology, 35,* 251-278. (Original work published 1963)

Desmurget, M., Epstein, C.M., Turner, R.S., Prablanc, C., Alexander, G.E., & Grafton, S.T. (1999). Role of the posterior parietal cortex in updating reaching movements to a visual target. *Nature Neuroscience, 2,* 563-567.

Desmurget, M., & Grafton, S. (2000). Forward modeling allows feedback control for fast reaching movements. *Trends in Cognitive Sciences, 4,* 423-431.

Elliott, D., & Allard, F. (1985). The utilization of visual feedback information during rapid pointing movements. *Quarterly Journal of Experimental Psychology A: Human Experimental Psychology, 37,* 407-425.

Elliott, D., Binsted, G., & Heath, M. (1999). The control of goal-directed limb movements: Correcting errors in the trajectory. *Human Movement Science, 8,* 121-136.

Elliott, D., Carson, R.G., Goodman, D., & Chua, R. (1991). Discrete vs. continuous visual control of manual aiming. *Human Movement Science, 10,* 393-418.

Elliott, D., Chua, R., Pollock, B.J., & Lyons, J. (1995). Optimizing the use of vision in manual aiming: The role of practice. *Quarterly Journal of Experimental Psychology A: Human Experimental Psychology, 48,* 72-83.

Elliott, D., Hansen, S., Mendoza, J., & Tremblay, L. (2004). Learning to optimize speed, accuracy, and energy expenditure: A framework for understanding speed-accuracy relations in goal-directed aiming. *Journal of Motor Behavior, 36,* 339-351.

Elliott, D., Helsen, W.F., & Chua, R. (2001). A century later: Woodworth's two-component model of goal directed aiming. *Psychological Bulletin, 127,* 342-357.

Elliott, D., & Lee, T.D. (1995). The role of target information on manual-aiming bias. *Psychological Research, 58,* 2-9.

Elliott, D., Welsh, T.N., Lyons, J., Hansen, S., & Wu, M. (2006). The visual regulation of goal-directed reaching movements in adults with Williams syndrome, Down syndrome and other developmental disabilities. *Motor Control, 10,* 34-54.

Engelbrecht, S.E., Berthier, N.E., & O'Sullivan, L.P. (2003). The undershooting bias: Learning to act optimally under uncertainty. *Psychological Science, 14,* 257-261.

Fitts, P.M. (1954). The information capacity of the human motor system in controlling the amplitude of movement. *Journal of Experimental Psychology, 47,* 381-391.

Fitts, P.M., & Peterson, J.R. (1964). Information capacity of discrete motor responses. *Journal of Experimental Psychology, 67,* 103-112.

Glover, S. (2004). Separate visual representations in the planning and control of action. *Behavioral and Brain Sciences, 27,* 3-24.

Grierson, L.E.M., & Elliott, D. (2008). Kinematic analysis of goal-directed aims made against early and late perturbations: An investigation of the relative influence of two online control processes. *Human Movement Science, 27,* 839-856.

Grierson, L.E.M., & Elliott, D. (2009). Goal-directed aiming and the relative contribution of two online control processes. *American Journal of Psychology, 122,* 309-324.

Guiard, Y. (1993). On Fitts' and Hooke's laws: Simple harmonic movement in upper-limb cyclical aiming. *Acta Psychologica, 82,* 139-159.

Hansen, S., Elliott, D., & Tremblay, L. (2007). Online control of discrete action following visual perturbation. *Perception, 36,* 268-287.

Hansen, S., Glazebrook, C., Anson, J.G., Weeks, D.J., & Elliott, D. (2006). The influence of advance information about target location and visual feedback on movement planning and execution. *Canadian Journal of Experimental Psychology, 60,* 200-208.

Hansen, S., Tremblay, L., & Elliott, D. (2005). Part and whole practice: Chunking and online control in the acquisition of a serial motor task. *Research Quarterly for Exercise and Sport, 76,* 60-67.

Heath, M. (2005). Role of limb and target vision in the online control of memory-guided reaches. *Motor Control, 9,* 281-309.

Heath, M., Neely, K., & Binsted, G. (2007). Allocentric visual cues influence online limb adjustments. *Motor Control, 11,* 54-70.

Helsen, W.F., Elliott, D., Starkes, J.L., & Ricker, K.L. (2000). Coupling of eye, finger, elbow and shoulder movements during manual aiming. *Journal of Motor Behavior, 32,* 241-248.

Hodges, N.J., Cunningham, S.J., Lyons, J., Kerr, T.L., & Elliott, D. (1995). Visual feedback processing and goal-directed movement in adults with Down syndrome. *Adapted Physical Activity Quarterly, 12,* 176-186.

Howarth, C.E., Beggs, W.D.A., & Bowden, J.M. (1971). The relationship between speed and accuracy of movements aimed at a target. *Acta Psychologica, 35,* 207-218.

Keele, S.W. (1968). Movement control in skilled motor performance. *Psychological Bulletin, 70,* 387-403.

Keele, S.W., & Posner, M.I. (1968). Processing visual feedback in rapid movements. *Journal of Experimental Psychology, 77,* 155-158.

Khan, M.A., Chua, R., Elliott, D., Coull, J., & Lyons, J. (2002). Optimal control strategies under different feedback schedules: Kinematic evidence. *Journal of Motor Behavior, 34,* 45-57.

Khan, M.A., & Franks, I.M. (2003). Online versus offline processing of visual feedback in the production of component submovements. *Journal of Motor Behavior, 35,* 285-295.

Khan, M.A., Franks, I.M., Elliott, D., Lawrence, G.P., Chua, R., Bernier, P., Hansen, S., & Weeks, D.J. (2006). Inferring online and offline processing of visual feedback in target-directed movements from kinematic data. *Neuroscience and Behavioral Reviews, 30,* 1106-1121.

Khan, M.A., Franks, I.M., & Goodman, D. (1998). The effect of practice on the control of rapid aiming movements: Evidence for an interdependence between programming and feedback processing. *Quarterly Journal of Experimental Psychology A: Human Experimental Psychology, 51,* 425-444.

Khan, M.A., Lawrence, G., Franks, I.M., & Buckolz, E. (2004). The utilization of peripheral and central vision in the control of movement direction. *Experimental Brain Research, 158,* 241-251.

Langolf, G.D., Chaffin, D.B., & Foulke, J.A. (1976). An investigation of Fitts' law using a wide range of movement amplitudes. *Journal of Motor Behavior, 8,* 113-128.

Lyons, J., Hansen, S., Hurding, S., & Elliott, D. (2006). Optimizing rapid aiming behaviour: Movement kinematics depend on the cost of corrective modifications. *Experimental Brain Research, 174,* 95-100.

Mendoza, J.E., Elliott, D., Meegan, D.V., Lyons, J., & Welsh, T.N. (2006). The effect of the Muller-Lyer illusion on the planning and control of manual aiming movements. *Journal of Experimental Psychology: Human Perception and Performance, 32,* 413-422.

Mendoza, J., Hansen, S., Glazebrook, C.M., Keetch, K.M., & Elliott, D. (2005). Visual illusions affect both movement planning and on-line control: A multiple cue position on bias and goal-directed action. *Human Movement Science, 24,* 760-773.

Meyer, D.E., Abrams, R.A., Kornblum, S., Wright, C.E., & Smith, J.E.K. (1988). Optimality in human motor performance: Ideal control of rapid aimed movements. *Psychological Review, 95,* 340-370.

Meyer, D.E., Smith, J.E.K., & Wright, C.E. (1982). Models for the speed and accuracy of aimed movements. *Psychological Review, 89,* 449-482.

Miall, R.C., & Wolpert, D.M. (1996). Forward models for physiological motor control. *Neural Networks, 9,* 1265-1279.

Milner, A.D., & Goodale, M.A. (1995). *The visual brain in action.* Oxford, UK: Oxford University Press.

Obhi, S.S., Lyons, J., Welsh, T.N., Glazebrook, C.M., Anson, G., & Elliott, D. (2007). The perceived time of voluntary action for adults with and without Down syndrome. *Down Syndrome Quarterly, 9,* 4-9.

Oliveira, F.T.P., Elliott, D., & Goodman, D. (2005). The energy minimization bias: Compensating for intrinsic influence of energy minimization mechanisms. *Motor Control, 9,* 101-114.

Paillard, J. (1982). The contribution of peripheral and central vision to visually guided reaching. In D. Ingle, M. Goodale, & R. Marsfield (Eds.), *Analysis of visual behavior (pp. 367-385).* Cambridge, MA: MIT Press.

Plamondon, R. (1995). A kinematic theory of rapid human movements. Part 1. Movement representation and generation. *Biological Cybernetics, 72,* 295-307.

Proteau, L. (1992). On the specificity of learning and the role of visual information for movement control. In L. Proteau & D. Elliott (Eds.), *Vision and motor control* (pp. 67-103). Amsterdam: North-Holland.

Proteau, L., & Masson, G. (1997). Visual perception modifies goal-directed movement control: Supporting evidence from a visual perturbation paradigm. *Quarterly Journal of Experimental Psychology A: Human Experimental Psychology, 50,* 726-741.

Schmidt, R.A., Zelaznik, H.N., & Frank, J.S. (1978). Sources of inaccuracy in rapid movement. In G.E. Stelmach (Ed.), *Information processing in motor control and learning* (pp. 183-203). New York: Academic Press.

Schmidt, R.A., Zelaznik, H.N., Hawkins, B., Frank, J.S., & Quinn, J.T. (1979). Motor output variability: A theory for the accuracy of rapid motor acts. *Psychological Review, 86*, 415-451.

Sternberg, S. (1969). The discovery of processing stages: Extensions of Donders' method. *Acta Psychologica, 30*, 276-315.

Von Holst, E. (1954). Relations between the central nervous system and the peripheral organs. *British Journal of Animal Behaviour, 2*, 89-94.

Wallace, S.A., & Newell, K.M. (1983). Visual control of discrete aiming movements. *Quarterly Journal of Experimental Psychology A: Human Experimental Psychology, 35*, 311-321.

Welsh, T.N., Higgins, L., & Elliott, D. (2007). Are there age-related differences in learning to optimize speed, accuracy and energy expenditure? *Human Movement Science, 26*, 892-912.

Wolpert, D.M., & Ghahramani, Z. (2000). Computational principles of movement neuroscience. *Nature Neuroscience, 3*, 1212-1217.

Woodworth, R.S. (1899). The accuracy of voluntary movement. *Psychological Review, Monograph Supplements, 3*(13), 1-119.

Zelaznik, H.N., Hawkins, B., & Kisselburgh, L. (1983). Rapid visual feedback processing in single-aiming movements. *Journal of Motor Behavior, 15*, 217-236.

CHAPTER 2

Abahnini, K, Proteau, L., & Temprado, J.J. (1997). Evidence supporting the importance of peripheral visual information for the directional control of aiming movement. *Journal of Motor Behavior, 29*, 230-242.

Abrams, R.A., & Pratt, J. (1993). Rapid aimed limb movements: Differential effects of practice on component submovements. *Journal of Motor Behavior, 25*, 288-298.

Bard, C., Hay, L., & Fleury, M. (1985). Role of peripheral vision in the directional control of rapid aiming movements. *Canadian Journal of Experimental Psychology, 39*, 151-161.

Bard, C., Paillard, J., Fleury, M., Hay, L., & Larue., J. (1990). Positional versus directional control loops in visuomotor pointing. *European Bulletin of Cognitive Psychology, 39*, 151-161.

Binsted, G., & Elliott, D. (1999). The Muller-Lyer illusion as a perturbation to the saccadic system. *Human Movement Science, 18*, 103-117.

Carson, R.G., Goodman, D., Chua, R., & Elliott, D. (1993). Asymmetries in the regulation of visually guided aiming. *Journal of Motor Behavior, 25*, 21-32.

Chua, R., & Elliott, D. (1993). Visual regulation of manual aiming. *Human Movement Science, 12*, 366-401.

de Oliveira, R.F., Huys, R., Oudejans, R.R.D., van de Langenberg, R., & Beek, P.J. (2007). Basketball jump shooting is controlled online by vision. *Experimental Psychology, 54*, 180-186.

Desmurget, M., & Grafton, S. (2000). Forward modeling allows feedback control for fast reaching movements. *Trends in Cognitive Sciences, 4*, 423-431.

Elliott, D., Binsted, G., & Heath, M. (1999). The control of goal-directed limb movements: Correcting errors in the trajectory. *Human Movement Science, 8*, 121-136.

Elliott, D., Carson, R.G., Goodman, D., & Chua, R. (1991). Discrete vs. continuous visual control of manual aiming. *Human Movement Science, 10*, 393-418.

Elliott, D., Chua, R., Pollock, B.J., & Lyons, J. (1995). Optimizing the use of vision in manual aiming: The role of practice. *Quarterly Journal of Experimental Psychology A: Human Experimental Psychology, 48*, 72-83.

Elliott, D., Hansen, S., Mendoza, J., & Tremblay, L. (2004). Learning to optimize speed, accuracy, and energy expenditure: A framework for understanding speed-accuracy relations in goal-directed aiming. *Journal of Motor Behavior, 36*, 339-351.

Elliott, D., Helsen, W.F., & Chua, R. (2001). A century later: Woodworth's two-component model of goal directed aiming. *Psychological Bulletin, 127*, 342-357.

Elliott, D., Lyons, J., & Dyson, K. (1997). Rescaling an acquired discrete aiming movement: Specific or general motor learning? *Human Movement Science, 16*, 81-96.

Engelbrecht, S.E., Berthier, N.E., & O'Sullivan, L.P. (2003). The undershooting bias: Learning to act optimally under uncertainty. *Psychological Science, 14,* 257-261.

Franks, I.M., Sanderson, D.J., & Van Donkelaar, P. (1990). A comparison of directly recorded and derived acceleration data in movement control research. *Human Movement Science, 9,* 573-582

Hansen, S., & Elliott, D. (2009). Three-dimensional manual responses to unexpected target perturbations during rapid aiming. *Journal of Motor Behavior, 41,* 16-29.

Hansen, S., Elliott, D., & Khan, M.A. (2007). Comparing derived and acquired acceleration profiles: Three dimensional optical electric data analysis. *Behavior Research Methods, 39,* 748-754.

Hansen, S., Elliott, D., & Khan, M.A. (2008). Quantifying the variability of three-dimensional aiming movements using ellipsoids. *Motor Control, 12,* 241-251.

Hansen, S., Elliott, D., & Tremblay, L. (2007). Online control of discrete action following visual perturbation *Perception, 36,* 268-287.

Hansen, S., Glazebrook, C., Anson, J.G., Weeks, D.J., & Elliott, D. (2006). The influence of advance information about target location and visual feedback on movement planning and execution. *Canadian Journal of Experimental Psychology, 60,* 200-208.

Hansen, S., Tremblay, L., & Elliott, D. (2005). Part and whole practice: Chunking and online control in the acquisition of a serial motor task. *Research Quarterly for Exercise and Sport, 76,* 60-67.

Heath, M. (2005). Role of limb and target vision in the online control of memory-guided reaches. *Motor Control, 9,* 281-309.

Heath, M., Neely, K., & Binsted, G. (2007). Allocentric visual cues influence online limb adjustments. *Motor Control, 11,* 54-70.

Jagacinski, R.J., Repperger, D.W., Moran, M.S., Ward, S.L., & Glass, D. (1980). Fitts' law and the microstructure of rapid discrete movements. *Journal of Experimental Psychology: Human Perception and Performance, 6,* 309-320.

Keele, S.W. (1968). Movement control in skilled motor performance. *Psychological Bulletin, 70,* 387-403.

Khan, M.A., Chua, R., Elliott, D., Coull, J., & Lyons, J. (2002). Optimal control strategies under different feedback schedules: Kinematic evidence. *Journal of Motor Behavior, 34,* 45-57.

Khan, M.A., & Franks, I.M. (2000). The effect of practice on component submovements is dependent on the availability of visual feedback. *Journal of Motor Behavior, 32,* 227-240.

Khan, M.A., & Franks, I.M. (2003). Online versus offline processing of visual feedback in the production of component submovements. *Journal of Motor Behavior, 35,* 285-295.

Khan, M.A., Franks, I.M., Elliott, D., Lawrence, G.P., Chua, R., Bernier, P., Hansen, S., & Weeks, D.J. (2006). Inferring online and offline processing of visual feedback in target-directed movements from kinematic data. *Neuroscience and Behavioral Reviews, 30,* 1106-1121.

Khan, M.A., Franks, I.M., & Goodman, D. (1998). The effect of practice on the control of rapid aiming movements: Evidence for an interdependence between programming and feedback processing. *Quarterly Journal of Experimental Psychology A: Human Experimental Psychology, 51,* 425-444.

Khan, M.A., Lawrence, G.P., Fourkas, A., Franks, I.M., Elliott, D., & Pembroke, S. (2003). Online versus offline processing of visual feedback in the production of movement distance. *Acta Psychologica, 113,* 83-97

Khan, M.A., Lawrence, G., Franks, I.M., Elliott, D (2003). The utilization of visual feedback in the control of movement direction. Evidence from a video aiming task. *Motor Control, 7,* 290-303.

Langolf, G.D., Chaffin, D.B., & Foulke, J.A. (1976). An investigation of Fitts' law using a wide range of movement amplitudes. *Journal of Motor Behavior, 8,* 113-128.

Lyons, J., Hansen, S., Hurding, S., & Elliott, D. (2006). Optimizing rapid aiming behaviour: movement kinematics depend on the cost of corrective modifications. *Experimental Brain Research , 174,* 95-100.

Meyer, D.E., Abrams, R.A., Kornblum, S., Wright, C.E., & Smith, J.E.K. (1988). Optimality in human motor performance: Ideal control of rapid aimed movements. *Psychological Review, 95,* 340-370.

Oliveira, F.T.P., Elliott, D., & Goodman, D. (2005). The energy minimization bias: Compensating for intrinsic influence of energy minimization mechanisms. *Motor Control, 9,* 101-114.

Pew, R.W. (1966). Acquisition of hierarchical control over the temporal organization of a skill. *Journal of Experimental Psychology, 71*, 764-771.

Pratt, J., & Abrams, R.A. (1996). Practice and component submovements: The role of programming and feedback in rapid aimed limb movements. *Journal of Motor Behavior, 28*, 149-156.

Proteau, L., Marteniuk, R.G., Girouard, Y., & Dugas, C. (1987). On the type of information used to control and learn an aiming movement after moderate and extensive practice. *Human Movement Science, 6*, 181-199.

Rabbitt, P.M.A. (1981). Sequential reactions. In D.H. Holding (Ed.), *Human skill* (pp. 147-170). London: Wiley.

Schmidt, R.A., & McCabe, J.F. (1976). Motor program utilization over extended practice. *Journal of Human Movement Studies, 2*, 239-247.

Schmidt, R.A., Zelaznik, H.N., Hawkins, B., Frank, J.S., & Quinn, J.T. (1979). Motor output variability: A theory for the accuracy of rapid motor acts. *Psychological Review, 86*, 415-451.

Sparrow, W.A., & Newell, K.M. (1998). Metabolic energy expenditure and the regulation of movement economy. *Psychonomic Bulletin & Review, 5*, 173-196.

Trommershauser, J., Gepshtein, S., Maloney, L.T., Landy, M.S., & Banks, M.S. (2005). Optimal compensation for changes in task-relevant movement variability. *Journal of Neuroscience, 25*, 7169-7178.

van Donkelaar, P., & Franks, I.M. (1991). The effects of changing movement velocity and complexity on response preparation: Evidence from latency, kinematic and EMG measure. *Experimental Brain Research, 83*, 618-632.

Walker, N., Philbin, D., Worden, A., & Smelcer, J.B. (1997). A program of parsing mouse movements into component submovements. *Behavior Research Methods, Instruments and Computers, 29*, 456-460.

Welsh, T.N., Higgins, L., & Elliott, D. (2007). Are there age-related differences in learning to optimize speed, accuracy, and energy expenditure? *Human Movement Science, 26*, 892-912.

Woodworth, R.S. (1899). The accuracy of voluntary movement. *Psychological Review, Monograph Supplements, 3*(13), 1-119.

Worringham, C.J. (1991). Variability effects on the internal structure of rapid aiming movements. *Journal of Motor Behavior, 23*, 75-85.

CHAPTER 3

Abrams, R.A., & Chirst, S.E. (2003). Motion onset captures attention. *Psychological Science, 14*, 427-432.

Allport, A. (1987). Selection for action: Some behavioral and neurophysiological considerations of attention and action. In H. Heuer & A.F. Sanders (Eds.), *Perspectives on perception and action* (pp. 395-419). Hillsdale, NJ: Erlbaum.

Bekkering, H., & Neggers, S.F.W. (2002). Visual search modulated by action intentions. *Psychological Science, 13*, 370-374.

Broadbent, D.E. (1958). Perception and communication. New York: Pergamon Press.

Buetti, S., & Kerzel, D. (2009). Conflicts during response selection affect response programming: Reactions towards the source of stimulation. *Journal of Experimental Psychology: Human Perception and Performance, 35*, 816-834.

Cheal, M.L., & Lyon, D.R. (1991). Central and peripheral precuing of forced-choice discrimination. *Quarterly Journal of Experimental Psychology A: Human Experimental Psychology, 43*, 859-880.

Cherry, E.C. (1953). Some experiments on the recognition of speech, with one and with two ears. *Journal of the Acoustical Society of America, 25*, 975-979.

Coles, M.G., Gratton, G., Bashore, T.R., Eriksen, C.W., & Donchin, E. (1985). A psychophysiological investigation of the continuous flow model of human informational processing. *Journal of Experimental Psychology: Human Perception and Performance, 11*, 529-553.

Cressman, E.K., Franks, I.M., Enns, J.T., & Chua, R. (2007). On-line control of pointing is modified by unseen visual shapes. *Consciousness and Cognition, 16*, 265-275.

Eriksen, B.A., & Eriksen, C.W. (1974). Effects of noise letters upon the identification of a target letter in a non-search task. *Perception & Psychophysics, 16*, 143-146.

Fagioli, S., Ferlazzo, F., & Hommel, B. (2007). Controlling attention through action: Observing actions primes action-related stimulus dimensions. *Neuropsychologia, 45,* 3351-3355.

Fagioli, S., Hommel, B., & Schubotz, R.I. (2007). Intentional control of attention: Action planning primes action-related stimulus dimensions. *Psychological Research, 71,* 22-29.

Fischer, M.H., & Adam, J.J. (2001). Distractor effects on pointing: The role of spatial layout. *Experimental Brain Research, 136,* 507-513.

Fisk, J.D., & Goodale, M.A. (1985). The organization of eye and limb movements during unrestricted reaching to targets in contralateral and ipsilateral visual space. *Experimental Brain Research, 60,* 159-178.

Fitts, P.M. (1954). The information capacity of the human motor system in controlling the amplitude of movement. *Journal of Experimental Psychology, 47,* 381-391.

Fitts, P.M., & Peterson, J.R. (1964). Information capacity of discrete motor responses. *Journal of Experimental Psychology, 67,* 103-112.

Folk, C.L., Remington, R.W., & Johnston, J.C. (1992). Involuntary covert orienting is contingent on attentional control settings. *Journal of Experimental Psychology: Human Perception and Performance, 18,* 1030-1044.

Folk, C.L., Remington, R.W., & Wright, J.H. (1994). The structure of attentional control: Contingent attentional capture by apparent motion, abrupt onset, and color. *Journal of Experimental Psychology: Human Perception and Performance, 20,* 317-329.

Georgeopolous, A.P. (1990). Neurophysiology of reaching. In M. Jeannerod (Ed.), *Attention and performance XIII* (pp. 227-263). Hillsdale, NJ: Erlbaum.

Georgeopoulos, A.P. (1995). Current issues in directional motor control. *Trends in Neurosciences, 18,* 506-510.

Gibson, B.S., & Kelsey, E.M. (1998). Stimulus-driven attentional capture is contingent on attentional set for displaywide visual features. *Journal of Experimental Psychology: Human Perception and Performance, 24,* 699-706.

Grosjean, M., Shiffrar, M., & Knoblich, G. (2007). Fitts's law holds in action perception. *Psychological Science, 18,* 95-99.

Higgins, L.A., & Welsh, T.N. (2009). *Attentional capture in selective reaching task: The influence of the to-be-performed action on the attentional set.* Manuscript in preparation.

Howard, L.A., & Tipper, S.P. (1997). Hand deviations away from visual cues: Indirect evidence for inhibition. *Experimental Brain Research, 113,* 144-152.

Johnson, J.D., Hutchinson, K.A., & Neill, W.T. (2001). Attentional capture by irrelevant color singletons. *Journal of Experimental Psychology: Human Perception and Performance, 27,* 841-847.

Jonides, J. (1981). Voluntary versus automatic control over the mind's eye's movement. In J.B. Long & A.D. Baddeley (Eds.), *Attention and performance IX* (pp. 187-203). Hillsdale, NJ: Erlbaum.

Keulen, R.F., Adam, J.J., Fischer, M.H., Kuipers, H., & Jolles, J. (2002). Selective reaching: Evidence for multiple frames of reference. *Journal of Experimental Psychology: Human Perception and Performance, 28,* 515-526.

Keulen, R.F., Adam, J.J., Fischer, M.H., Kuipers, H., & Jolles, J. (2003). Distractor interference in selective reaching: Dissociating distance and grouping effects. *Journal of Motor Behavior, 35,* 119-126.

Keulen, R.F., Adam, J.J., Fischer, M.H., Kuipers, H., & Jolles, J. (2004). Selective reaching: Distracter effects on movement kinematics as a function of target-distracter separation. *Journal of General Psychology, 131,* 345-363.

Khan, M.A., Franks, I.M., Elliott, D., Lawrence, G.P., Chua, R., Bernier, P.M., Hansen, S., & Weeks, D.J. (2006). Inferring online and offline processing of visual feedback in target-directed movements from kinematic data. *Neuroscience and Biobehavioral Reviews, 30,* 1106-1121.

Maljkovic, V., & Nakayama, K. (1994). Priming of pop-out. 1. Role of features. *Memory and Cognition, 22,* 657-672.

McKinstry, C., Dale, R., & Spivey, M.J. (2008). Action dynamics reveal parallel competition in decision making. *Psychological Science, 19,* 22-24.

Meegan, D.V., & Tipper, S.P. (1998). Reaching into cluttered environments: Spatial and temporal influences of distracting objects. *Quarterly Journal of Experimental Psychology A: Human Experimental Psychology, 51,* 225-249.

Meegan, D.V., & Tipper, S.P. (1999). Visual search and target-directed action. *Journal of Experimental Psychology: Human Perception and Performance, 25,* 1347-1362.

Müller, H.J., & Rabbitt, P.M.A. (1989). Reflexive and voluntary orienting of visual-attention: Time course of activation and resistance to interruption. *Journal of Experimental Psychology: Human Perception and Performance, 15,* 315-330.

Posner, M.I., & Cohen, Y. (1984). Components of visual orienting. In H. Bouma & D.G. Bouwhuis (Eds.), *Attention and performance X.* (pp. 531-556). Hillsdale, NJ: Erlbaum.

Posner, M.I., Nissen, M.J., & Ogden, W.C. (1978). Attended and unattended processing modes: The role of set for spatial location. In H. Pick & E. Saltzman (Eds.), *Modes of perceiving and processing information* (pp. 137-157). Hillsdale, NJ: Erlbaum.

Pratt, J., & Arnott, S.R. (2008). Modulating the attentional repulsion effect. *Acta Psychologica, 127,* 137-145.

Pratt, J., & Abrams, R.A. (1994). Action-centred inhibition: Effects of distractors on movement planning and execution. *Human Movement Science, 13,* 245-254.

Pratt, J., & McAuliffe, J. (2001). The effects of onsets and offsets on visual attention. *Psychological Research, 65,* 185-191.

Proffitt, D.R., Stefanucci, J., Banton, T., & Epstein, W. (2003). The role of effort in perceiving distance. *Psychological Science, 14,* 106-112.

Rizzolatti, G., Riggio, L., & Sheliga, B.M. (1994). Space and selective attention. In C. Umilta & M. Moscovitch, *Attention and performance XV* (pp. 231-265). Cambridge, MA: MIT Press.

Rizzolatti, G., Riggio, L., Dascola, J., & Umilta, C. (1987). Reorienting attention across the horizontal and vertical meridians: Evidence in favor of a premotor theory of attention. *Neuropsychologia, 25,* 31-40.

Sailer, U., Eggert, T., Ditterich, J., & Straube, A. (2002). Global effect of a nearby distractor on targeting eye and hand movements. *Journal of Experimental Psychology: Human Perception and Performance, 28,* 1432-1446.

Tipper, S.P. (1985). The negative priming effect: Inhibitory priming by ignored objects. *Quarterly Journal of Experimental Psychology A: Human Experimental Psychology, 37,* 571-590.

Tipper, S.P., Howard, L.A., & Houghton, G. (1999). Behavioral consequences of selection form neural population codes. In S. Monsell & J. Driver (Eds.), *Attention and performance XVIII* (pp. 223-245). Cambridge, MA: MIT Press.

Tipper, S.P., Lortie, C., & Baylis, G.C. (1992). Selective reaching: Evidence for action-centered attention. *Journal of Experimental Psychology: Human Perception and Performance, 18,* 891-905.

Tipper, S.P., Meegan, D.V., & Howard, L.A. (2002). Action-centred negative priming: Evidence for reactive inhibition. *Visual Cognition, 9,* 591-614.

Treisman, A.M., & Gelade, G. (1980). A feature-integration theory of attention. *Cognitive Psychology, 12,* 97-136.

Welsh, T.N., & Elliott, D. (2001). The processing of visual and verbal movement information by adults with and without Down syndrome. *Adapted Physical Activity Quarterly, 18,* 156-167.

Welsh, T.N., & Elliott, D. (2004a). Movement trajectories in the presence of a distracting stimulus: Evidence for a response activation model of selective reaching. *Quarterly Journal of Experimental Psychology A: Human Experimental Psychology, 57,* 1031-1057.

Welsh, T.N., & Elliott, D. (2004b). The effects of response priming and inhibition on movement planning and execution. *Journal of Motor Behavior, 36,* 200-211.

Welsh, T.N., & Elliott, D. (2005). The effects of response priming on the planning and execution of goal-directed movements in the presence of a distracting stimulus. *Acta Psychologica, 119,* 123-142.

Welsh, T.N., Elliott, D., & Weeks, D.J. (1999). Hand deviations toward distractors. Evidence for response competition. *Experimental Brain Research, 127,* 207-212.

Welsh, T.N., & Pratt, J. (2008). Actions modulate attentional capture. *Quarterly Journal of Experimental Psychology, 61*, 968-976.

Welsh, T.N., Ray, M., Weeks, D.J., Dewey, D., & Elliott, D. (2009). Does Joe influence Fred's action? Not if Fred has autism spectrum disorder. *Brain Research, 1248*, 141-148.

Welsh, T.N., Weeks, D.J., Chua, R., & Goodman, D. (2007). Perceptual-motor interaction: Some implications for human-computer interaction. In A. Sears & J.A. Jacko (Eds.), *Human-computer interaction handbook* (2nd ed., pp. 27-41). Hillsdale, NJ: Erlbaum.

Welsh, T.N., & Zbinden, M. (2009). Fitts' Law and action-centred reference frames in selective reaching: The "proximity-to-hand" effect revisited. *Motor Control, 13*, 100-112.

Witt, J.K., Proffitt, D.R., & Epstein, W. (2005). Tool use affects perceived distance but only when you intend to use it. *Journal of Experimental Psychology: Human Perception and Performance, 31*, 880-888.

Woodworth, R.S., (1899). The accuracy of voluntary movement. *Psychological Review, Monograph Supplements, 3*(13), 1-119.

CHAPTER 4

Abraham, W.C., & Bear, M.F. (1996). Metaplasticity: The plasticity of synaptic plasticity. *Trends in Neurosciences, 19*, 126-130.

Anson, J.G., Scott, R.L., & Hyland, B.I. (2007). Neuromotor programming of simultaneous bilateral upper limb movements. *Society for Neuroscience Abstracts.* . http://www.sfn.org/index.cfm?pagename=abstracts_ampublications.

Binsted, G., & Heath, M. (2005). No evidence of a lower visual field specialization for visuomotor control. *Experimental Brain Research, 162*, 89-94.

Binsted, G., Rolheiser, T.M., & Chua, R. (2006). Decay in visuomotor representations during manual aiming. *Journal of Motor Behavior, 38*, 82-87.

Bliss, T.V.P., & Collingridge, G.L. (1993). A synaptic model of memory: Long-term potentiation in the hippocampus. *Nature, 361*(6407), 31-39.

Chieffi, S., Allport, D.A., & Woodin, M. (1999). Hand-centred coding of target location in visuo-spatial working memory. *Neuropsychologia, 37*, 495-502.

Coles, M.G.H. (1997). Neurons and reaction times. *Science, 275*(5297), 142-143.

Compte, A., Constantinidis, C., Tegner, J., Raghavachari, S., Chafee, M.V., Goldman-Rakic, P.S., & Wang, X-J. (2003). Temporally irregular mnemonic persistent activity in prefrontal neurons of monkeys during a delayed response task. *Journal of Neurophysiology, 90*, 3441-3454.

Danckert, J.A., Sharif, N., Haffenden, A.M., Schiff, K.C., & Goodale, M.A. (2002). A temporal analysis of grasping in the Ebbinghaus illusion: Planning versus online control. *Experimental Brain Research, 144*, 275-280.

Darling, W.G., & Rizzo, M. (2001). Developmental lesions of visual cortex influence control of reaching. *Neuropsychologia, 39*, 346-351.

Desmurget, M., Pelisson, D., Rossetti, Y., & Prablanc, C. (1998). From eye to hand: Planning goal-directed movements. *Neuroscience and Biobehavioral Reviews, 22*, 761-788.

Elliott, D., & Calvert, R. (1990). The influence of uncertainty and premovement visual information on manual aiming. *Canadian Journal of Psychology, 44*, 501-511.

Eversheim, U., & Bock, O. (2002). The role of precues in the preparation of motor responses in humans. *Journal of Motor Behavior, 34*, 271-276.

Gail, A., & Andersen, R.A. (2006). Neural dynamics in monkey parietal reach region reflect context-specific sensorimotor transformations. *Journal of Neuroscience, 26*, 9376-9384.

Gazzaniga, M.S., Ivry, R.B., & Mangun, G.R. (2002). *Cognitive neuroscience.* London: Norton.

Georgopoulos, A.P., Ashe, J., Smyrnis, N., & Taira, M. (1992). The motor cortex and the coding of force. *Science, 256*, 1692-1695.

Georgopoulos, A.P., Crutcher, M.D., & Schwartz, A.B. (1989). Cognitive spatial-motor processes. 3. Motor cortical prediction of movement direction during an instructed delay period. *Experimental Brain Research, 75*, 183-194.

Georgopoulos, A. P., Kalaska, J. F., Caminiti, R., & Massey, J.T. (1982). On the relations between the direction of two-dimensional arm movements and cell discharge in primate motor cortex. *Journal of Neuroscience, 2,* 1527-1537.

Ghez, C., Gordon, J., & Ghilardi, M.F. (1995). Impairments of reaching movements in patients without proprioception. 2. Effects of visual information on accuracy. *Journal of Neurophysiology, 73,* 361-372.

Gleick, J. (1999). Faster: The acceleration of just about everything. New York: Pantheon.

Goodale, M.A., & Milner, A.D. (1992). Separate visual pathways for perception and action. *Trends in Neuroscience, 15,* 20-25.

Goodale, M.A., Westwood, D.A., & Milner, A.D. (2003). Two distinct modes of control for object-directed action. *Progress in Brain Research, 144,* 131-144.

Hanes, D.P., & Schall, J.D. (1996). Neural control of voluntary movement initiation. *Science, 274,* 427-430.

Hansen, S., Glazebrook, C.M., Anson, J.G., Weeks, D.J., & Elliott, D. (2006). The influence of advance information about target location and visual feedback on movement planning and execution. *Canadian Journal of Experimental Psychology, 60,* 200-208.

Heath, M. (2005). Role of limb and target vision in the online control of memory-guided reaches. *Motor Control, 9,* 281-311.

Heath, M., & Westwood, D.A. (2003). Can a visual representation support the online control of memory-dependent reaching? Evidence from a variable spatial mapping paradigm. *Motor Control, 7,* 346-361.

Heath, M., Westwood, D.A., & Binsted, G. (2004). The control of memory-guided reaching movements in peripersonal space. *Motor Control, 8,* 76-106.

Hebb, D.O. (1949). The organisation of behaviour: A neuropsychological theory. New York: Wiley.

Heekeren, H.R., Marrett, S., Ruff, D.A., Bandettini, P.A., & Ungerleider, L.G. (2006). Involvement of human left dorsolateral prefrontal cortex in perceptual decision making is independent of response modality. *Proceedings of the National Academy of Sciences of the United States of America, 103,* 10023-10028.

Jaeger, D., Gilman, S., & Aldridge, J.W. (1993). Primate basal ganglia activity in a precued reaching task: Preparation for movement. *Experimental Brain Research, 95,* 51-64.

Jordan, K., Hyland, B.I., Wickens, J.R., & Anson, J.G. (2005). Motor preparation in a memorised delay task. *Experimental Brain Research, 166,* 102-108.

Khan, M.A., Elliot, D., Coull, J., Chua, R., & Lyons, J. (2002). Optimal control strategies under different feedback schedules: Kinematic evidence. *Journal of Motor Behavior, 34,* 45-57.

Krigolson, O., & Heath, M. (2004). Background visual cues and memory-guided reaching. *Human Movement Science, 23,* 861-877.

Labutta, R.J., Miles, R.B., Sanes, J.N., & Hallett, M. (1994). Motor program memory storage in Parkinson's disease patients tested with a delayed response task. *Movement Disorders, 9,* 218-222.

Latash, M. (2007). No, we don't need internal models. *Motor Control, 11*(Suppl.), S10-S11.

Lawrence, G.P., Khan, M.A., Buckolz, E., & Oldham, A.R.H. (2006). The contribution of peripheral and central vision in the control of movement amplitude. *Human Movement Science, 25,* 326-338.

Lemay, M., Bertram, C.P., & Stelmach, G.E. (2004). Pointing to an allocentric and egocentric remembered target. *Motor Control, 8,* 16-32.

Lemay, M., & Stelmach, G.E. (2005). Multiple frames of reference for pointing to a remembered target. *Experimental Brain Research, 164,* 301-310.

Mazzoni, P., Bracewell, R.M., Barash, S., & Andersen, R.A. (1996). Motor intention activity in the macaque's lateral intraparietal area. 1. Dissociation of motor plan from sensory memory. *Journal of Neurophysiology, 76,* 1439-1456.

McIntyre, J., Stratta, F., & Lacquaniti, F. (1998). Short-term memory for reaching to visual targets: Psychophysical evidence for body-centered reference frames. *Journal of Neuroscience, 18,* 8423-8435.

Meegan, D.V., Glazebrook, C.M., Dhillon, V.P., Tremblay, L., Welsh, T.N., & Elliott, D. (2004). The Muller-Lyer illusion affects the planning and control of manual aiming movements. *Experimental Brain Research, 155,* 37-47.

Mohagheghi, A.A., Anson, J.G., Hyland, B.I., Parr-Brownlie, L., & Wickens, J.R. (1998). Foreperiod length, but not memory, affects human reaction time in a precued, delayed response. *Motor Control, 2*, 133-141.

Morasso, P. (2007). Yes, we need internal models. *Motor Control, 11*(Suppl.), S9-S10.

Parr-Brownlie, L., Wickens, J., Anson, J.G., & Hyland, B. (1998). Does having to remember the position of a target improve reaction time? *Motor Control, 2*, 142-147.

Pellizzer, G., Hedges, J.H., & Villaneuva, R.R. (2006). Time-dependent effects of discrete spatial cues on the planning of directed movements. *Experimental Brain Research, 172*, 22-34.

Porter, R. (1987). Introduction. In G. Bock, M. O'Connor, & J. Marsh (Eds.), *Motor areas of the cerebral cortex: Ciba foundation symposium 132* (pp. 1-4). Chichester, UK: Wiley.

Prabhu, G., Lemon, R., & Haggard, P. (2007). On-line control of grasping actions: Object-specific motor facilitation requires sustained visual input. *Journal of Neuroscience, 27*, 12651-12654.

Proteau, L., & Carnahan, H. (2001). What causes specificity of practice in a manual aiming movement: Vision dominance or transformation errors? *Journal of Motor Behavior, 33*, 226-234.

Reynolds, J.N., Hyland, B.I., & Wickens, J.R. (2001). A cellular mechanism of reward-related learning. *Nature, 413*, 67-70.

Sawaguchi, T., & Yamane, I. (1999). Properties of delay-period neuronal activity in the monkey dorsolateral prefrontal cortex during a spatial delayed matching-to-sample task. *Journal of Neurophysiology, 82*, 2070-2080.

Schall, J.D. (2001). Neural basis of deciding, choosing and acting. *Nature Reviews Neuroscience, 2*, 33-42.

Sherrington, C. (1947). *The integrative action of the nervous system* (2nd ed.). New Haven, CT: Yale University Press.

Smyrnis, N., Taira, M., Ashe, J., & Georgopoulos, A.P. (1992). Motor cortical activity in a memorized delay task. *Experimental Brain Research, 92*, 139-151.

Sober, S.J., & Sabes, P.N. (2005). Flexible strategies for sensory integration during motor planning. *Nature Neuroscience, 8*, 490-497.

Sommer, M.A., & Wurtz, R.H. (2001). Frontal eye field sends delay activity related to movement, memory, and vision to the superior colliculus. *Journal of Neurophysiology, 85*, 1673-1685.

Swinnen, S.P. (2002). Intermanual coordination: From behavioural principles to neural-network interactions. *Nature Reviews Neuroscience, 3*, 350-361.

Theleritis, C., Smyrnis, N., Mantas, A., & Evdokimidis, I. (2004). The effects of increasing memory load on the directional accuracy of pointing movements to remembered targets. *Experimental Brain Research, 157*, 518-525.

Trommershäuser, J., Mattis, J., Maloney, L.T., & Landy, M.S. (2006). Limits to human movement planning with delayed and unpredictable onset of needed information. *Experimental Brain Research, 175*, 276-284.

Vaziri, S., Diedrichsen, J., & Shadmehr, R. (2006). Why does the brain predict sensory consequences of oculomotor commands? Optimal integration of the predicted and the actual sensory feedback. *Journal of Neuroscience, 26*, 4188-4197.

Westwood, D.A., Heath, M., & Roy, E.A. (2003). No evidence for accurate visuomotor memory: Systematic and variable error in memory-guided reaching. *Journal of Motor Behavior, 35*, 127-133.

Westwood, D.A., McEachern, T., & Roy, E.A. (2001). Delayed grasping of a Muller-Lyer figure. *Experimental Brain Research, 141*, 166-173.

CHAPTER 5

Adamovich, S.V., Berkinblit, M.B., Fookson, O., & Poizner, H. (1999). Pointing in 3D space to remembered targets. II. Effects of movement speed toward kinesthetically defined targets. *Experimental Brain Research, 125*, 200-210.

Aglioti, S., DeSouza, J.F.X., & Goodale, M.A. (1995). Size-contrast illusions deceive the eye but not the hand. *Current Biology, 5*, 679-685.

Berkinblit, M.B., Fookson, O.I., Smetanin, B., Adamovich, S.V., & Poizner, H. (1995). The interaction of visual and proprioceptive inputs in pointing to actual and remembered targets. *Experimental Brain Research, 107,* 326-330.

Binsted, G., Brownell, K., Vorontsova, Z., Heath, M., & Saucier, D. (2007). Visuomotor system uses target features unavailable to conscious awareness. *Proceedings of the National Academy of Sciences of the United States of America, 104,* 12669-12672.

Bridgeman, B., Lewis, S., Heit, G., & Nagle, M. (1979). Relation between cognitive and motor-oriented systems of visual position perception. *Journal of Experimental Psychology: Human Perception and Performance, 5,* 692-700.

Bridgeman, B., Peery. S., & Anand, S. (1997). Interaction of cognitive and sensorimotor maps of visual space. *Perception and Psychophysics, 59,* 456-469.

Buneo, C.A., Jarvis, M.R., Batista, A.P., & Andersen, R.A. (2002). Direct visuomotor transformations for reaching. *Nature, 416,* 632-636.

Chua, R., & Elliott, D. (1993). Visual regulation of manual aiming. *Human Movement Science, 12,* 365-401.

Coello, Y., Richaud, S., Magne, P., & Rossetti, Y. (2003). Vision for spatial perception and vision for action: A dissociation between the left-right and near-far dimensions. *Neuropsychologia, 41,* 622-633.

Cressman, E.K., Franks, I.M., Enns, J.T., & Chua, R. (2007). On-line control of pointing is modified by unseen visual shapes. *Consciousness and Cognition, 16,* 265-275.

Cui, R.Q., & Deecke, L. (1999). High resolution DC-EEG of the Bereitschaftspotential preceding anatomically congruent versus spatially congruent bimanual finger movements. *Brain Topography, 12,* 117-127.

Danckert, J., & Rossetti, Y. (2005). Blindsight in action: What can the different sub-types of blindsight tell us about the control of visually guided actions? *Neuroscience and Biobehavioral Review, 29,* 1035-1046.

Di Lollo, V., Enns, J.T., & Rensink, R.A. (2000). Competition for consciousness among visual events: The psychophysics of reentrant visual processes. *Journal of Experimental Psychology: General, 129,* 481-507.

Ehresman, C., Saucier, D., Heath, M., & Binsted, G. (2008). Online corrections can produce illusory bias during closed-loop pointing. *Experimental Brain Research, 188,* 371-378..

Elliott, D. (1988). The influence of visual target and limb information on manual aiming. *Canadian Journal of Psychology, 42,* 57-68.

Elliott, D. (1990). Intermittent visual pickup and goal-directed movement: A review. *Human Movement Science, 9,* 531-548.

Elliott, D., & Allard, F. (1985). The utilization of visual feedback information during rapid pointing movements. *Quarterly Journal of Experimental Psychology, 37,* 407-425.

Elliott, D., Binsted, G., & Heath, M. (1999). The control of goal-directed limb movements: Correcting errors in the trajectory. *Human Movement Science, 18,* 121-136.

Elliott, D., & Calvert, R. (1990). The influence of uncertainty and premovement visual information on manual aiming. *Canadian Journal of Psychology, 44,* 501-511.

Elliott, D., Calvert, R., Jaeger, M., & Jones, R. (1990). A visual representation and the control of manual aiming movements. *Journal of Motor Behavior, 22,* 327-346.

Elliott, D., Helsen, W.F., & Chua, R. (2001). A century later: Woodworth's (1899) two-component model of goal-directed aiming. *Psychological Bulletin, 127,* 342-357.

Elliott, D., & Lee, T.D., (1995). The role of target information on manual-aiming bias. *Psychological Research, 58,* 2-9.

Elliott, D., & Madalena, J. (1987). The influence of premovement visual information on manual aiming. *Quarterly Journal of Experimental Psychology, 39,* 541-559.

Enns, J.T., & Di Lollo, V. (2000). What's new in visual masking? *Trends in Cognitive Science, 4,* 345-352.

Felleman, D.J., & Van Essen, D.C. (1991). Distributed hierarchical processing in the primate cerebral cortex. *Cerebral Cortex, 1,* 1-47.

Fitts, P.M. (1954). The information capacity of the human motor system in controlling the amplitude of movement. *Journal of Experimental Psychology, 47,* 381-391.

Flanders, M., Helms Tillery, S.I., & Soechting, J.F. (1992). Early stages in a sensorimotor transformation. *Behavioral and Brain Sciences, 15,* 309-362.

Gerloff, C., Uenishi, N., & Hallett, M. (1998). Cortical activation during fast repetitive finger movements in humans: Dipole sources of steady-state movement-related cortical potentials. *Journal of Clinical Neurophysiology, 15,* 502-512.

Glover, S. (2004). Separate visual representations in the planning and control of action. *Behavioral and Brian Sciences, 27,* 3-78.

Goodale, M.A., Jakobson, L.S., & Keillor, J.M. (1994). Differences in the visual control of pantomimed and natural grasping movements. *Neuropsychologia, 32,* 1159-1178.

Goodale, M.A., & Milner, A.D. (1992). Separate visual pathways for perception and action. *Trends in Neurosciences, 15,* 20-25.

Goodale, M.A., Pelisson, D., & Prablanc. C. (1986). Large adjustments in visually guided reaching do not depend on vision of the hand or perception of target displacement. *Nature, 320,* 748-750.

Haffenden, A.M., & Goodale, M.A. (1998). The effect of pictorial illusion on prehension and perception. *Journal of Cognitive Neuroscience, 10,* 122-136.

Heath, M. (2005). Role of limb and target vision in the online control of memory-guided reaches. *Motor Control, 9,* 281-311.

Heath, M., & Binsted, G. (2007). Visuomotor memory for target location in near and far reaching space. *Journal of Motor Behavior, 39,* 169-177.

Heath, M., Maraj, A., Goldbolt, B., & Binsted, G. (2008). Action without awareness: reaching to an object you do not remember seeing. *Public Library of Science, 3,* e3539.

Heath, M., Neely, K.A., & Binsted, G. (2007). Allocentric visual cues influence on-line limb adjustments. *Motor Control, 11,* 54-70.

Heath, M., Neely, N., Yakimishyn, J., & Binsted, G. (2008). Visuomotor memory is independent of conscious awareness of target features. *Experimental Brain Research, 188,* 517-527.

Heath, M., & Rival, C. (2005). Role of the visuomotor system in online attenuation of a premovement illusory bias in grip aperture. *Brain and Cognition, 57,* 111-114.

Heath, M., Rival, C., & Binsted, G. (2004). Can the motor system resolve a premovement bias in grip aperture? Online analysis of grasping the Müller-Lyer illusion. *Experimental Brain Research, 158,* 378-384.

Heath, M., Rival, C., & Neely, K. (2006). Visual feedback schedules influence visuomotor resistance to the Müller-Lyer figures. *Experimental Brain Research, 168,* 348-356.

Heath, M., Rival, C., Neely, K., & Krigolson, O. (2006). Müller-Lyer illusions influence the online reorganization of visually guided grasping movements. *Experimental Brain Research, 169,* 473-481.

Heath, M., Rival, C., Westwood, D.A, & Neely, K. (2005). Time course analysis of closed- and open-loop grasping of the Müller-Lyer illusion. *Journal of Motor Behavior, 37,* 179-185.

Heath, M., & Westwood, D.A. (2003). Can a visual representation support the online control of memory-dependent reaching? Evidence from a variable spatial mapping paradigm. *Motor Control, 7,* 346-361.

Heath, M., Westwood, D.A., & Binsted, G. (2004). The control of memory-guided reaching movements in peripersonal space. *Motor Control, 8,* 76-106.

Henriques, D.Y., Klier, E.M., Smith, M.A., Lowy, D., & Crawford, J.D. (1998). Gaze-centered remapping of remembered visual space in an open-loop pointing task. *Journal of Neuroscience, 18,* 1583-1594.

Henry, F.M., & Rogers, D.E. (1960). Increased response latency for complicated movements and a "memory drum" theory of neuromotor reaction. *Research Quarterly for Exercise and Sport, 31,* 448-458.

Himmelbach, M., & Karnath, H.O. (2005). Dorsal and ventral stream interaction: Contributions from optic ataxia. *Journal of Cognitive Neuroscience, 17,* 632-40.

Hu, Y., Eagleson, R., & Goodale, M.A. (1999). The effects of delay on the kinematics of grasping. *Experimental Brain Research, 126,* 109-116.

Hu, Y., & Goodale, M.A. (2000). Grasping after a delay shifts size-scaling from absolute to relative metrics. *Journal of Cognitive Neuroscience, 12,* 856-868.

Jakobson, L.S., & Goodale, M.A. (1991). Factors affecting higher-order movement planning: A kinematic analysis of human prehension. *Experimental Brain Research, 86,* 199-208.

James, T.W., Culham, J., Humphrey, G.K., Milner, A.D., & Goodale, M.A. (2003). Ventral occipital lesions impair object recognition but not object-directed grasping: An fMRI study. *Brain, 126,* 2463-2475.

Keele, S.W., & Posner, M.I. (1968). Processing of visual feedback in rapid movements. *Journal of Experimental Psychology, 77,* 155-158.

Khan, M.A., Elliott, D., Coull, J., Chua, R., & Lyons, J. (2002). Optimal control strategies under different feedback schedules: Kinematic evidence. *Journal of Motor Behavior, 34,* 45-57.

Krigolson, O., Clark, N., Heath, M., & Binsted, G. (2007). The proximity of visual landmarks impacts reaching performance. *Spatial Vision, 20,* 317-336.

Krigolson, O., & Heath, M. (2004). Background visual cues and memory-guided reaching. *Human Movement Science, 23,* 861-877.

Krigolson, O., Heath, M., & Holroyd, C. *Reduced cortical motor potentials reflect the contraction of remembered visual space.* Manuscript submitted for publication.

Lemay, M., & Proteau, L. (2001). A distance effect in a manual aiming task to remembered targets: A test of three hypotheses. *Experimental Brain Research, 140,* 357-368.

McIntyre, J., Stratta, F., & Lacquaniti, F. (1997). Viewer-centered frame of reference for pointing to memorized targets in three-dimensional space. *Journal of Neurophysiology, 78,* 1601-1618.

Merigan, W.H., & Maunsell, J.H. (1993). How parallel are the primate visual pathways? *Annual Review of Neuroscience, 16,* 369-402.

Messier, J., & Kalaska, J.F. (1997). Differential effect of task conditions on errors of direction and extent of reaching movements. *Experimental Brain Research, 115,* 469-478.

Milner, A.D., Dijkerman, H.C., McIntosh, R.D., Rossetti, Y., & Pisella, L. (2003). Delayed reaching and grasping in patients with optic ataxia. *Progress in Brain Research, 142,* 225-242.

Milner, A.D., Paulignan, Y., Dijkerman, H.C., Michel, F., & Jeannerod, M. (1999). A paradoxical improvement of misreaching in optic ataxia: New evidence for two separate neural systems for visual localization. *Proceedings: Biological Science, 7,* 2225-2229.

Neely, K.A., Binsted, G., & Heath, M. (2008). Allocentric and egocentric visual cues influence the specification of movement distance and direction. *Journal of Motor Behavior, 40,* 203-213.

Neely, K.A, Tessmer, A., Binsted, G., & Heath, M. (2008). Goal-directed reaching: Movement strategies influence the weighting of allocentric and egocentric visual cues. *Experimental Brain Research, 186,* 375-384.

Pisella, L., Grea, H., Tilikete, C., Vighetto, A., Desmurget, M., Rode, G., Boisson, D., & Rossetti, Y. (2000). An "automatic pilot" for the hand in human posterior parietal cortex: Toward reinterpreting optic ataxia. *Nature Neuroscience, 3,* 729-736.

Rice, N.J., Cross, E.S., Tunik, E., Grafton, S.T., & Culham, J.C. *Ventral and dorsal stream contributions to immediate and delayed grasping.* Manuscript submitted for publication.

Rice, N.J., McIntosh, R.D., Schindler, I., Mon-Williams, M., Démonet, J.F., & Milner, A.D. (2006). Intact automatic avoidance of obstacles in patients with visual form agnosia. *Experimental Brain Research, 174,* 176-188.

Schindler, I., Rice, N.J., McIntosh, R.D., Rossetti, Y., Vighetto, A., & Milner, A.D. (2004). Automatic avoidance of obstacles is a dorsal stream function: Evidence from optic ataxia. *Nature Neuroscience, 7,* 779-784.

Shibasaki, H., Barrett, G., Halliday, E., & Halliday, A.M. (1980). Cortical potentials following voluntary and passive finger movements. *Electroencephalography and Clinical Neurophysiology, 50,* 201-213.

Shibasaki, H., & Hallett, M. (2006). What is the Bereitschaftspotential? *Clinical Neurophysiology, 117,* 2341-2356.

Singhal, A., Kaufman, L., Valyear, K., & Culham, J.C. (2006). fMRI reactivation of the human lateral occipital complex during delayed actions to remembered targets. *Visual Cognition, 14,* 122-125.

Thomson, J.A. (1983). Is continuous visual monitoring necessary in visually guided locomotion? *Journal of Experimental Psychology: Human Perception and Performance, 9,* 427-443.

Ungerleider, L.G., Courtney, S.M., & Haxby, J.V. (1998). A neural system for human visual working memory. *Proceedings of the National Academy of Sciences of the United States of America, 3,* 883-890.

Weiskrantz, L. (2008). Is blindsight just degraded normal vision? *Experimental Brain Research, 192,* 413-416.

Weiskrantz, L., Warrington, E.K., Sanders, M.D., & Marshall, J. (1974). Visual capacity in the hemianopic field following a restricted occipital ablation. *Brain, 97,* 709-728.

Westwood, D.A., & Goodale, M.A. (2003). Perceptual illusion and the real-time control of action. *Spatial Vision, 16,* 243-254.

Westwood, D.A., Heath, M., & Roy, E.A. (2000). The effect of a pictorial illusion on closed-loop and open-loop prehension. *Experimental Brain Research, 134,* 456-463.

Westwood, D.A., Heath, M., & Roy, E.A. (2001). The accuracy of reaching movements in brief delay conditions. *Canadian Journal of Experimental Psychology, 55,* 304-310.

Westwood, D.A., Heath, M., & Roy, E.A. (2003). No evidence for accurate visuomotor memory: Systematic and variable error in memory-guided reaching. *Journal of Motor Behavior, 35,* 127-133.

Wheaton, L.A., Yakota, S., & Hallett, M. (2005). Posterior parietal negativity preceding self-paced praxis movements. *Experimental Brain Research, 163,* 535-539.

Woodworth, R.S. (1899). The accuracy of voluntary movement. *Psychological Review, Monograph Supplements, 3*(13), 1-119.

Yazawa, S., Ikeda, A., Kunieda, T., Ohara, S., Mima, T., Nagamine, T., Taki, W., Kimura, J., Hori, T., & Shibasaki, H. (2000). Human presupplementary motor area is active before voluntary movement: Subdural recording of Bereitschaftspotential from medial frontal cortex. *Experimental Brain Research, 131,* 165-177.

Zelaznik, H.Z., Hawkins, B., & Kisselburgh, L. (1983). Rapid visual feedback processing in single-aiming movements. *Journal of Motor Behavior, 15,* 217-236.

CHAPTER 6

Adam, J.J., Helsen, W.F., Elliott, D., & Buekers, M.J. (2001). The one-target advantage in the control of rapid sequential aiming movements: The effect of practice. *Journal of Human Movement Studies, 41,* 301-313.

Adam, J.J., Nieuwenstein, J.H., Huys, R., Paas, F.G.W.C., Kingma, H., Willems, P., & Werry, M. (2000). Control of rapid aimed hand movements: The one-target advantage. *Journal of Experimental Psychology: Human Perception and Performance, 26,* 295-312.

Adam, J.J., & Paas, F.G.W. C. (1996). Dwell time in reciprocal aiming tasks. *Human Movement Science, 15,* 1-24.

Adam, J.J., Paas, F.G.W.C., Eyssen, I.C.J.M., Slingerland, H., Bekkering, H., & Drost, M.R. (1995). The control of two element, reciprocal aiming movements: Evidence for chunking. *Human Movement Science, 14,* 1-11.

Adam, J.J., van der Bruggen, D.P.W., & Bekkering, H. (1993). The control of discrete and reciprocal target aiming responses: Evidence for the exploitation of mechanics. *Human Movement Science, 12,* 353-364.

Cameron, B.D., Franks, I.M., Enns, J.T., & Chua, R. (2007). Dual-target interference for the automatic pilot in the dorsal stream. *Experimental Brain Research, 181,* 297-305.

Canic, M., & Franks, I.M. (1989). Response preparation and latency patterns of tapping movements. *Human Movement Science, 8,* 123-139.

Chamberlin, C.J., & Magill, R.A. (1989). Preparation and control of rapid multisegmented responses in simple and choice environments. *Research Quarterly for Exercise and Sport, 60,* 256-267.

Fischman, M.G. (1984). Programming time as a function of number of parts and changes in movement direction. *Journal of Motor Behavior, 16,* 405-423.

Fischman, M.G., & Reeve, T.G. (1992). Slower movement times may not necessarily imply on-line programming. *Journal of Human Movement Studies, 22,* 131-144.

Glencross, D.J. (1980). Response planning and the organisation of speed movements. In R.S. Nickerson (Ed.), *Attention and performance VIII* (pp. 107-125). Hillsdale, NJ: Erlbaum.

Guiard Y (1993). On Fitts's and Hooke's laws: Simple harmonic movement in upper-limb cyclical aiming. Acta Psychologica 82: 139-159

Helsen, W.F., Adam, J.J., Elliott, D., & Buekers, M.J. (2001). The one-target advantage: A test of the movement integration hypothesis. *Human Movement Science, 20,* 643-674.

Henry, F.M. (1980). Use of simple reaction time in motor programming studies: A reply to Klapp, Wyatt and Lingo. *Journal of Motor Behavior, 12,* 163-168.

Henry, F.M., & Rogers, D.E. (1960). Increased response latency for complicated movements and a "memory drum" theory of neuromotor reaction. *Research Quarterly, 31,* 448-458.

Ketelaars, M.A.C., Garry, M.I., & Franks, I.M. (1997). On-line programming of simple movement sequences. *Human Movement Science, 16,* 461-483.

Ketelaars, M.A.C., Khan, M.A., & Franks, I.M. (1999). Dual-task interference as an indicator of online programming in simple movement sequences. *Journal of Experimental Psychology: Human Perception and Performance, 25,* 1302-1315.

Khan, M.A., Lawrence, G.P., Buckolz, E., & Franks, I.M. (2006). Programming strategies for rapid aiming movements under simple and choice reaction time conditions. *Quarterly Journal of Experimental Psychology, 59,* 524-542.

Khan, M.A., Mourton, S., Buckolz, E., & Franks, I.M. (2007). The influence of advance information on the response complexity effect in manual aiming movements. *Acta Psychologica, 127,* 154-162.

Khan, M.A., Tremblay, L., Cheng, D.T., Luis, M., & Mourton, S.J. (2008). The preparation and control of reversal movements as a single unit of action. *Experimental Brain Research, 187,* 33-40.

Klapp, S.T. (1995). Motor response programming during simple and choice reaction time: The role of practice. *Journal of Experimental Psychology: Human Perception and Performance, 21,* 1015-1027.

Klapp, S.T. (1996). Reaction time analysis of central motor control. In H.N. Zelaznik (Ed.), *Advances in motor learning and control* (pp. 13-35). Champaign, IL: Human Kinetics.

Klapp, S.T. (2003). Reaction time analysis of two types of motor preparation for speech articulation: Action as a sequence of chunks. *Journal of Motor Behavior, 35,* 135-150.

Klapp, S.T., Abbott, J., Coffman, K., Snider, R., & Young, F. (1979). Simple and choice reaction time methods in the study of motor programming. *Journal of Motor Behavior, 11,* 91-101.

Klapp, S.T., & Erwin, C.I. (1976). Relation between programming time and the duration of the response being programmed. *Journal of Experimental Psychology: Human Perception and Performance, 2,* 591-598.

Klapp, S.T., Wyatt, E.P., & Lingo, W.M. (1974). Response programming in simple and choice reactions. *Journal of Motor Behavior, 6,* 263-271.

Lajoie, J.M., & Franks, I.M. (1997). The control of rapid aiming movements: Variations in response accuracy and complexity. *Acta Psychologica, 97,* 289-305.

Lavrysen, A., Helsen, W.F., Elliott, D., & Adam, J.J. (2002). The one-target advantage: Advance preparation or on-line processing? *Motor Control, 6,* 230-245.

Lavrysen, A., Helsen, W.F., Tremblay, L., Elliott, D., Adam, J.J., Feys, P., & Beukers, M. (2003). The control of sequential aiming movements: The influence of practice and manual asymmetries on the one-target advantage. *Cortex, 39,* 307-325.

McGarry, T., & Franks, I.M. (1997). A horse race between independent processes: Evidence for a phantom point of no return in the preparation of a speeded motor response. *Journal of Experimental Psychology: Human Perception and Performance, 23,* 1533-1542.

McGarry, T., Chua, R., & Franks, I.M. (2003). Stopping and starting an unfolding action at various times. *Quarterly Journal of Experimental Psychology A: Human Experimental Psychology, 56,* 601-620.

Paulignan, Y., Mackenzie, C.L., Marteniuk, R.G., & Jeannerod, M. (1990). The coupling of arm and finger movements during prehension. *Experimental Brain Research, 79,* 431-435.

Rand, M.K., Alberts, J.L., Stelmach, G.E., & Bloedel, J.R., (1997). The influence of segment difficulty on movements with two stroke sequence. *Experimental Brain Research, 115,* 137-146.

Rand, M.K., & Stelmach, G.E. (2000). Segment interdependency and difficulty in two-stroke sequences. *Experimental Brain Research, 134,* 228-236.

Ricker, K.L., Elliott, D., Lyons, J., Gauldie, D., Chua, R., & Byblow, W. (1999). The utilization of visual information in the control of rapid sequential aiming movements. *Acta Psychologica, 103,* 103-123.

Savelberg, H.H.C.M., Adam, J.J., Verhaegh, R.H.J., & Helsen, W.F. (2002). Electromyographic pattern in fast goal-directed arm movements. *Journal of Human Movement Studies, 43,* 121-133.

Schmidt, R.A., Zelaznik, H.N., Hawkins, B., Frank, J.S., & Quinn, J.T. (1979). Motor output variability: A theory for the accuracy of rapid motor acts. *Psychological Review, 86,* 415-451.

Sidaway, B. (1991). Motor programming as a function of constraints of movement initiation. *Journal of Motor Behavior, 23,* 120-130.

Sidaway, B., Sekiya, H., & Fairweather, M. (1995). Movement variability as a function of accuracy demand in programmed serial aiming aiming responses. *Journal of Motor Behavior, 27,* 67-76.

Smiley-Oyen, A.L., & Worringham, C.J. (1996). Distribution of programming in a rapid aimed sequential movement. *Quarterly Journal of Experimental Psychology A: Human Experimental Psychology, 49,* 379-397.

Sternberg, S., Monsell, S., Knoll, R.R., & Wright, C.E. (1978). The latency and duration of rapid movement sequences: Comparisons of speech and typewriting. In G.E. Stelmach (Ed.), *Information processing in motor control and learning* (pp. 117-152). New York: Academic Press.

Van Donkelaar, P., & Franks, I.M. (1991). The effects of changing movement velocity and complexity on response preparation: Evidence from latency, kinematic and EMG measures. *Experimental Brain Research, 83,* 618-632.

Vindras, P., & Viviani, P. (2005). Planning short pointing sequences. *Experimental Brain Research, 160,* 141-153.

CHAPTER 7

Aglioti, S., DeSouza, J.F.X., & Goodale, M.A. (1995). Size-contrast illusions deceive the eye but not the hand. *Current Biology, 5,* 679-685.

Binsted, G., & Elliott, D. (1999). Ocular perturbations and retinal/extraretinal information: The coordination of saccadic and manual movements. *Experimental Brain Research, 127,* 193-206.

Carlton, L.G. (1981a). Processing visual feedback information for movement control. *Journal of Experimental Psychology: Human Perception and Performance, 7,* 1019-1030.

Carlton, L.G. (1981b). Visual information: The control of aiming movements. *Quarterly Journal of Experimental Psychology, 33,* 87-93.

Chua, R., & Elliott, D. (1993). Visual regulation of manual aiming. *Human Movement Science, 12,* 365-401.

Coren, S. (1986). An efferent component in the visual perception of direction and extent. *Psychological Review, 93,* 391-410.

Crossman, E.R.F.W., & Goodeve, P.J. (1983). Feedback control of hand movement and Fitts' law. *Quarterly Journal of Experimental Psychology A: Human Experimental Psychology, 37,* 251-278. (Original work published 1963)

Darling, W.G., & Cooke, J.D. (1987). Changes in the variability of movement trajectories with practice. *Journal of Motor Behavior, 19,* 291-309.

Desmurget, M., Epstein, C.M., Turner, R.S., Prablanc, C., Alexander, G.E., & Grafton, S.T. (1999). Role of the posterior parietal cortex in updating reaching movements to a visual target. *Nature Neuroscience, 2,* 563-567.

Desmurget, M., Turner, R.S., Pranblanc, C., Russo, G.S., Alexander, G.E., & Grafton, S.T. (2005). Updating target location at the end of an orienting saccade affects the characteristics of simple point to point movements. *Journal of Experimental Psychology: Human Perception and Performance, 31*, 1510-1536.

Elliott, D. (1988). The influence of visual target and limb information on manual aiming. *Canadian Journal of Psychology, 42*, 57-68.

Elliott, D., & Allard, F. (1985). The utilization of visual feedback information during rapid pointing movements. *Quarterly Journal of Experimental Psychology, 37*, 407-425.

Elliott, D., Binsted, G., & Heath, M. (1999). The control of goal directed aiming movements: Correcting errors in the trajectory. *Human Movement Science, 18*, 121-136.

Elliott, D., & Calvert, R. (1990). The influence of uncertainty and pre-movement visual information on manual aiming. *Canadian Journal of Psychology, 44*, 501-511.

Elliott, D., Calvert, R., Jaeger, M., & Jones, R. (1990). A visual representation and the control of manual aiming movements. *Journal of Motor Behavior, 22*, 327-346.

Elliott, D., Carson, R.G., Goodman, D., & Chua, R. (1991). Discrete versus continuous visual control of manual aiming. *Human Movement Science, 10*, 393-418.

Elliott, D., Chua, R., Pollock, B.J., & Lyons, J. (1995). Optimizing the use of vision in manual aiming: The role of practice. *Quarterly Journal of Experimental Psychology, 48*, 72-83.

Elliott, D., Hansen, S., Mendoza, J., & Tremblay, L. (2004). Learning to optimize speed, accuracy, and energy expenditure: A framework for understanding speed-accuracy relations in goal-directed aiming. *Journal of Motor Behavior, 36*, 339-351.

Elliott, D., Helsen, W.F., & Chua, R. (2001). A century later: Woodworth's (1899) two-component model of goal directed aiming. *Psychological Bulletin, 3*, 342-357.

Elliott, D., & Jaeger, M. (1988). Practice and the visual control of manual aiming movements. *Journal of Human Movement Studies, 14*, 279-291.

Elliott, D., & Lee, T.D. (1995). The role of target information on manual-aiming bias. *Psychological Research, 58*, 2-9.

Elliott, D., Lyons, J., Chua, R., Goodman, D., & Carson, R.G. (1995). The influence of target perturbation on manual asymmetries in right-handers. *Cortex, 31*, 685-697.

Elliott, D., Lyons, J., & Dyson, K. (1997). Rescaling an acquired aiming movement: Specific or general motor learning? *Human Movement Science, 16*, 81-96.

Elliott, D., & Madalena, J. (1987). The influence of pre-movement visual information on manual aiming. *Quarterly Journal of Experimental Psychology, 39*, 541-559.

Fernandez, L., Warren, W.H., & Bootsma, R.J. (2006). Kinematic adaptation to sudden changes in visual task constraints during reciprocal aiming. *Human Movement Science, 25*, 695-717.

Fitts, P.M. (1954). The information capacity of the human motor system in controlling the amplitude of movement. *Journal of Experimental Psychology, 47*, 381-391.

Fitts, P.M., & Peterson, J.R. (1964). Information capacity of discrete motor responses. *Journal of Experimental Psychology, 67*, 103-112.

Franz, V.H., Gegenfurtner, K.R., Bülthoff, H.H., & Fahle, M. (2000). Grasping visual illusions: No evidence for a dissociation between perception and action. *Psychological Science, 11*, 20-25.

Gibson, J.J. (1977). The theory of affordances. In R. Shaw & J. Bradsford (Eds.), *Perceiving, acting, and knowing* (pp. 67-82). Hillsdale, NJ: Erlbaum.

Glover, S.R., & Dixon, P. (2002). Dynamic effects of the Ebbinghaus illusion in grasping: Support for a planning/control model of action. *Perception & Psychophysics, 64*, 266-278.

Grierson, L.E.M., & Elliott, D. (2008). Kinematic analysis of goal-directed aims made against early and late perturbations: An investigation of the relative influence of two online control processes. *Human Movement Science, 27*, 839-856.

Grierson, L.E.M., & Elliott, D. (2009). Goal-directed aiming and the relative contribution of two online control processes. *American Journal of Psychology, 122*, 309-324.

Haffenden, A.M., & Goodale, M.A. (1998). The effect of pictorial illusion on prehension and perception. *Journal of Cognitive Neuroscience, 10*, 122-136.

Handlovsky, I., Hansen, S., Lee, T.D., & Elliott, D. (2004). The Ebbinghaus illusion affects on-line movement control. *Neuroscience Letters, 366,* 308-311.

Hansen, S., Cullen, J.D., & Elliott, D. (2005). Self-selected visual information during discrete manual aiming. *Journal of Motor Behavior, 37,* 343-347.

Hansen, S., & Elliott, D. (2009). Three-dimensional manual responses to unexpected target perturbations during rapid aiming. *Journal of Motor Behavior, 41,* 16-29.

Hansen, S., Elliott, D., & Khan, M.A. (2008). Quantifying the variability of three-dimensional aiming movements using ellipsoids. *Motor Control, 12,* 241-251.

Hansen, S., Elliott, D., & Tremblay, L. (2007). Gender differences in discrete action following visual perturbation. *Perception, 36,* 268-287.

Hansen, S., Glazebrook, C.M., Anson, J.G., Weeks, D.J., & Elliott, D. (2006). The influence of advance information about target knowledge and visual feedback on movement planning and execution. *Canadian Journal of Experimental Psychology, 60,* 200-208.

Hansen, S., Tremblay, L., & Elliott, D. (2008). Real time manipulation of visual displacement during manual aiming. *Human Movement Science, 27,* 1-11.

Hay, L. (1979). Spatial-temporal analysis of movements in children: Motor programs versus feedback in the development of reaching. *Journal of Motor Behavior, 11,* 189-200.

Heath, M., Hodges, N.J., Chua, R., & Elliott, D. (1998). On-line control of rapid aiming movements: Unexpected target perturbations and movement kinematics. *Canadian Journal of Experimental Psychology, 52,* 163-173.

Heath, M., Westwood, D.A., & Binsted, G. (2004). The control of memory-guided reaching movements in peripersonal space. *Motor Control, 8,* 76-106.

Jüngling, S., Bock, O., & Girgenrath, M. (2002). Speed-accuracy trade-off of grasping movements during microgravity. *Aviation, Space, and Environmental Medicine, 73,* 430-435.

Keele, S.W., & Posner, M.I. (1968). Processing of visual feedback in rapid movements. *Journal of Experimental Psychology, 77,* 155-158.

Ketelaars, M.A.C., Khan, M.A., & Franks, I.M. (1999). Dual-task interference as an indicator of on-line programming in simple movement sequences. *Journal of Experimental Psychology: Human Perception and Performance, 25,* 1302-1315.

Kerr, R. (1978). Diving, adaptation, and Fitts law. *Journal of Motor Behavior, 10,* 255-260.

Khan, M.A., Elliott, D., Coull, J., Chua, R., & Lyons, J. (2002). Optimal control strategies under different feedback schedules: Kinematic evidence. *Journal of Motor Behavior, 34,* 45-57.

Khan, M.A., & Franks, I.M. (2000). The effect of practice on component sub-movements is dependent on visual feedback. *Journal of Motor Behavior, 32,* 227-240.

Khan, M.A., & Franks, I.M. (2003). Online versus offline processing of visual feedback in the production of component sub movements. *Journal of Motor Behavior, 35,* 285-295.

Khan, M.A., Franks, I.M., Elliott, D., Lawrence, G.P., Chua, R., Bernier, P.-M., Hansen, S., & Weeks, D.J. (2006). Inferring online and offline processing of visual feedback in target directed movements from kinematic data. *Neuroscience and Biobehavioral Reviews, 30,* 1106-1121.

Khan, M.A., Franks, I.M., & Goodman, D. (1998). The effect of practice on the control of rapid aiming movements: Evidence for an interdependency between programming and feedback processing. *Quarterly Journal of Experimental Psychology, 51,* 425-444.

Langolf, G.D., Chaffin, D.B., & Foulke, J.A. (1976). An investigation of Fitts' law using a wide range of movement amplitudes. *Journal of Motor Behavior, 8,* 113-128.

Lhuisset, L., & Proteau, L. (2002). Developmental aspects of the control of manual aiming movements in aligned and non-aligned visual displays. *Experimental Brian Research, 146,* 293-306.

MacKenzie, C.L., Marteniuk, R.G., Dugas, C., Liske, D., & Eickmeier, B. (1987). Three dimensional movement trajectory in a Fitts' task: Implications for control. *Quarterly Journal of Experimental Psychology, 39,* 629-647.

Maruff, P., Wilson, P.H., De Fazio, J., Cerritelli, B., Hedt, A., & Currie, J. (1999). Asymmetries between dominant and non-dominant hands in real and imagined motor task performance. *Neuropsychologia, 37,* 379-384.

Mendoza, J.E., Elliott, D., Meegan, D.V., Lyons, J., & Welsh, T.N. (2006). The effect of the Müller-Lyer illusion on the planning and control of manual aiming movements. *Journal of Experimental Psychology: Human Perception and Performance, 32,* 413-422.

Mendoza, J., Hansen, S., Glazebrook, C.M., Keetch, K.M., & Elliott, D. (2005). Visual illusions affect both movement planning and on-line control: A multiple cue position. *Human Movement Science, 24,* 760-773.

Messier, J., & Kalaska, J.F. (1999). Comparison of variability of initial kinematics and endpoints of reaching movements. *Experimental Brain Research, 125,* 139-152.

Meyer, D.E., Abrams, R.A., Kornblum, S., Wright, C.E., & Smith, J.E.K. (1988). Optimality in human motor performance: Ideal control of rapid aimed movements. *Psychological Review, 95,* 340-370.

Milner, A.D., & Goodale, M.A. (1995). *The visual brain in action.* Oxford, UK: Oxford University Press.

Paulignan, Y., MacKenzie, C., Marteniuk, R., & Jeannerod, M. (1991). Selective perturbation of visual input during prehension movements. *Experimental Brain Research, 83,* 502-512.

Pélisson, D., Prablanc, C., Goodale, M.A., & Jeannerod, M. (1986). Visual control of reaching movements without vision of the limb: II. Evidence of fast unconscious processes correcting the trajectory of the hand to the final position of a double-step stimulus. *Experimental Brain Research, 62,* 303-313.

Plamondon, R. (1995). A kinematic history of rapid human movements: Part I. Movement representation and generation. *Biological Cybernetics, 72,* 295-307.

Prablanc, C., Echallier, J.F., Komilis, E., & Jeannerod, M. (1979). Optimal responses of the eye and hand motor systems in pointing to a visual target (I). *Biological Cybernetics, 35,* 113-124.

Prablanc, C., Pélisson, D., & Goodale, M.A. (1986). Visual control of reaching movements without vision of the limb. *Experimental Brain Research, 62,* 293-302.

Pratt, J., & Abrams, R.A. (1996). Practice and component sub-movements: The roles of programming and feedback in rapid aimed limb movements. *Journal of Motor Behavior, 28,* 149-156.

Proteau, L. (1995) Sensory integration in the learning of an aiming task. *Canadian Journal of Experimental Psychology, 49,* 113-120.

Proteau, L. (1992). On the specificity of learning and the role of visual information for movement control. In L. Proteau and D. Elliott (Eds.), *Vision and motor control* (pp. 67-103). Amsterdam: North-Holland.

Proteau, L., & Cournoyer, J. (1990). Vision of the stylus in a manual aiming task: The effects of practice. *Quarterly Journal of Experimental Psychology, 42A,* 811-828.

Proteau, L., & Masson, G. (1997). Visual perception modifies goal-directed movement control: Supporting evidence from a visual perturbation paradigm. *Quarterly Journal of Experimental Psychology, 50,* 726-741.

Proteau, L., Marteniuk, R.G., & Levesque, L. (1992). A sensorimotor basis for motor learning: Evidence indicating the specificity of practice. *Quarterly Journal of Experimental Psychology A: Human Experimental Psychology, 44,* 557-575.

Rabbitt, P.M.A. (1981). Sequential reactions. In D.H. Holding (Ed.), *Human skill.* London: Wiley.

Redding, G.M., & Wallace, B. (2001). Calibration and alignment are separable: Evidence from prism adaptation. *Journal of Motor Behavior, 33,* 401-412.

Redding, G.M., & Wallace, B. (2002). Strategic calibration and spatial alignment: A model from prism adaptation. *Journal of Motor Behavior, 34,* 126-138.

Redding, C.M., & Wallace, B. (2003). First-trial adaptation to prism exposure. *Journal of Motor Behavior, 35,* 229-245.

Schmidt, R.A., Zelaznik, H., Hawkins, B., Frank, J.S., & Quinn, J.T., Jr. (1979). Motor output variability: A theory for the accuracy of rapid motor acts. *Psychological Review, 86,* 415-451.

Smith, W.M., & Bowen, K.F. (1980). The effects of delayed and displaced visual feedback on motor control. *Journal of Motor Behavior, 12,* 91-101.

Tremblay, L., & Proteau, L. (1998). Specificity of practice: The case of powerlifting. *Research Quarterly for Exercise and Sport, 69,* 284-289.

Tremblay, L., Welsh, T.N., & Elliott, D. (2001). Specificity versus variability: Effects of practice conditions on the use of afferent information for manual aiming. *Motor Control, 5,* 347-360.

Trommershäuser, J., Gepshtein, S., Maloney, L.T., Landy, M.S., & Banks, M.S. (2005). Optimal compensation for changes in task relevant movement variability. *Journal of Neuroscience, 25,* 7178-7169.

Trommershäuser, J., Matis, J., Maloney, L.T., & Landy, M.S. (2006). Limits to human movement planning with delayed and unpredictable onset of needed information. *Experimental Brain Research, 175,* 276-284.

Ungerleider, L.G., & Mishkin, M. (1982). Two cortical visual systems. In D.J. Ingle, M.A. Goodale, & R.J.W. Mansfield (Eds.), *Analysis of visual behavior* (pp. 549-586). Cambridge, MA: MIT Press.

Westwood, D.A., Chapman, C.D., & Roy, E.A. (2000). Pantomimed actions may be controlled by the ventral visual stream. *Experimental Brain Research, 130,* 545-548.

Westwood, D.A. & Goodale, M.A. (2003). Perceptual illusion and the real-time control of action. *Spatial Vision, 16,* 243-254.

Westwood, D.A., Heath, M., & Roy, E.A. (2000). The effect of a pictorial illusion on closed-loop and open-loop prehension. *Experimental Brain Research, 141,* 166-173.

Welch, R.B. (1978). *Perceptual modification: Adapting to altered sensory environments.* New York: Academic Press.

Whiting, H.T.A., & Sharp, R.H. (1974). Visual occlusion factors in a discrete ball-catching task. *Journal of Motor Behavior, 6,* 11-16.

Wolpert, D.M., & Miall, R.C. (1996). Forward models for physiological motor control. *Neural Networks, 9,* 1265-1279.

Woodworth, R.S. (1899). The accuracy of voluntary movement. *Psychological Review, Monograph Supplements, 3*(13), 1-119.

Zelaznik, H.N., Hawkins, B., & Kisselburgh, L. (1983). Rapid visual feedback processing in single-aiming movements. *Journal of Motor Behavior, 15,* 217-236.

CHAPTER 8

Abahnini, K., & Proteau, L. (1999). The role of peripheral and central visual information for the directional control of manual movements. *Canadian Journal of Experimental Psychology, 53,* 160-175.

Abahnini, K., Proteau, L., & Temprado, J.J. (1997). Evidence supporting the importance of peripheral visual information for the directional control of aiming movement. *Journal of Motor Behavior, 29,* 230-242.

Abrams, R.A., Meyer, D.E., & Kornblum, S. (1990). Eye-hand coordination: Oculomotor control in rapid aimed limb movements. *Journal of Experimental Psychology: Human Perception and Performance, 16,* 248-267.

Bard, C., Hay, L., & Fleury, M. (1985). Role of peripheral vision in the directional control of rapid aiming movements. *Canadian Journal of Psychology, 39,* 151-161.

Bard, C., Paillard, J., Fleury, M., Hay, L., & Larue, J. (1990). Positional versus directional control loops in visuomotor pointing. *European Bulletin of Cognitive Psychology, 39,* 151-161.

Beaubaton, D., & Hay, L. (1986). Contribution of visual information to feedforward and feedback processes in rapid pointing movements. *Human Movement Science, 5,* 19-34.

Bédard, P., & Proteau, L. (2001). On the role of static and dynamic visual afferent information in goal directed aiming movements. *Experimental Brain Research, 138,* 419-431.

Bédard, P., & Proteau, L. (2003). On the role of peripheral visual afferent information for the control of rapid video-aiming movements. *Acta Psychologica, 113,* 99-117.

Bédard, P., & Proteau, L. (2004). On-line versus off-line utilization of peripheral visual afferent information to ensure spatial accuracy of goal-directed movements. *Experimental Brain Research, 158,* 75-85.

Binsted, G., & Heath, M. (2005). No evidence of a lower visual field specialization for visuomotor control. *Experimental Brain Research, 162,* 89-94.

Binsted, G., Brownell, K., Vorontsova, Z., Heath, M., & Saucier, D. (2007). Visuomotor system uses target features unavailable to conscious awareness. *Proceedings of National Academy of Sciences, 104,* 12669-12672.

Blouin, J., Bard, C., Teasdale, N., & Fleury, M. (1993). On-line versus off-line control of rapid aiming movements. *Journal of Motor Behavior, 25,* 275-279.

Bock, O. (1986). Contribution of retinal versus extraretinal signals towards visual localization in goal directed movements. *Experimental Brain Research, 64,* 476-482.

Carlton, L.G. (1981). Processing visual feedback information for movement control. *Journal of Experimental Psychology: Human Perception and Performance, 7,* 1019-1032.

Danckett, J., & Goodale, M.A. (2001). Superior performance for visually guided pointing in the lower visual field. *Experimental Brain Research, 137,* 303-308.

Danckert, J., & Goodale, M.A. (2004). Ups and downs in the visual control of action. In S.H. Johnson-Frey (Ed.), *Taking action: Cognitive neuroscience perspectives on intentional actions* (pp. 29-64). Cambridge, MA: MIT Press.

Fitts, P.M. (1954). The information capacity of the human motor system in controlling the amplitude of movement. *Journal of Experimental Psychology, 47,* 381-391.

Fleury, M., Bard, C., Audiffren, M., Teasdale, N., & Blouin, J. (1994). The attentional cost of amplitude and directional requirements when pointing to targets. *Quarterly Journal of Experimental Psychology A: Human Experimental Psychology, 47,* 481-495.

Galletti, C., Fattori, P., Gamberini, M., & Kutz, D.F. (1999). The cortical visual area V6: brain location and visual topography. *European Journal of Neuroscience, 11,* 3922-3936.

Khan, M.A., & Lawrence, G.P. (2005). Differences in visuomotor control between the upper and lower visual fields. *Experimental Brain Research, 164,* 395-398.

Khan, M.A., Lawrence, G.P., Fourkas, A., Franks, I.M., Elliott, D., & Pembroke, S. (2003). Online versus offline processing of visual feedback in the control of movement amplitude. *Acta Psychologica, 113,* 83-97.

Khan, M.A., Lawrence, G.P., Franks, I.M., & Buckolz, E. (2004). The utilization of peripheral and central vision in the control of movement direction. *Experimental Brain Research, 158,* 241-251.

Krigolson, O., & Heath, M. (2006). A lower visual field advantage for endpoint stability but no advantage for online movement precision. *Experimental Brain Research, 170,* 127-135.

Lawrence, G.P., Khan, M.A., Buckolz, E., & Oldham, A.R.H. (2006). The contribution of peripheral and central vision in the control of movement amplitude. *Human Movement Science, 25,* 326-338.

Maunsell, J.H., & van Essen, D.C. (1987). Topographic organization of the middle temporal visual area in the macaque monkey: Representational biases and the relationship to callosal connections and myeloarchitectonic boundaries. *Journal of Comparative Neurology, 266,* 535-555.

Paillard, J., & Amblard, B. (1985). Static versus kinetic visual cues for the processing of spatial relationships. In D.J Ingle, M. Jeannerod, & D.N. Lee (Eds.), *Brain mechanism in spatial vision* (pp. 367-385). The Hague, Netherlands: Martinus Nijhoff.

Popovic, Z., & Sjöstrand, J. (2001). Resolution, separation of retinal ganglion cells, and cortical magnification in humans. *Vision Research, 41,* 1313-1319.

Previc, F.H. (1990). Functional specialization in the lower and upper visual fields in humans: Its ecological origins and neurophysiological implications. *Behavioral and Brain Science, 13,* 519-575.

Previc, F.H. (1996). Attentional and oculomotor influences on visual field anisotropies in visual search performance. *Visual Cognition, 3,* 277-301.

Proteau, L., Boivin, K., Linossier, S., & Abahnini, K. (2000). Exploring the limits of peripheral vision for the control of movement. *Journal of Motor Behavior, 32,* 277-286.

Rovamo, J. (1978). Receptive field density of retinal ganglion cells and cortical magnification in man. *Medical Biology, 56,* 97-102.

Temprado, J.J., Vieilledent, S., & Proteau, L. (1996). Afferent information for motor control: The role of visual information in different portions of the movement. *Journal of Motor Behavior, 28,* 280-287.

Spijkers, W., & Lochner, P.M. (1994). Partial visual feedback and spatial endpoint accuracy of discrete aiming movements. *Journal of Motor Behavior, 26*, 283-295.

Spijkers, W., & Spellerberg, S. (1995). On-line visual control of aiming movements? *Acta Psychologica, 90*, 333-348.

Wässle, H., Grünert, U., Röhrenbeck, J., & Boycott, B.B. (1989). Cortical magnification factor and the ganglion cell density of the primate retina. *Nature, 341*, 643-646.

Woodworth, R.S. (1899). The accuracy of voluntary movement. *Psychological Review, Monograph Supplements, 3*(13), 1-119.

CHAPTER 9

Anderson, S.J., & Burr, D.C. (1985). Spatial and temporal selectivity of the human motion detection system. *Vision Research, 25*, 1147-1154.

Andersen, R.A., & Buneo, C.A. (2002). Intentional maps in posterior parietal cortex. *Annual Reviews of Neuroscience, 25*, 189-220.

Bahill, A.T., Clark, M., & Stark, L. (1975). The Main Sequence, a tool for studying human eye movements. *Mathematical Biosciences, 24*, 191-204.

Barborica, A., & Ferrera, V.P. (2003). Estimating invisible object speed from neuronal activity in monkey frontal eye field. *Nature Neuroscience, 6*, 66-74.

Barborica, A., & Ferrera, V.P. (2004). Modification of saccades evoked by simulation of frontal eye field during invisible target tracking. *Journal of Neuroscience, 24*, 3260-3267.

Barnes, G.R. (1993). Visual-vestibular interaction in the control of head and eye movement: The role of visual feedback and predictive mechanisms. *Progress in Neurobiology, 41*, 435-472.

Barnes, G.R. (1994). A model of predictive processes in oculomotor control based on experimental results in humans. In J.M. Delgado-Garcia, E. Godaux, & P.-P. Vidal (Eds.), *Information processing underlying gaze control* (pp. 279-290). Oxford: Elsevier.

Barnes, G.R., & Asselman, P.T. (1991). The mechanism of prediction in human smooth pursuit eye movements. *Journal of Physiology, 439*, 439-461.

Barnes, G.R., & Collins, S. (2008). The influence of briefly presented randomized target motion on the extraretinal component of ocular pursuit. *Journal of Neurophysiology, 99*, 831-842.

Barnes, G.R., Collins, C.J., & Arnold, L.R. (2005). Predicting the duration of ocular pursuit in humans. *Experimental Brain Research, 160*, 10-21.

Barnes, G.R. & Crombie, J.W. (1985). The interaction of conflicting retinal motion stimuli in oculomotor control. *Experimental Brain Research, 59*, 548-558. 40

Barnes, G.R., Donnelly, S.F., & Eason, R.D. (1987). Predictive velocity estimation in the pursuit reflex response to pseudo-random and step displacement stimuli in man. *Journal of Physiology, 389*, 111-136.

Barnes, G.R., Goodbody, S.J., & Collins, S. (1995). Volitional control of anticipatory ocular pursuit responses under stabilised image conditions in humans. *Experimental Brain Research, 106*, 301-317.

Barnes, G.R., Grealy, M.A., & Collins, C.J.S. (1997). Volitional control of anticipatory ocular smooth pursuit after viewing, but not pursuing, a moving target:evidence for a re-afferent velocity store. *Experimental Brain Research, 116*, 445-455.

Barnes, G.R., & Smith, R. (1981). The effects on visual discrimination of image movement across the stationary retina. *Aviation, Space, and Environmental Medicine, 52*, 466-472.

Barnes, G.R., & Wells, S.G. (1999). Modelling prediction in ocular pursuit: The importance of short-term storage. In W. Becker, H. Deubel, & T. Mergner (Eds.), *Current oculomotor research: Physiological and psychological aspects* (pp. 97-107). New York: Plenum Press.

Basso, M.A., Pokorny, J.J., & Liu, P. (2005). Activity of substantia nigra pars reticulata neurons during smooth pursuit eye movements in monkeys. *European Journal of Neuroscience, 22*, 448-464.

Batista, A.P., Buneo, C.A., Snyder, L.H., & Andersen, R.A. (1999). Reach plans in eye-centered coordinates. *Science, 285*, 257-260.

Becker, W., & Fuchs, A.F. (1985). Prediction in the oculomotor system: Smooth pursuit during transient disappearance of a visual object. *Experimental Brain Research, 57*, 562-575.

Bennett, S.J., & Barnes, G.R. (2003). Human ocular pursuit during the transient disappearance of a visual object. *Journal of Neurophysiology, 90,* 2504-2520.

Bennett, S.J., & Barnes, G.R. (2004). Predictive smooth ocular pursuit during the transient disappearance of a visual object. *Journal of Neurophysiology, 92,* 578-590.

Bennett, S.J., & Barnes, G.R. (2005a). Timing the anticipatory recovery in smooth ocular pursuit during the transient disappearance of a visual object. *Experimental Brain Research, 163,* 198-203.

Bennett, S.J., & Barnes, G.R. (2005b). Combined smooth and saccadic ocular pursuit during the transient occlusion of a moving visual object. *Experimental Brain Research, 168,* 313-321.

Bennett, S.J., & Barnes, G.R. (2006). Smooth ocular pursuit during the transient disappearance of an accelerating visual target: The role of reflexive and voluntary control. *Experimental Brain Research, 175,* 1-10.

Bennett, S.J., Orban de Xivry, J.J., Barnes, G.R., Lefevre, P. (2007). Target acceleration can be extracted and represented within the predictive drive to ocular pursuit. *Journal of Neurophysiology 98,* 1405-1414

Berryhill, M.E., Chiu, T., & Hughes, H.C. (2006). Smooth pursuit of nonvisual motion. *Journal of Neurophysiology, 96,* 461-465.

Blohm, G., Missal, M., & Lefèvre, P. (2003). Interaction between smooth anticipation and saccades during ocular orientation in darkness. *Journal of Neurophysiology, 89,* 1423-1433.

Bremmer, F., Distler, C., & Hoffmann, K.P. (1997). Eye position effects in monkey cortex: II. Pursuit- and fixation-related activity in posterior parietal areas LIP and 7A. *Journal of Neurophysiology, 77,* 962-977.

Brouwer, A., Brenner, E., & Smeets, J.B.J. (2002). Perception of acceleration with short presentation times: Can acceleration be used in interception? *Perception & Psychophysics, 64,* 1160-1168.

Carl, J.R., & Gellman, R.S. (1987). Human smooth pursuit: Stimulus-dependent responses. *Journal of Neurophysiology, 57,* 1446-1463.

Chakraborti, S.R., Barnes, G.R., & Collins, C.J. (2002). Factors affecting the longevity of a short-term velocity store for predictive oculomotor tracking. *Experimental Brain Research, 144,* 152-158.

Churchland, M.M., Chou, I.-H., & Lisberger, S.G. (2003). Evidence for object permanence in the smooth-pursuit eye movements of monkeys. *Journal of Neurophysiology, 90,* 2205-2218.

Coe, B., Tomihara, K., Matsuzawa, M., & Hikosaka, O. (2002). Visual and anticipatory bias in three cortical eye fields of the monkey during an adaptive decision-making task. *Journal of Neuroscience, 22,* 5081-5090.

Cui, D.M., Yan, Y.J., & Lynch, J.C. (2003). Pursuit subregion of the frontal eye field projects to the caudate nucleus in monkeys. *Journal of Neurophysiology, 89,* 2678-2684.

Dallos, P.J., & Jones, R.W. (1963). Learning behavior of the eye fixation control system. *IEEE Engineering in Medicine and Biology Magazine, 8,* 218-227.

De Brouwer, S., Yuksel, D., Blohm, G., Missal, M., & Lefèvre, P. (2002). What triggers catch-up saccades during visual tracking? *Journal of Neurophysiology, 87,* 1646-1650.

Duhamel, J.R., Colby, C.L., & Goldberg, M.E. (1992). The updating of the representation of visual space in parietal cortex by intended eye movements. *Science, 255*(5040), 90-92.

Dürsteler, M.R., & Wurtz, R.H. (1988). Pursuit and optokinetic deficits following chemical lesions of cortical areas MT and MST. *Journal of Neurophysiology, 60,* 940-965.

Epelboim, J., Steinman, R.M., Kowler, E., Pizlo, Z., Erkelens, C.J., & Collewijn, H. (1997). Gaze-shift dynamics in two kinds of sequential looking tasks. *Vision Research, 37,* 2597-2607.

Erkelens, C.J. (2006). Coordination of smooth pursuit and saccades. *Vision Research, 46,* 163-170.

Gauthier, G.M., & Hofferer, J.M. (1976). Eye tracking of self-moved targets in the absence of vision. *Experimental Brain Research, 26,* 121-139.

Gauthier, G.M., Vercher, J.L., Mussa Ivaldi, F., & Marchetti, E. (1988). Oculo-manual tracking of visual targets: Control learning, coordination control and coordination model. *Experimental Brain Research, 73,* 127-137.

Goltz, H.C., & Whitney, D. (2004). The influence of background motion on smooth pursuit: Separation matters. *Journal of Vision, 4,* 649a.

Gottlieb, J.P., Bruce, C.J., & MacAvoy, M.G. (1993). Smooth eye movements elicited by microstimulation in the primate frontal eye field. *Journal of Neurophysiology, 69*, 786-799.

Grzywacz, N.M., Watamaniuk, S.N.J., & McKee, S.P. (1995). Temporal coherence theory for the detection and measurement of visual motion. *Vision Research, 35*, 3183-3203.

Greenlee, M.W., Lang, H.J., Mergner, T., & Seeger, W. (1995). Visual short term memory of stimulus velocity in patients with unilateral posterior brain damage. *Journal of Neuroscience, 15*, 2287-2300.

Heide,W., Binkofski, F., Seitz, R.J., Posse, S., Nitschke, M.F., Freund, H.J., & Kompf, D. (2001). Activation of frontoparietal cortices during memorized triple-step sequences of saccadic eye movements: An fMRI study. *European Journal of Neuroscience, 13*, 1177-1189.

Heinen, S.J., & Liu, M. (1997). Single-neuron activity in the dorsomedial frontal cortex during smooth-pursuit eye movements to predictable target motion. *Visual Neuroscience, 14*, 853-865.

Heywood, S., & Churcher, J. (1971). Eye movements and the afterimage. I. Tracking the afterimage. *Vision Research, 11*, 1163-1168.

Hollands, M.A., & Marple-Horvat, D.E. (1996). Visually guided stepping under conditions of step cycle-related denial of visual information. *Experimental Brain Research, 109*, 343-356.

Howard, I.P., & Marton, C. (1992). Visual pursuit over textured backgrounds in different depth planes. *Vision Research, 90*, 625-629.

Ilg, U.J., & Their, P. (2003). Visual tracking neurons in primate area MST are activated by smooth pursuit eye movements of an "imaginary" target. *Journal of Neurophysiology, 90*, 1489-502.

Jarrett, C.B., & Barnes, G.R. (2001). Volitional selection of direction in the generation of anticipatory smooth pursuit in humans. *Neuroscience Letters, 312*, 25-28.

Jarrett, C.B., & Barnes, G.R. (2002). Volitional scaling of anticipatory ocular pursuit velocity using precues. *Cognitive Brain Research, 14*, 383-388.

Jarrett, C.B., & Barnes, G.R. (2005). The use of non-motion-based cues to pre-programme the timing of ocular pursuit reversal in human smooth pursuit. *Experimental Brain Research, 164*, 423-430.

Kao, G.W., & Morrow, M.J. (1994). The relationship of anticipatory smooth eye movement to smooth pursuit initiation. *Vision Research, 34*, 3027-3036.

King, W.M., & Zhou, W.U. (1995). Initiation of disjunctive smooth pursuit in monkeys: Evidence that Hering's law of equal innervation is not obeyed by the smooth pursuit system. *Vision Research, 35*, 3389-3400.

Komatsu, H., & Wurtz, R.H. (1989). Modulation of pursuit eye movements by stimulation of cortical areas MT and MST. *Journal of Neurophysiology, 62*, 31-47.

Kommerell, G., & Taumer, R. (1972). Investigations of the eye tracking system through stabilised retinal images. *Bibliotheca Ophthalmologica, 82*, 288-297.

Kowler, E., & Steinman, R.M. (1979a). The effect of expectations on slow oculomotor control. I. Periodic target steps. *Vision Research, 19*, 619-632.

Kowler, E., & Steinman, R.M. (1979b). The effect of expectations on slow oculomotor control. II. Single target displacements. *Vision Research, 19*, 633-646.

Kowler, E. (1989). Cognitive expectations, not habits, control anticipatory smooth oculomotor pursuit. *Vision Research, 29*, 1049-1057.

Krauzlis, R.J. (2004). Recasting the smooth pursuit eye movement system. *Journal of Neurophysiology, 91*, 591-603.

Krauzlis, R.J. (2005). The control of voluntary eye movements: New perspectives. *Neuroscientist, 11*, 124-137.

Krauzlis, R.J., & Miles, F.A. (1996). Transitions between pursuit eye movements and fixation in the monkey: Dependence on context. *Journal of Neurophysiology, 76*, 1622-1638.

Krauzlis RJ, Lisberger SG (1994) A model of visually-guided smooth pursuit eye movements based on behavioral observations. *Journal of Computational Neuroscience 1*, 265-283

Krauzlis, R.J., & Stone, L.S. (1999). Tracking with the mind's eye. *Trends in Neuroscience, 22*, 544-550.

Leigh, R.J., & Zee, D.S. (2006). *The neurology of eye movements.* Philadelphia: Davis.

Leist, A., Freund, H.-J., & Cohen, B. (1987). Comparative characteristics of predictive eye-hand tracking. *Human Neurobiology, 6*, 19-26.

Lencer, R., Nagel, M., Sprenger, A., Zapf, S., Erdmann, C., Heide, W., & Binkofski, F. (2004). Cortical mechanisms of smooth pursuit eye movements with object blanking: An fMRI study. *European Journal of Neuroscience, 19*, 1430-1436.

Levy, R., & Goldman-Rakic, P.S. (2000). Segregation of working memory functions within the dorsolateral prefrontal cortex. *Experimental Brain Research, 133*, 23-32.

Lindner, A., & Ilg, U.J. (2006). Suppression of optokinesis during smooth pursuit eye movements revisited: The role of extra-retinal information. *Vision Research, 46*, 761-767.

Lindner, A., Schwarz, U., & Ilg, U.J. (2001). Cancellation of self-induced retinal image motion during smooth pursuit eye movements. *Vision Research, 41*, 1685-1694.

Lisberger, S.G. (1998). Postsaccadic enhancement of initiation of smooth pursuit eye movements in monkeys. *Journal of Neurophysiology, 79*, 1918-1930.

Lisberger, S.G., & Fuchs, A.F. (1978). Role of primate flocculus during rapid behavioral modification of vestibuloocular reflex. I. Purkinje cell activity during visually guided horizontal smooth-pursuit eye movements and passive head rotation. *Journal of Neurophysiology, 41*, 733-763.

Lisberger, S.G., Morris, E.J., & Tychsen, L. (1981). Visual motion processing and sensory-motor integration for smooth pursuit eye movements. *Annual Reviews of Neuroscience, 10*, 97-129.

Lisberger, S.G., & Movshon, J.A. (1999). Visual motion analysis for pursuit eye movements in area MT of macaque monkeys. *Journal of Neuroscience, 19*, 2222-2246.

Lisberger, S.G., & Westbrook, L.E. (1985). Properties of visual inputs that initiate horizontal smooth pursuit eye movements in monkeys. *Journal of Neuroscience, 5*, 1662-1673.

Madelain, L., & Krauzlis, R.J. (2003). Pursuit of the ineffable: Perceptual and motor reversals during the tracking of apparent motion. *Journal of Vision, 3*, 642-653.

MacAvoy, M.G., Gottlieb, J.P., & Bruce, C.J. (1991). Smooth-pursuit eye movement representation in the primate frontal eye field. *Cerebral Cortex, 1*, 95-102.

Marple-Horvat, D.E., Chattington, M., Anglesea, M., Ashford, D.G., Wilson, M., & Keil, D. (2005). Prevention of coordinated eye movements and steering impairs driving performance. *Experimental Brain Research, 163*, 411-420.

Masson, G., Proteau, L., & Mestre, D.R. (1993). Effects of stationary and moving textured backgrounds on the visuo-oculo-manual tracking in humans. *Vision Research, 35*, 837-852.

Medendorp, W.P., Goltz, H.C., Vilis, T., & Crawford, J.D. (2003). Gaze centered updating of visual space in human parietal cortex. *Journal of Neuroscience, 23*, 6209-6214.

Meyer, C.H., Lasker, A.G., & Robinson, D.A. (1985). The upper limit of human smooth pursuit velocity. *Vision Research, 25*, 561-563.

Miall, R.C., Reckess, G.Z., & Imamizu, H. (2001). The cerebellum coordinates eye and hand tracking movements. *Nature Neuroscience, 4*, 638-644.

McKee, S.P. (1981). A local mechanism for differential velocity detection. *Vision Research, 21*, 491-500.

Missal, M., & Heinen, S.J. (2004). Supplementary eye fields stimulation facilitates anticipatory pursuit. *Journal of Neurophysiology, 92*, 1257-1262.

Mitrani, L., & Dimitrov, G. (1978). Pursuit eye movements of a disappearing moving target. *Vision Research, 18*, 537-539.

Morris, E.J., & Lisberger, S.G. (1987). Different responses to small visual errors during initiation and maintenance of smooth-pursuit eye movements in monkeys. *Journal of Neurophysiology, 58*, 1351-1369.

Morrow, M.J. & Sharpe, J.A. (1993). Smooth pursuit initiation in young and elderly subjects. *Vision Research, 33*, 203-210.

Mrotek, L.A., & Soechting, J.F. (2006). Predicting curvilinear target motion through an occlusion. *Experimental Brain Research, 178*, 99-114.

Nagel, M., Sprenger, A., Zapf, S., Erdmann, C., Kompf, D., Heide, W., Binkofski, F., & Lencer, R. (2006). Parametric modulation of cortical activation during smooth pursuit with and without target blanking. An fMRI study. *NeuroImage, 29*, 1319-1325.

Newsome, W.T., Wurtz, R.H., & Komatsu, H. (1988). Relation of cortical areas MT and MST to pursuit eye movements. II. Differentiation of retinal from extraretinal inputs. *Journal of Neurophysiology, 60,* 604-620.

Olson, I.R., Gatenby, J.C., Leung, H., Skudlarski, P., & Gore, J.C. (2003). Neuronal representation of occluded objects in the human brain. *Neuropsychologia, 42,* 95-104.

Orban de Xivry, J.J., Bennett, S.J., Lefèvre, P., & Barnes, G.R. (2006). Evidence for synergy between saccades and smooth pursuit during transient target disappearance. *Journal of Neurophysiology, 95,* 418-427.

Orban de Xivry, J.J., & Lefèvre, P., (2007). Saccades and pursuit: two outcomes of a single sensorimotor process. *Journal of Physiology, 584,* 11-23.

Ono, S., & Mustari, M.J. (2006). Extraretinal signals in MSTd neurons related to volitional smooth pursuit. *Journal of Neurophysiology, 96,* 2819-2825.

Passingham, D., & Sakai, K. (2004). The prefrontal cortex and working memory: Physiology and brain imaging. *Current Opinions in Neurobiology, 14,* 163-168.

Pasternak, T., & Zaksas, D. (2003). Stimulus specificity and temporal dynamics of working memory for visual motion. *Journal of Neurophysiology, 90,* 2752-2757.

Pierrot-Deseilligny, C., Milea, D., & Müri, R.M. (2004). Eye movement control by the cerebral cortex. *Current Opinion in Neurology, 17,* 17-25.

Pola, J., & Wyatt, H. (1997). Offset dynamics of human smooth pursuit eye movements: Effects of target presence and subject attention. *Vision Research, 37,* 2579-2595.

Rashbass, C. (1961). The relationship between saccadic and smooth tracking eye movements. *Journal of Physiology, 159,* 326-338.

Robinson, D.A. (1975). Oculomotor control signals. In F. Lennerstand & P. Bach-y-Rita (Eds.), *Basic mechanisms of ocular motility and their clinical implications* (pp. 337-374). Oxford: Pergamon Press.

Robinson, D.A., Gordon, J.L., & Gordon, S.E. (1986). A model of the smooth eye pursuit eye movement system. *Biological Cybernetics, 55,* 43-57.

Rosander, K., & von Hofsten, C. (2004). Infants' emerging ability to represent occluded object motion. *Cognition, 91,* 1-22.

Segraves, M.A., & Goldberg, M.E. (1994). Effect of stimulus position and velocity upon the maintenance of smooth pursuit eye velocity. *Vision Research, 34,* 2477-2482.

Schlack, A., Hoffmann, K.P., & Bremmer, F. (2003). Selectivity of macaque area VIP for smooth pursuit eye movements. *Journal of Physiology, 551,* 551-561.

Schweigart, G., Mergner, T., Barnes, G. (1999). Eye movements during combined pursuit, optokinetic and vestibular stimulation in macaque monkey. *Experimental Brain Research, 127:*54-66.

Schweigart, G., Mergner, T., & Barnes, G.R. (2003). Object motion perception is shaped by the motor control mechanism of ocular pursuit. *Experimental Brain Research, 148,* 350-365.

Snyder, L.H., Calton, J.L., Dickinson, A.R., & Lawrence, B.M. (2002). Eye-hand coordination: Saccades are faster when accompanied by a coordinated arm movement. *Journal of Neurophysiology, 87,* 2279-2286.

Tanaka, M., & Fukushima, K. (1988). Neuronal responses related to smooth pursuit eye movements in the periarcuate cortical area of monkeys. *Journal of Neurophysiology, 80,* 28-47.

Tanaka, M., & Lisberger, S.G. (2000). Context-dependent smooth eye movements evoked by stationary visual stimuli in trained monkeys. *Journal of Neurophysiology, 84,* 1748-1762.

Tanaka, M., & Lisberger, S.G. (2001). Regulation of the gain of visually guided smooth-pursuit eye movements by frontal cortex. *Nature, 409,* 191-194.

Their, P., & Ilg, U.J. (2005). The neural basis of smooth-pursuit eye movements. *Current Opinions in Neurobiology, 15,* 645-652.

Watamaniuk, S.N.J., & Heinen, S.J. (1999). Human smooth pursuit direction discrimination. *Vision Research, 39,* 59-70.

Watamaniuk, S.N., Heinen, S.J. (2003). Perceptual and oculomotor evidence of limitations on processing accelerating motion. *Jounral of Vision, 3,* 698-709.

Werkhoven, P., Snippe, H.P., & Toet, A. (1992). Visual processing of optic acceleration. *Vision Research, 32,* 2313-2329.

Westheimer, G., & McKee, S.P. (1975). Visual acuity in the presence of retinal-image motion. *Journal of the Optical Society of America, 65,* 847-850.

Wilkie, R.M., & Wann, J.P. (2003). Eye-movements aid the control of locomotion. *Journal of Vision, 3,* 677-684.

Worfolk, R., & Barnes, G.R. (1992). Interaction of active and passive slow eye movement systems. *Experimental Brain Research, 90,* 589-598.

Wyatt, H.J., & Pola, J. (1981). Slow eye movements to eccentric targets. *Investigative Ophthalmology and Visual Science, 21,* 477-483.

Wyatt, H.J., & Pola, J. (1987). Smooth eye movements with step ramp stimuli: The influence of attention and stimulus extent. *Vision Research, 27,* 1565-1580.

Xiao, Q., Barborica, A., & Ferrera, V.P. (2007). Modulation of visual responses in macaque frontal eye field during covert tracking of invisible targets. *Cerebral Cortex, 17,* 918-928.

Yasui, S., & Young, L.R. (1975). Perceived visual motion as effective stimulus to pursuit eye movement system. *Science, 190*(4217), 906-908.

Yasui, S., & Young, L.R. (1984). On the predictive control of foveal eye tracking and slow phases of optokinetic and vestibular nystagmus. *Journal of Physiology, 347,* 17-33.

Young, L.R., & Stark, L. (1963). Variable feedback experiments testing a sampled data model for eye tracking movements. *IEEE Transactions on Human Factors in Electronics, HFE-4,* 28-51.

Zee, D.S., FitzGibbon, E.J., & Optican, L.M. (1992). Saccade-vergence interactions in humans. *Journal of Neurophysiology, 68,* 1624-1641.

CHAPTER 10

Andersen, R.A., & Buneo, C.A. (2002). Intentional maps in posterior parietal cortex. *Annual Review of Neuroscience, 25,* 189-220.

Avillac, M., Denève, S., Olivier, E., Pouget, A., & Duhamel, J.R. (2005). Reference frames for representing visual and tactile locations in parietal cortex. *Nature Neuroscience, 8,* 941-949.

Batista, A.P., Buneo, C.A., Snyder, L.H., & Anderson, R.A. (1999). Reach plans in eye-centered coordinates. *Science, 285,* 257-260.

Battaglia-Mayer, A., Archambault, P.S., & Caminiti R. (2006). The cortical network for eye-hand coordination and its relevance to understanding motor disorders of parietal patients. *Neuropsychologia, 44,* 2607-2620.

Bernardis, P., Knox, P., & Bruno, N. (2005). How does action resist visual illusion? Uncorrected oculomotor information does not account for accurate pointing in peripersonal space. *Experimental Brain Research, 162,* 133-144.

Biguer, B., Jeannerod, M., & Prablanc, C. (1982). The coordination of eye, head, and arm movements during reaching at a single visual target. *Experimental Brain Research, 46,* 301-304.

Biguer, B., Prablanc, C., & Jeannerod, M. (1984). The contribution of coordinated eye and head movements in pointing accuracy. *Experimental Brain Research, 55,* 462-469.

Binsted, G., & Elliott, D. (1999a). The Muller-Lyer illusion as a perturbation to the saccadic system. *Human Movement Science, 18,* 103-117.

Binsted, G., & Elliott, D. (1999b). Ocular perturbations and retinal/extraretinal information: The coordination of saccadic and manual movements. *Experimental Brain Research, 127,* 193-206.

Binsted, G., Brownell, K., Vorontsova, Z., Heath, M., & Saucier, D. (2007). Visuomotor system uses target features unavailable to conscious awareness. *Proceedings of the National Academy of Sciences of the United States of America, 104,* 12669-12672.

Binsted, G., Chua, R., Helsen, W., & Elliott, D. (2001). Eye hand coordination in goal-directed aiming. *Human Movement Science, 20,* 563-585.

Bizzi, E., Kalil, R.E., & Tagliasco, V. (1971). Eye-hand coordination in monkeys: Evidence for centrally patterned organization. *Science, 173,* 452-454.

Bock, O. (1986). Contributions of retinal versus extraretinal signals toward visual localization in goal-directed movements. *Experimental Brain Research, 64,* 476-482.

Bock, O. (1993). Localization of objects in the peripheral visual field. *Behavioral Brain Research, 56,* 77-84.

Buneo, C.A., & Andersen, R.A. (2006). The posterior parietal cortex: Sensorimotor interface for the planning and online control of visually guided movements. *Neuropsychologia, 44,* 2594-2606.

Carey, D.P. (2000). Eye-hand coordination: Eye to hand or hand to eye? *Current Biology, 10,* R416-419.

Carey, D.P., Coleman, R.J., Della Salla, S. (1997). Magnetic misreaching. *Cortex, 33,* 639-652.

Carlton, L.G. (1981). Processing visual feedback information for movement control. *Journal of Experimental Psychology: Human Perception and Performance, 33,* 403-418.

Carnahan, H., & Marteniuk, R.G. (1991). The temporal organization of hand, eye, and head movements during reaching and pointing. *Journal of Motor Behavior, 23,* 109-119.

Chouinard, P.A., & Paus, T. (2006). The primary motor and premotor areas of the human cerebral cortex. *Neuroscientist, 12,* 143-152.

Cohen, Y.E., & Anderson, R.A. (2000). Reaches to sounds encoded in an eye-centered reference frame. *Neuron, 27,* 647-652.

Crawford, J.D., Henriques, D.Y., Medendorp, W.P., & Khan, A.Z. (2003). Ocular kinematics and eye-hand coordination. *Strabismus, 11,* 33-47.

Desmurget, M., & Grafton, S. (2000). Forward modeling allows feedback control for fast reaching. *Trends in Cognitive Science, 4,* 423-431.

Desmurget, M., Pélisson, D., Rossetti, Y., & Prablanc, C. (1998). From eye to hand: Planning goal-directed movements. *Neuroscience Biobehavioral Reviews, 22,* 761-788.

Desmurget, M., Turner, R.S., Prablanc, C., Russo, G.S., Alexander, G.E., & Grafton, S.T. (2005). Updating target location at the end of an orienting saccade affects the characteristics of simple point-to-point movements. *Journal of Experimental Psychology: Human Perception and Performance, 31,* 1510-1536.

Deubel, H., Wolf, W., & Hauske, G. (1982). Corrective saccades: Effect of shifting the saccade goal. *Vision Research, 22,* 353-364.

Ehresman, C., Saucier, D., Heath, M., & Binsted, G. (2008). Online corrections can produce illusory bias during closed-loop pointing. *Experimental Brain Research, 188,* 371-378.

Elliott, D., Heath, M., Binsted, G., Ricker, K.L., Roy, E.A., Chua, R. (1999). Goal-directed aiming: Correcting a force specification error with the right and left hands. *Jouranl of Motor Behavior, 31,* 309-324.

Enright, J.T. (1995). The non-visual impact of eye-orientation on eye-hand coordination. *Vision Research, 35,* 1611-1618.

Findlay, J.M., & Walker, R. (1999). A model of saccade generation based on parallel processing and competitive inhibition. *Behavioral Brain Science, 22,* 661-721.

Fisk, J.D., & Goodale, M.A. (1985). The organization of eye and limb movement during unrestricted reaching to targets in contralateral and ipsilateral space. *Experimental Brain Research, 60,* 159-178.

Flanders, M., Daghestani, L., & Berthoz, A. (1999). Reaching beyond reach. *Experimental Brain Research, 126,* 19-30.

Furneaux, S., & Land, M.F. (1999). The effects of skill on the eye-hand span during musical sight-reading. *Proceedings of the Royal Society of London. Series B, Biological Sciences, 266,* 2435-2440.

Gauthier, G.M., Nommay, D., & Vercher, J.L. (1990). The role of ocular muscle proprioception in visual localization of targets. *Science, 249,* 58-61.

Girard, G., & Berthoz, A. (2005). From brainstem to cortex: Computational models of saccadic generation circuitry. *Progress in Neurobiology, 77,* 215-251.

Glover, S. (2004). Separate visual representations in the planning and control of action. *Behavioral and Brain Sciences, 27,* 3-24.

Goodale, M.A., Pélisson, D., & Prablanc, C. (1986). Large adjustments in visually guided reaching do not depend on vision of the hand or perception of target displacement. *Nature, 320,* 748-750.

Graziano, M.S.A. (2006). Progress in understanding spatial coordinate systems in the primate brain. *Neuron, 51,* 7-9.

Grea, H., Pisella, L., Rosetti, Y., Desmurget, M., Tilikete, C., Grafton, S., Prablanc, C., & Vighetto, A. (2002). A lesion of the posterior parietal cortex disrupts on-line adjustments during aiming movements. *Neuropsychologia, 40,* 2471-2480.

Gribble, P.L., Everling, S., Ford, K., & Mattar, A. (2002). Hand-eye coordination for rapid pointing movements. Arm movement direction and distance are specified prior to saccade onset. *Experimental Brain Research, 145,* 372-382.

Heath, M. (2005). Role of limb and target vision in the online control of memory-guided reaches. *Motor Control, 9,* 281-311.

Heath, M., & Binsted, G. (2007). Visuomotor memory for target location in near and far reaching spaces. *Journal of Motor Behavior, 39,* 169-177.

Heath, M., Neely, K.A., Yakimishyn, J., & Binsted, G. (2008). Visuomotor memory is independent of conscious awareness of target features. *Experimental Brain Research, 188,* 517-527

Heath, M., Westwood, D.A., & Binsted, G. (2004). The control of memory-guided reaching movements in peripersonal space. *Motor Control, 8,* 76-106.

Helsen, W.F., Elliott, D., Starkes, J.L., & Ricker, K.L. (2000). Coupling of eye, finger, elbow, and shoulder movements during manual aiming. *Journal of Motor Behavior, 32,* 241-248.

Helsen, W.F., Starkes, J.L., Elliott, D., & Buekers, M.J. (1998). Manual asymmetries and saccadic eye movements in right-handers during single and reciprocal aiming movements. *Cortex, 34,* 513-529.

Henriques, D.Y., & Crawford, J.D. (2000). Direction-dependent distortions of retinotopic space in the visuomotor transformation of pointing. *Experimental Brain Research, 132,* 179-194.

Herst, A.N., Epelboim, J., & Steinman, R.M. (2001). Temporal coordination of the human head and eye during sequential tapping. *Vision Research, 41,* 3307-3309.

Hore, J., Watts, S., & Vilis, T. (1992). Constraints on arm position when pointing in three-dimensions: Donders' law and the Fick gimbal strategy. *Journal of Neurophysiology, 68,* 374-383.

Johansson, R.S., Westling, G., Bäckström, A., Flanagan, J.R. (2001). Eye-hand coordination in object manipulation. *Journal of Neuroscience, 21,* 6917-6932.

Land, M.F. (2005). Eye-hand coordination: Learning a new trick. *Current Biology, 15,* R955-R956.

Land, M.F., & McLeod, P. (2000). From eye movements to actions: How batsmen hit the ball. *Nature Neuroscience, 3,* 1340-1345.

Lyons, J., Hansen, S., Hurding, S., Elliott, D. (2006). Optimizing rapid aiming behaviour: Movement kinematics depend on the cost of corrective modifications. *Experimental Brain Research, 174,* 95-100.

McIntyre, J., Stratta, F., & Lacquaniti, F. (1997). Viewer-centered frame of reference for pointing to memorized targets in three-dimensional space. *Journal of Neurophysiology, 78,* 1601-1618.

Medendorp, W.P., Goltz, H.C., Vilis, T., & Crawford J.D. (2003). Integration of target and effector information in human posterior parietal cortex for the planning of action. *Journal of Neurophysiology, 23,* 6209-6214.

Medendorp, W.P., Smith, M.A., Tweed, D.B., & Crawford, J.D. (2001). Rotational remapping in human spatial memory during eye and head motion. *Journal of Neuroscience, 21,* 1-4.

Mennie, N., Hayhoe, M., & Sullivan, B. (2007). Look-ahead fixations: Anticipatory eye movements in natural tasks. *Experimental Brain Research, 179,* 427-442.

Merriam, E.P., Genovese, C.R., & Colby, C.L. (2003). Spatial updating in human parietal cortex. *Neuron, 39,* 361-373.

Miall, R.C., Reckess, G.Z., & Imamizu, H. (2001). The cerebellum coordinates eye and hand tracking movements. *Nature Neuroscience, 4,* 638-644.

Miller, L.E., Theeuwen, M., & Gielen, C.C. (1992). The control of arm pointing in three dimensions. *Experimental Brain Research, 90,* 415-426.

Milner, A.D., & Goodale, M.A. (1995). *The visual brain in action.* Oxford: Oxford University Press.

Milner, A.D., Dijkerman, H.C., Pisella, L., McIntosh, R.D., Tilikete, C., Vighetto, A., & Rossetti, Y. (2001). Grasping the past: Delay can improve visuomotor performance. *Current Biology, 11,* 1896-1901.

Mullette-Gillman, O.A., Cohen, Y.E., & Groh, J.M. (2005). Eye-centered, head-centered, and complex coding of visual and auditory targets in the intraparietal sulcus. *Journal of Neurophysiology, 94,* 2331-2352.

Naranjo, J.R., Brovelli, A., Longo, R., Budai, R., Kristeva, R., & Battaglini, P.P. (2007). EEG dynamics of frontoparietal network during reaching preparation in humans. *NeuroImage, 34,* 1673-1682.

Neggers, S.F., & Bekkering, H. (2000). Ocular gaze in anchored to the target of an ongoing pointing movement. *Journal of Neurophysiology, 83,* 639-651.

Neggers, S.F., & Bekkering, H. (2001). Gaze anchoring to a pointing target is present during the entire pointing movement and is driven by a non-visual signal. *Journal of Neurophsiology, 86,* 961-970.

Pélisson, D., Prablanc, C., Goodale, M.A., & Jeannerod, M. (1986). Visual control of reaching without vision of the limb. II. Evidence of fast unconscious processes correcting the trajectory of the hand to the final position of a double-step stimulus. *Experimental Brain Research, 62,* 303-311.

Perenin, M.T., & Vighetto, A. (1988). Optic ataxia: A specific disruption in visuomotor mechanisms. *Brain, 111,* 643-674.

Prablanc, C., & Jeannerod, M. (1975). Corrective saccades: Dependence on retinal reafferent signals. *Vision Research, 15,* 465-469.

Prablanc, C., & Martin, O. (1992). Automatic control during hand reaching at undetected two-dimensional target displacements. *Journal of Neurophysiology, 67,* 455-569.

Prablanc, C., Echallier, J.F., Jeannerod, M., & Komilis, E. (1979). Optimal response of eye and hand motor systems in pointing at a visual target. II. Static and dynamic visual cues in the control of hand movement. *Biological Cybernetics, 35,* 183-187.

Prablanc, C., Echallier, J.F., Komilis, E., & Jeannerod, M. (1979). Optimal response of eye and hand motor systems in pointing at a visual target. I. Spatio-temporal characteristics of eye and hand movements and their relationships when varying the amount of visual information. *Biological Cybernetics, 35,* 113-124.

Prablanc, C., Pélisson, D., & Goodale, M.A. (1986). Visual control of reaching without vision of the limb. I. Role of retinal feedback of target position in guiding the hand. *Experimental Brain Research, 62,* 293-302.

Regan, D., & Gray, R. (2001). Hitting what one wants to hit and missing what one wants to miss. *Vision Research, 41,* 3321-3329.

Revol, P., Rossetti, Y., Vighetto, A., Rode, G., Boisson, D., & Pisella, L. (2003). Pointing errors in immediate and delayed conditions in unilateral optic ataxia. *Spatial Vision, 16,* 347-364.

Rodgers, C.K., Munoz, D.P., Scott, S.H., & Pare, M. (2006). Discharge properties of tectoreticular neurons. *Journal of Neurophysiology, 95,* 3502-3511.

Rolheiser, T.M., Binsted, G., & Brownell, K.J. (2006). Visuomotor representation decay: Influence on motor systems. *Experimental Brain Research, 173,* 698-707.

Romanelli, P., Esposito, V., Schaal, D.W., & Heit, G. (2005). Somatotopy in the basal ganglia: Experimental and clinical evidence for segregated sensorimotor channels. *Brain Research Reviews, 48,* 112-128.

Sailer, A., Eggert, T., & Straube, A. (2005). Impaired temporal prediction and eye-hand coordination in patients with cerebellar lesions. *Behavioral Brain Research, 160,* 72-87.

Sarlegna, F., Blouin, J., Bresciani, J.P., Bourdin, C., Vercher, J.L., & Gauthier, G.M. (2003). Target and hand position information in the online control of goal-directed arm movements. *Experimental Brain Research, 151,* 524-535.

Schlack, A., Sterbing-D'Angelo, S.J., Hartung, K., Hoffmann, K.P., & Bremmer, F. (2005). Multisensory space representations in the macaque ventral intraparietal area. *Journal of Neuroscience, 25,* 4616-4625.

Schieber, M.H. (2001). Constraints on somatotopic organization in the primary motor cortex. *Journal of Neurophysiology, 86,* 2125-2143.

Schneider, G.E. (1969). Two visual systems: Brain mechanisms for localization and discrimination are dissociated by tectal and cortical lesions. *Science, 163,* 895-902.

Snyder, L.H., Calton, J.L., Dickinson, A.R., & Lawrence, B.M. (2002). Eye-hand coordination: Saccades are faster when accompanied by a coordinated arm movement. *Journal of Neurophysiology, 87,* 2279-2286.

Soechting J.F., Engel, K.C., & Flanders, M. (2001). The Duncker illusion and eye-hand coordination. *Journal of Neurophysiology, 85,* 843-854.

Soechting, J.F., & Lacquaniti, F. (1981). Invariant characteristics of a pointing movement in man. *Journal of Neuroscience, 1,* 710-720.

Steinman, R.M., Pizlo, Z., Forofonova, T.I., & Epelboim, J. (2003). One fixates accurately in order to see clearly not because one sees clearly. *Spatial Vision, 16,* 225-241.

Stricane, B., Anderson, R.A., & Mazzoni, P. (1996). Eye-centered, head-centered, and intermediate coding of remembered sound locations in area LIP. *Journal of Neurophysiology, 76,* 2071-2076.

Terao, Y., Andersson, N.E., Flanagan, J.R., & Johansson, R.S. (2002). Engagement of gaze in capturing targets for future sequential actions. *Journal of Neurophysiology, 88,* 1716-1725.

Thompson, A.A., & Westwood, D.A. (2007). The hand knows something that the eye does not: Reaching movements resist the Muller-Lyer illusion whether or not the target is foveated. *Neuroscience Letters, 426,* 111-116.

Thura, D., Hadj-Bouziane, F., Meunier, M., & Boussaoud, D. (2008). Hand position modulates saccadic activity in the frontal eye field. *Behavioral Brain Research, 186,* 148-153.

Turner, R.S., Owens, J.W., & Anderson, M.E. (1995). Directional variation of spatial and temporal characteristics of limb movements made by monkeys in a two-dimensional work space. *Journal of Neurophysiology, 74,* 684-697.

Ungerleider, L.G., & Mishkin, M. (1982). Two cortical visual systems. In D.J. Ingle, M.A. Goodale, & R.J.W. Mansfield (Eds.), *Analysis of visual behaviour* (pp. 549-586). Cambridge, MA: MIT Press.

van Donkelaar, P. (1998). Saccadic amplitude influences pointing movement kinematics. *Neuroreport, 9,* 2015-2018.

van Donkelaar, P., Lee, J.H., & Drew, A.S. (2000). Transcranial magnetic stimulation disrupts eye-hand interactions in the posterior parietal cortex. *Journal of Neurophysiology, 84,* 1677-1680.

van Donkelaar, P., Lee, J.H., & Drew, A.S. (2002). Eye-hand interactions differ in the human premotor and parietal cortices. *Human Movement Science, 21,* 377-386.

Vercher, J.L., Magenes, G., Prablanc, C., & Gauthier, G.M. (1994). Eye-hand coordination in pointing at visual targets: Spatial and temporal analysis. *Experimental Brain Research, 99,* 507-523.

Westwood, D.A., & Goodale, M.A. (2003). Perceptual illusion and the real-time control of action. *Spatial Vision, 16,* 243-254.

Wilmut, K., Wann, J.P., & Brown J.H. (2006). How active gaze informs the hand in sequential pointing movements. *Experimental Brain Research, 175,* 654-666.

Woodworth, R.S. (1899). The accuracy of voluntary movement. *Psychological Review, Monograph Supplements, 3*(13), 1-119.

CHAPTER 11

Alusi, S.H., Glickman, S., Aziz, T.Z., & Bain, P.G. (1999). Tremor in multiple sclerosis. *Journal of Neurology, Neurosurgery, and Psychiatry, 66,* 131-134.

Alusi, S.H., Worthington, J., Glickman, S., & Bain, P.G. (2001). A study of tremor in multiple sclerosis. *Brain, 124,* 720-730.

Armstrong, R.A. (1999). Multiple sclerosis and the eye. *Ophthalmic and Physiological Optics, 19,* S32-42.

Averbuch-Heller, L., & Leigh, R.J. (1996). Eye movements. *Current Opinion in Neurology, 9,* 26-31.

Averbuch-Heller, L. (2001). Supranuclear control of ocular motility. *Ophthalmology Clinics of North America, 14,* 187-204.

Bastian, A.J., & Thach, W.T. (1995). Cerebellar outflow lesions: A comparison of movement deficits resulting from lesions at the levels of the cerebellum and thalamus. *Annals of Neurology, 38,* 881-892.

Bogousslavsky, J., Fox, A.J., Carey, L.S., Vinitski, S., Bass, B., Noseworthy, J.H., Ebers, G.C., & Barnett, H.J. (1986). Correlates of brain-stem oculomotor disorders in multiple sclerosis. *Archives of Neurology, 43,* 460-463.

Bonnefoi-Kyriacou, B., Legallet, E., Lee, R.G., & Trouche, E. (1998). Spatio-temporal and kinematic analysis of pointing movements performed by cerebellar patients with limb ataxia. *Experimental Brain Research, 119,* 460-466.

Brown, R.G., & Marsden, C.D. (1988). Internal versus external cues and the control of attention in Parkinson's disease. *Brain, 111,* 323-345.

Brown, S.H., Kessler, K.R., Hefter, H., Cooke, J.D., & Freund, H.J. (1993). Role of the cerebellum in visuomotor coordination. I. Delayed eye and arm initiation in patients with mild cerebellar ataxia. *Experimental Brain Research, 94,* 478-488.

Buekers, M.J., & Helsen, W.F. (2000). Vision and laterality: Does occlusion disclose a feedback processing advantage for the right hand system? *Cortex, 36,* 507-519.

Carnahan, H., & Marteniuk, R.G. (1991). The temporal organization of hand, eye, and head movements during reaching and pointing. *Journal of Motor Behavior, 23,* 109-119.

Clanet, M.G., & Brassat, D. (2000). The management of multiple sclerosis patients. *Current Opinion in Neurology, 13,* 263-270.

Cody, F., Lovgreen, B., & Schady, W. (1993). Increased dependence upon visual information of movement performance during visuo-motor tracking in cerebellar disorders. *Electroencephalography and Clinical Neurophysiology, 89,* 399-407.

Crammond, D.J. (1997). Motor imagery: Never in your wildest dream. *Trends in Neurosciences, 20,* 54-57.

Crowdy, K.A., Hollands, M.A., Ferguson, I.T., & Marple-Horvat, D.E. (2000). Evidence for interactive locomotor and oculomotor deficits in cerebellar patients during visually guided stepping. *Experimental Brain Research, 135,* 437-454.

Crowdy, K.A., Kaur-Mann, D., Cooper, H.L., Mansfield, A.G., Offord, J.L., & Marple-Horvat, D.E. (2002). Rehearsal by eye movement improves visuomotor performance in cerebellar patients. *Experimental Brain Research, 146,* 244-247.

Danckert, J., Ferber, S., Doherty, T., Steinmetz, H., Nicolle, D., & Goodale, M.A. (2002). Selective, non-lateralized impairment of motor imagery following right parietal damage. *Neurocase, 8,* 194-204.

Day, B.L., Thompson, P.D., Harding, A.E., & Marsden, C.D. (1998). Influence of vision on upper limb reaching movements in patients with cerebellar ataxia. *Brain, 121,* 357-372.

De'Sperati, C. (2003). Precise oculomotor correlates of visuospatial mental rotation and circular motion imagery. *Journal of Cognitive Neuroscience, 15,* 1244-1259.

Debaere, F., Wenderoth, N., Sunaert, S., Van Hecke, P., & Swinnen, S.P. (2003). Internal vs external generation of movements: Differential neural pathways involved in bimanual coordination performed in the presence or absence of augmented visual feedback. *NeuroImage, 19,* 764-776.

Desmurget, M., Grea, H., Grethe, J.S., Prablanc, C., Alexander, G.E., & Grafton, S.T. (2001). Functional anatomy of nonvisual feedback loops during reaching: A positron emission tomography study. *Journal of Neuroscience, 21,* 2919-2928.

Deuschl, G., Bain, P., & Brin, M. (1998). Consensus statement of the Movement Disorder Society on Tremor. Ad Hoc Scientific Committee. *Movement Disorders, 13,* 2-23.

Deuschl, G., Raethjen, J., Lindemann, M., & Krack, P. (2001). The pathophysiology of tremor. *Muscle & Nerve, 24,* 716-735.

Deuschl, G., Wenzelburger, R., Loffler, K., Raethjen, J., & Stolze, H. (2000). Essential tremor and cerebellar dysfunction clinical and kinematic analysis of intention tremor. *Brain, 123,* 1568-1580.

Diener, H.C., & Dichgans, J. (1992). Pathophysiology of cerebellar ataxia. *Movement Disorders, 7,* 95-109.

Downey, D.L., Stahl, J.S., Bhidayasiri, R, Derwenskus, J., Adams, N.L., Ruff, R.L., & Leigh, R.J. (2002). Saccadic and vestibular abnormalities in multiple sclerosis: Sensitive clinical signs of brainstem and cerebellar involvement. *Annals of the New York Academy of Sciences, 956,* 438-440.

Eggenberger, E. (1996). Neuro-ophthalmology of multiple sclerosis. *Current Opinion in Ophthalmology, 7*, 19-29.

Elliott, D., Binsted, G., & Heath, M. (1999). The control of goal-directed limb movements: Correcting errors in the trajectory. *Human Movement Science, 18*, 121-136.

Elliott, D., Helsen, W.F., & Chua, R. (2001). A century later: Woodworth's (1899) two-component model of goal-directed aiming. *Psychological Bulletin, 127*, 342-357.

Elliott, D. (1992). Intermittent versus continuous control of manual aiming movements. In L. Proteau & D. Elliott (Eds.), *Vision and motor control* (pp. 33-48). Amsterdam: Elsevier.

Feys, P., Helsen, W., Buekers, M., Ceux, T., Heremans, E., Nuttin, B., Ketelaer, P., & Liu, X. (2006). The effect of changed visual feedback on intention tremor in multiple sclerosis. *Neuroscience Letters, 394*, 17-21.

Feys, P., Helsen, W., Liu, X., Nuttin, B., Lavrysen, A., Swinnen, S.P., & Ketelaer, P. (2005). Interaction between eye and hand movements in MS patients with intention tremor. *Movement Disorders, 20*, 705-713.

Feys, P., Helsen, W., Nuttin, B., Lavrysen, A., Ketelaer, P., Swinnen, S.P., & Liu, X. (2008). Unsteady gaze fixation enhances the severity of MS intention tremor. *Neurology, 70*, 106-113.

Feys, P., Helsen, W.F., Lavrysen, A., Nuttin, B., & Ketelaer, P. (2003). Intention tremor during manual aiming: A study of eye and hand movements. *Multiple Sclerosis, 9*, 44-54.

Feys, P., Helsen, W.F., Liu, X., Lavrysen, A., Loontjes, V., Nuttin, B., & Ketelaer, P. (2003). Effect of visual information on step-tracking movements in patients with intention tremor due to multiple sclerosis. *Multiple Sclerosis, 9*, 492-502.

Feys, P., Helsen, W.F., Verschueren, S., Swinnen, S.P., Klok, I., Lavrysen, A., Nuttin, B., Ketelaer, P., & Liu, X. (2006). Online movement control in multiple sclerosis patients with tremor: Effects of tendon vibration. *Movement Disorders, 21*, 1148-1153.

Feys, P., Maes, F., Nuttin, B., Helsen, W.F., Malfait, V., Nagels, G., Lavrysen, A., & Liu, X. (2005). Relationship between multiple sclerosis intention tremor severity and lesion load in the brainstem. *Neuroreport, 16*, 1379-1382.

Frak, V., Cohen, H., & Pourcher, E. (2004). A dissociation between real and simulated movements in Parkinson's disease. *Neuroreport, 15*, 1489-1492.

Gao, J.H., Parsons, L.M., Bower, J.M., Xiong, J., Li, J., & Fox, P.T. (1996). Cerebellum implicated in sensory acquisition and discrimination rather than motor control. *Science, 272*, 545-547.

Gerardin, E., Sirigu, A., Lehéricy, S., Poline, J.B., Gaymard, B., Marsault, C., Agid, Y., & Le Bihan, D. (2000). Partially overlapping neural networks for real and imagined hand movements. *Cerebral Cortex, 10*, 1093-1104.

Glickstein, M. (2000). How are visual areas of the brain connected to motor areas for the sensory guidance of the movement? *Trends in Cognitive Sciences, 23*, 613-617.

Grill, S.E., Hallett, M., Marcus, C., & McShane, L. (1994). Disturbances of kinaesthesia in patients with cerebellar disorders. *Brain, 117*, 1433-1447.

Grill, S.E., Hallett, M., & McShane, L.M. (1997). Timing of onset of afferent responses and of use of kinesthetic information for control of movement in normal and cerebellar-impaired subjects. *Experimental Brain Research, 113*, 33-47.

Helsen, W.F., Elliott, D., Starkes, J.L., & Ricker, K.L. (2000). Coupling of eye, finger, elbow, and shoulder movements during manual aiming. *Journal of Motor Behavior, 32*, 241-248.

Helsen, W.F., Elliott, D., Starkes, J.L., & Ricker, K.L. (1998a). Temporal and spatial coupling of point of gaze and hand movements in aiming. *Journal of Motor Behavior, 30*, 249-259.

Helsen, W.F., Starkes, J.L., & Buekers, M.J. (1997). Effects of target eccentricity on temporal costs of point of gaze and the hand in aiming. *Motor Control, 1*, 161-177.

Helsen, W.F, Starkes, J.L., Elliott, D., & Buekers, M.J. (1998). Manual asymmetries and saccadic eye movements in right-handers during single and reciprocal aiming movements. *Cortex, 34*, 513-529.

Helsen, W.F., Starkes, J.L., Elliott, D., & Ricker, K.L. (1998b). Sampling frequency and the study of eye-hand coordination in aiming. *Behavior Research Methods, Instruments, & Computers, 30*, 617-623.

Helsen, W.F., Tremblay, L., Van den Berg, M., & Elliott, D. (2004). The role of oculomotor information in the learning of sequential aiming movements. *Journal of Motor Behavior, 36,* 82-90.

Heremans, E., Helsen, W.F., De Poel, H.J., Alaerts, K., Meyns, P., Feys, P. (2009). Facilitation of motor imagery through movement-related cueing. *Brain Research, 1278,* 50-58.

Heremans, E., Helsen, W.F., & Feys, P. (2008). The eyes as a mirror of our thoughts: Quantification of motor imagery through eye movement registration. *Behavioural Brain Research, 187,* 351-360.

Hore, J., Wild, B., & Diener, H.C. (1991). Cerebellar dysmetria at the elbow, wrist, and fingers. *Journal of Neurophysiology, 65,* 563-571.

Hotson, J.R. (1982). Cerebellar control of fixation eye movements. *Neurology, 32,* 31-36.

Huettel, S.A., Song, A.W., & McCarthy, G. (2004). Functional magnetic resonance imaging. Sunderland, MA: Sinauer Associates.

Jackson, P.L., Lafleur, M.F., Malouin, F., Richards, C., & Doyon, J. (2001). Potential role of mental practice using motor imagery in neurologic rehabilitation. *Archives of Physical Medicine and Rehabilitation, 82,* 1133-1141.

Johnson, S.H., Sprehn, G., & Saykin, A.J. (2002). Intact motor imagery in chronic upper limb hemiplegics: Evidence for activity-independent action representations. *Journal of Cognitive Neuroscience, 14,* 841-852.

Jueptner, M., Ottinger, S., Fellows, S.J., Adamschewski, J., Flerich, L., Müller, S.P., Diener, H.C., Thilmann, A.F., & Weiller, C. (1997). The relevance of sensory input for the cerebellar control of movements. *NeuroImage, 5,* 41-48.

Lavrysen, A. (2005). *The role of visual afferences in goal-directed upper limb movements: Control and learning issues.* Unpublished doctoral dissertation, Katholieke Universiteit Leuven, Leuven, Belgium.

Lavrysen, A., Elliott, D., Buekers, M.J., Feys, P., & Helsen, W.F. (2007). Eye-hand coordination asymmetries in manual aiming. *Journal of Motor Behavior, 39,* 9-18.

Lavrysen, A., Helsen, W.F., Elliott, D., Buekers, M.J., Feys, P., & Heremans, E. (2006). The type of visual information mediates eye and hand movement bias when aiming to a Muller-Lyer illusion. *Experimental Brain Research, 174,* 544-554.

Lavrysen, A., Heremans, E., Peeters, R., Wenderoth, N., Helsen, W.F., Feys, P., & Swinnen, S.P. (2008). Hemispheric asymmetries in eye-hand coordination. *NeuroImage, 39,* 1938-1949.

Li, C.R. (2000). Impairment of motor imagery in putamen lesions in humans. *Neuroscience Letters, 287,* 13-16.

Liu, X., Ingram, H.A., Palace, J.A., & Miall, R.C. (1999). Dissociation of 'on-line' and 'off-line' visuomotor control of the arm by focal lesions in the cerebellum and brainstem. *Neuroscience Letters, 264,* 121-124.

Liu, X., Miall, C., Aziz, T.Z., Palace, J.A., Haggard, P.N., & Stein, J.F. (1997). Analysis of action tremor and impaired control of movement velocity in multiple sclerosis during visually guided wrist-tracking tasks. *Movement Disorders, 12,* 992-999.

Liu, X., Robertson, E., & Miall, R.C. (2003). Neuronal activity related to the visual representation of arm movements in the lateral cerebellar cortex. *Journal of Neurophysiology, 89,* 1223-1237.

Lopez, L.I., Bronstein, A.M., Gresty, M.A., Du Boulay, E.P., & Rudge, P. (1996). Clinical and MRI correlates in 27 patients with acquired pendular nystagmus. *Brain, 119,* 465-472.

Maschke, M., Gomez, C.M., Tuite, P.J., & Konczak, J. (2003). Dysfunction of the basal ganglia, but not the cerebellum, impairs kinaesthesia. *Brain, 126,* 2312-2322.

Meister, I.G., Krings, T., Foltys, H., Boroojerdi, B., Muller, M., Topper, R., & Thron, A. (2004). Playing piano in the mind—an fMRI study on music imagery and performance in pianists. *Brain Research. Cognitive Brain Research, 19,* 219-228.

Miall, R.C., & Jenkinson, E.W. (2005). Functional imaging of changes in cerebellar activity related to learning during a novel eye-hand tracking task. *Experimental Brain Research, 166,* 170-183.

Miall, R.C., Reckess, G.Z., & Imamizu, H. (2001). The cerebellum coordinates eye and hand tracking movements. *Nature Neuroscience, 4,* 638-644.

Miall, R.C., Weir, D.J, Wolpert, D.M., & Stein, J.F. (1993). Is the cerebellum a Smith predictor? *Journal of Motor Behavior, 25,* 203-216.

Mieschke, P.E., Elliott, D., Helsen, W.F., Carson, R.G., & Coull, J.A. (2001). Manual asymmetries in the preparation and control of goal-directed movements. *Brain and Cognition, 45,* 129-140.

Murphy, S.M. (1994). Imagery interventions in sport. *Medicine and Science in Sports and Exercise, 26,* 486-494.

Nakashima, I., Fujihara, K., Okita, N., Takase, S., & Itoyama, Y. (1999). Clinical and MRI study of brain stem and cerebellar involvement in Japanese patients with multiple sclerosis. *Journal of Neurology, Neurosurgery, and Psychiatry, 67,* 153-157.

Neggers, S.F., & Bekkering, H. (2000). Ocular gaze is anchored to the target of an ongoing pointing movement. *Journal of Neurophysiology, 83,* 639-651.

Pittock, S.J., McClelland, R.L., Mayr, W.T., Rodriguez, M., & Matsumoto, J.Y. (2004). Prevalence of tremor in multiple sclerosis and associated disability in the Olmsted County population. *Movement Disorders, 19,* 1482-1485.

Proteau, L., & Elliott, D. (1992). *Vision and motor control.* Amsterdam: Elsevier.

Quintern, J., Immisch, I., Albrecht, H., Pollmann, W., Glasauer, S., & Straube, A. (1999). Influence of visual and proprioceptive afferences on upper limb ataxia in patients with multiple sclerosis. *Journal of the Neurological Sciences, 163,* 61-69.

Rand, M.K., Shimansky, Y., Stelmach, G.E., Bracha, V., & Bloedel, J.R. (2000). Effects of accuracy constraints on reach-to-grasp movements in cerebellar patients. *Experimental Brain Research, 135,* 179-188.

Rogers, R.G. (2006). Mental practice and acquisition of motor skills: Examples from sports training and surgical education. *Obstetrics and Gynecology Clinics of North America, 33,* 297-304.

Sailer, U., Eggert, T., & Straube, A. (2005). Impaired temporal prediction and eye-hand coordination in patients with cerebellar lesions. *Behavioral Brain Research, 160,* 72-87.

Serra, A., Derwenskus, J., Downey, D.L., & Leigh, R.J. (2003). Role of eye movement examination and subjective visual vertical in clinical evaluation of multiple sclerosis. *Journal of Neurology, 250,* 569-575.

Siegert, R.J., Harper, D.N., Cameron, F.B., Abernethy, D. (2002). Self-initiated versus externally cued reaction times in Parkinson's disease. *Journal of Clinical & Experimental Neuropsychology, 24,* 146-153.

Sharma, N., Pomeroy, V.M., & Baron, J.C. (2006). Motor imagery: A backdoor to the motor system after stroke? *Stroke, 37,* 1941-1952.

Shimansky, Y., Saling, M., Wunderlich, D.A., Bracha, V., Stelmach, G.E., & Bloedel, J.R. (1997). Impaired capacity of cerebellar patients to perceive and learn two-dimensional shapes based on kinesthetic cues. *Learning & Memory, 4,* 36-48.

Starkes, J., Helsen, W., & Elliott, D. (2002). A menage a trois: The eye, the hand and on-line processing. *Journal of Sports Sciences, 20,* 217-224.

Stein, J.F., & Glickstein, M. (1992). Role of the cerebellum in visual guidance of movement. *Physiological Reviews, 72,* 967-1017.

Tamir, R., Dickstein, R., & Huberman, M. (2007). Integration of motor imagery and physical practice in group treatment applied to subjects with Parkinson's disease. *Neurorehabilitation and Neural Repair, 21,* 68-75.

Topka, H., Konczak, J., & Dichgans, J. (1998). Coordination of multi-joint arm movements in cerebellar ataxia: Analysis of hand and angular kinematics. *Experimental Brain Research, 119,* 483-492.

Van Donkelaar, P., & Lee, R.G. (1994). Interactions between the eye and hand motor systems: Disruptions due to cerebellar dysfunction. *Journal of Neurophysiology, 72,* 1674-1685.

Vercher, J.L., Magenes, G., Prablanc, C., & Gauthier, G.M. (1994). Eye-head-hand coordination in pointing at visual targets: Spatial and temporal analysis. *Experimental Brain Research, 99,* 507-523.

Verschueren, S.M., Cordo, P.J., & Swinnen, S.P. (1998). Representation of wrist joint kinematics by the ensemble of muscle spindles from synergistic muscles. *Journal of Neurophysiology, 79,* 2265-2276.

Versino, M., Hurko, O., & Zee, D.S. (1996). Disorders of binocular control of eye movements in patients with cerebellar dysfunction. *Brain, 119,* 1933-1950.

Wolpert, D.M., Miall, R.C., & Kawato, M. (1998). Internal models in the cerebellum. *Trends in Cognitive Sciences, 2,* 338-347.

Woodworth, R.S. (1899). The accuracy of voluntary movement. *Psychological Review, Monograph Supplements, 3*(13), 1-119.

CHAPTER 12

Amunts, K., Schlaug, G., Schleicher, A., Steinmetz, H., Dabringhaus, A., Roland, P.E., & Zilles, K (1996). Asymmetry in the human motor cortex and handedness. *NeuroImage, 4*(3, Pt. 1), 216-222.

Annett, J., Annett, M., & Hudson, P.T.W. (1979). The control of movement in the preferred and non-preferred hands. *Quarterly Journal of Experimental Psychology, 31,* 641-652.

Annett, M. (2003). Cerebral asymmetry in twins: Predictions of the right shift theory. *Neuropsychologia, 41,* 469-479.

Anzola, G.P. (1980). Effect of unilateral right hemisphere lesions upon recognition of faces tachistoscopically presented to the left hemisphere. *Bollettino della Società Italiana di Biologia Sperimentale, 56,* 1433-1439.

Bagesteiro, L.B., & Sainburg, R.L. (2002). Handedness: Dominant arm advantages in control of limb dynamics. *Journal of Neurophysiology, 88,* 2408-2421.

Bagesteiro, L.B., & Sainburg, R.L. (2003). Nondominant arm advantages in load compensation during rapid elbow joint movements. *Journal of Neurophysiology, 90,* 1503-1513.

Bagesteiro, L.B., & Sainburg, R.L. (2005). Interlimb transfer of load compensation during rapid elbow joint movements. *Experimental Brain Research, 161,* 155-165.

Blackburn, A., & Knusel, C.J. (2006). Hand dominance and bilateral asymmetry of the epicondylar breadth of the humerus—a test in a living sample. *Current Anthropology, 47,* 377-382.

Boles, D.B., & Karner, T.A. (1996). Hemispheric differences in global versus local processing: Still unclear. *Brain and Cognition, 30,* 232-243.

Bowers D., Bauer R.M., Coslett H.B., & Heilman, K.M.. (1985). Processing of faces by patients with unilateral hemisphere lesions. I. Dissociation between judgments of facial affect and facial identity. *Brain and Cognition, 4,* 258-72.

Brinkman, J., Kuypers, H.G., & Lawrence, D.G. (1970). Ipsilateral and contralateral eye-hand control in split-brain rhesus monkeys. *Brain Research, 24,* 559.

Buonomano, D.V., & Merzenich, M.M. (1998). Cortical plasticity: From synapses to maps. *Annual Review of Neuroscience, 21,* 149-186.

Carey, J.R., Baxter, T.L., & Di Fabio, R.P. (1998). Tracking control in the nonparetic hand of subjects with stroke. *Archives of Physical Medicine and Rehabilitation, 79,* 435-441.

Carson, R.G. (1993). Manual asymmetries: Old problems and new directions. *Human Movement Science, 12,* 479-506.

Carson, R.G., Chua, R., Elliott, D., & Goodman, D. (1990). The contribution of vision to asymmetries in manual aiming. *Neuropsychologia, 28,* 1215-1220.

Cauraugh, J.H., & Summers, J.J. (2005). Neural plasticity and bilateral movements: A rehabilitation approach for chronic stroke. *Progress in Neurobiology, 75,* 309-320.

Chen, A.C., German, C., & Zaidel, D.W. (1997). Brain asymmetry and facial attractiveness: Facial beauty is not simply in the eye of the beholder. *Neuropsychologia, 35,* 471-476.

Chua, R., Carson, R.G., Goodman, D., & Elliott, D. (1992). Asymmetries in the spatial localization of transformed targets. *Brain and Cognition, 20,* 227-235.

Corballis, M.C. (1983). *Human laterality.* London: Academic Press.

Corballis, M.C. (1997). The genetics and evolution of handedness. *Psychological Review, 104,* 714-727.

Corballis, M.C. (2003). From mouth to hand: Gesture, speech, and the evolution of right-handedness. *Behavioral and Brain Sciences, 26,* 199-208.

Dassonville, P., Zhu, X.H., Uurbil, K., Kim, S.G., & Ashe, J. (1997). Functional activation in motor cortex reflects the direction and the degree of handedness. *Proceedings of the National Academy of Sciences of the United States of America, 94*(25), 14015-14018.

Derakhshan, I. (2004). Hugo Liepmann revisited, this time with numbers. *Journal of Neurophysiology, 91*, 2.

Desrosiers, J., Bourbonnais, D., Bravo, G., Roy, P.M., & Guay, M. (1996). Performance of the 'unaffected' upper extremity of elderly stroke patients. *Stroke, 27*, 1564-1570.

Domkin, D., Laczko, J., Jaric, S., Johansson, H., & Latash, M.L. (2002). Structure of joint variability in bimanual pointing tasks. *Experimental Brain Research, 143*, 11-23.

Duff, S.V., & Sainburg, R.L. (2007). Lateralization of motor adaptation reveals independence in control of trajectory and steady-state position. *Experimental Brain Research, 179*, 551-561.

Elliott, D., Lyons, J., Chua, R., Goodman, D., & Carson, R.G. (1995). The influence of target perturbation on manual aiming asymmetries in right-handers. *Cortex, 31*, 685-697.

Elliott, D., Roy, E. A., Goodman, D., Carson, R. G., Chua, R., & Maraj, B. K. V. (1993). Asymmetries in the preparation and control of manual aiming movements. *Canadian Journal of Experimental Psychology, 47*, 570-589.

Fitts, P.M. (1954). The information capacity of the human motor system in controlling the amplitude of movement. *Journal of Experimental Psychology, 47*, 381-391.

Fitts, P.M. (1966). Cognitive aspects of information processing. 3. Set for speed versus accuracy. *Journal of Experimental Psycholology, 71*, 849-857.

Fitts, P.M., & Radford, B.K. (1966). Information capacity of discrete motor responses under different cognitive sets. *Journal of Experimental Psychology, 71*, 475-482.

Flowers, K. (1975). Handedness and controlled movement. *British Journal of Psychology, 66*, 39-52.

Francks, C., Maegawa, S., Lauren, J., Abrahams, B. S., Velayos-Baeza, A., Medland, S. E., Colella, S., Groszer, M., McAuley, E. Z., Caffrey, T. M., Timmusk, T., Pruunsild, P., Koppel, I., Lind, P. A., Matsumoto-Itaba, N., Nicod, J., Xiong, L., Joober, R., Enard, W., Krinsky, B., Nanba, E., Richardson, A. J., Riley, B. P., Martin, N. G., Strittmatter, S. M., Moller, H. J., Rujescu, D., St Clair, D., Muglia, P. & Roos, J. L. (2007). LRRTM1 on chromosome 2p12 is a maternally suppressed gene that is associated paternally with handedness and schizophrenia. *Molecular Psychiatry, 12*, 1129-1139.

Friel, K.M., Drew, T., & Martin, J.H. (2007). Differential activity-dependent development of corticospinal control of movement and final limb position during visually guided locomotion. *Journal of Neurophysiology, 97*, 3396-3406.

Friel, K.M., & Martin, J.H. (2005). Role of sensory-motor cortex activity in postnatal development of corticospinal axon terminals in the cat. *Journal of Comparative Neurology, 485*, 43-56.

Gazzaniga, M.S. (1998). The split brain revisited. *Scientific American, 279*, 50-55.

Gentilucci, M., & Corballis, M.C. (2006). From manual gesture to speech: A gradual transition. *Neuroscience and Biobehavioral Reviews, 30*, 949-960.

Geschwind, N. (1975). The apraxias: Neural mechanisms of disorders of learned movement. *American Scientist, 63*(2), 188-195.

Ghez, C., Gordon, J., Ghilardi, M.F., Christakos, C.N., & Cooper, S.E. (1990). Roles of proprioceptive input in the programming of arm trajectories. *Cold Spring Harbor Symposia on Quantitative Biology, 55*, 837-847.

Ghez, C., & Sainburg, R. (1995). Proprioceptive control of interjoint coordination. *Canadian Journal of Physiology and Pharmacology, 73*, 273-284.

Gitelman, D.R., Alpert, N.M., Kosslyn S., Daffner, K., Scinto,L., Thompson, W., & Mesulam, M. (1996). Functional imaging of human right hemispheric activation for exploratory movements. *Annals of Neurology, 39*, 174-179.

Gonzalez, C.L., Gharbawie, O.A., Williams, P.T., Kleim, J.A., Kolb, B., & Whishaw, I.Q. (2004). Evidence for bilateral control of skilled movements: Ipsilateral skilled forelimb reaching deficits and functional recovery in rats follow motor cortex and lateral frontal cortex lesions. *European Journal of Neuroscience, 20*, 3442-3452.

Grabowski, M., Brundin, P., & Johansson, B.B. (1993). Paw-reaching, sensorimotor, and rotational behavior after brain infarction in rats. *Stroke, 24,* 889-895.

Gribble, P.L., & Ostry, D.J. (1999). Compensation for interaction torques during single- and multijoint limb movement. *Journal of Neurophysiology, 82,* 2310-2326.

Grimshaw, G.M. (1998). Integration and interference in the cerebral hemispheres: Relations with hemispheric specialization. *Brain and Cognition, 36,* 108-127.

Haaland, K.Y., Cleeland, C.S., & Carr, D. (1977). Motor performance after unilateral hemisphere damage in patients with tumor. *Archives of Neurology, 34,* 556-559.

Haaland, K.Y., & Delaney, H.D. (1981). Motor deficits after left or right hemisphere damage due to stroke or tumor. *Neuropsychologia, 19,* 17-27.

Haaland, K.Y., & Harrington, D.L. (1996). Hemispheric asymmetry of movement. *Current Opinion in Neurobiology, 6,* 796-800.

Haaland, K.Y., Prestopnik, J.L., Knight, R.T., & Lee, R.R. (2004). Hemispheric asymmetries for kinematic and positional aspects of reaching. *Brain, 127*(Pt. 5), 1145-1158.

Haaland, K.Y., Temkin, N., Randahl, G., & Dikmen, S. (1994). Recovery of simple motor skills after head injury. *Journal of Clinical and Experimental Neuropsychology, 16,* 448-456.

Haridas, C., & Zehr, E.P. (2003). Coordinated interlimb compensatory responses to electrical stimulation of cutaneous nerves in the hand and foot during walking. *Journal of Neurophysiology, 90,* 2850-2861.

Harrington, D.L., & Haaland, K.Y. (1991). Hemispheric specialization for motor sequencing: Abnormalities in levels of programming. *Neuropsychologia, 29,* 147-163.

Harris-Love, M.L., McCombe Waller, S., & Whitall, J. (2005). Exploiting interlimb coupling to improve paretic arm reaching performance in people with chronic stroke. *Archives of Physical Medicine and Rehabilitation, 86,* 2131-2137.

Hasan, Z. (1986). Optimized movement trajectories and joint stiffness in unperturbed, inertially loaded movements. *Biological Cybernetics, 53,* 373-382.

Hauser, M.D. (1993). Right hemisphere dominance for the production of facial expression in monkeys. *Science, 261*(5120), 475-477.

Heilman, K.M., Bowers, D., Valenstein, E., & Watson, R.T. (1986). The right hemisphere: neuropsychological functions. *Journal of Neurosurgery, 64,* 693-704.

Hellige, J.B. (1996). Hemispheric asymmetry for visual information processing. *Acta Neurobiologiae Experimentalis, 56,* 485-497.

Holstege, J.C., & Kuypers, H.G. (1982). Brain stem projections to spinal motoneuronal cell groups in rat studied by means of electron microscopy autoradiography. *Progress in Brain Research, 57,* 177-183.

Hopkins, W.D. (2006). Chimpanzee right-handedness: Internal and external validity in the assessment of hand use. *Cortex, 42,* 90-93.

Hopkins, W.D., Russell, J.L., Cantalupo, C., Freeman, H., & Schapiro, S.J. (2005). Factors influencing the prevalence and handedness for throwing in captive chimpanzees (Pan troglodytes). *Journal of Comparative Psychology, 119,* 363-370.

Hopkins, W.D., Stoinski, T.S., Lukas, K.E., Ross, S.R., & Wesley, M.J. (2003). Comparative assessment of handedness for a coordinated bimanual task in chimpanzees (Pan troglodytes), gorillas (Gorilla gorilla) and orangutans (Pongo pygmaeus). *Journal of Comparative Psychology, 117,* 302-308.

Hunt, A.L., Orrison, W.W., Yeo, R.A., Haaland , K.Y., Rhyne, R.L., Garry, P.J., & Rosenberg, G.A. (1989). Clinical significance of MRI white matter lesions in the elderly. *Neurology, 39,* 1470-1474.

Jansen, A., Lohmann, H., Scharfe, S., Sehlmeyer, C., Deppe, M., & Knecht, S. (2007). The association between scalp hair-whorl direction, handedness and hemispheric language dominance: Is there a common genetic basis of lateralization? *NeuroImage, 35,* 853-861.

Kawashima, R., Roland, P.E., & O'Sullivan, B.T. (1994). Activity in the human primary motor cortex related to ipsilateral hand movements. *Brain Research, 663,* 251-256.

Kelso, J.A., Southard, D.L., & Goodman, D. (1979a). On the coordination of two-handed movements. *Journal of Experimental Psychology: Human Perception and Performance, 5,* 229-238.

Kelso, J.A., Southard, D.L., & Goodman, D. (1979b). On the nature of human interlimb coordination. *Science, 203*(4384), 1029-1031.

Kim, S.G., Ashe, J., Hendrich, K., Ellermann, J.M., Merkle, H., Uğurbil, K., & Georgopoulos, A.P.. (1993). Functional magnetic resonance imaging of motor cortex: Hemispheric asymmetry and handedness. *Science, 261*(5121), 615-617.

Kimura, T., Haggard, P., & Gomi, H. (2006). Transcranial magnetic stimulation over sensorimotor cortex disrupts anticipatory reflex gain modulation for skilled action. *Journal of Neuroscience, 26*, 9272-9281.

Klar, A.J. (1999). Genetic models for handedness, brain lateralization, schizophrenia, and manic-depression. *Schizophrenia Research, 39*, 207-218.

Klar, A.J. (2003). Human handedness and scalp hair-whorl direction develop from a common genetic mechanism. *Genetics, 165*, 269-276.

Kooistra, C.A., & Heilman, K.M. (1988). Motor dominance and lateral asymmetry of the globus pallidus. *Neurology, 38*, 388-390.

Kutas, M., & Donchin, E. (1974). Studies of squeezing: Handedness, responding hand, response force, and asymmetry of readiness potential. *Science, 186*(4163), 545-548.

Kuypers, H.G. (1982). A new look at the organization of the motor system. *Progress in Brain Research, 57*, 381-403.

Kuypers, H.G.M.J., & Laurence, D.G. (1967). Cortical projections to the red nucleus and the brain stem in the rhesus monkey. *Brain Research, 4*, 151-188.

Kuypers, H.G.M.J., Fleming, W.R., & Farinholt, J.W. (1962). Subcorticospinal projections in the rhesus monkey. *Journal of Comparative Neurology, 118*, 107-137.

Kuypers, H.G.M.J., & Maisky, V.A. (1975). Retrograde axonal transport of horseradish peroxidase from spinal cord to brain stem cell groups in the cat. *Neuroscience Letters, 1*, 9-14.

Lacquaniti, F., Carrozzo, M., & Borghese, N.A. (1993). Time-varying mechanical behavior of multi-jointed arm in man. *Journal of Neurophysiolology, 69*, 1443-1464.

Lawrence, D.G., & Kuypers, H.G. (1968). The functional organization of the motor system in the monkey. I. The effects of bilateral pyramidal lesions. *Brain, 91*, 1-14.

Levy, J. (1977). A reply to Hudson regarding the Levy-Nagylaki model for the genetics of handedness. *Neuropsychologia, 15*, 187-190.

Levy, J., & Nagylaki, T. (1972). A model for the genetics of handedness. *Genetics, 72*, 117-128.

Liepmann, H. (1905). Die linke Hemisphäre und das Handeln. *Münchener Medizinische Wochenschrift, 49*, 2375-2378.

Liu, D., & Todorov, E. (2007). Evidence for the flexible sensorimotor strategies predicted by optimal feedback control. *Journal of Neuroscience, 27*, 9354-9368.

Lonsdorf, E.V., & Hopkins, W.D. (2005). Wild chimpanzees show population-level handedness for tool use. *Proceedings of the National Academy of Sciences of the United States of America, 102*(35), 12634-12638.

Loring, D.W., Meador, K.J., Lee, G.P., Murro, A.M., Smith, J.R., Flanigin, H.F., Gallagher, B.B., & King, D.W. (1990). Cerebral language lateralization: Evidence from intracarotid amobarbital testing. *Neuropsychologia, 28*, 831-838.

Macdonell, R.A., Shapiro, B.E., Chiappa, K.H., Helmers, S.L., Cros, D., Day, B.J., & Shahani, B.T. (1991). Hemispheric threshold differences for motor evoked potentials produced by magnetic coil stimulation. *Neurology, 41*, 1441-1444.

Martin, J.H. (2005). The corticospinal system: From development to motor control. *Neuroscientist, 11*, 161-173.

Martin, J.H., Friel, K.M., Salimi, I., & Chakrabarty, S. (2007). Activity- and use-dependent plasticity of the developing corticospinal system. *Neuroscience and Biobehavior Reviews, 31*, 1125-1135.

Marzke, M.W. (1971). Origin of the human hand. *American Journal of Physical Anthropology, 34*, 61-84.

Marzke, M.W. (1988). Man's hand in evolution. *Journal of Hand Surgery (Edinburgh, Scotland), 13*, 229-230.

Marzke, M.W. (1997). Precision grips, hand morphology, and tools. *American Journal of Physical Anthropology, 102,* 91-110.

McManus, I.C. (1985). Handedness, language dominance and aphasia: A genetic model. *Psychological Medicine Monograph Supplement, 8,* 1-40.

Medland, S.E., Perelle, I., De Monte, V., & Ehrman, L. (2004). Effects of culture, sex, and age on the distribution of handedness: An evaluation of the sensitivity of three measures of handedness. *Laterality, 9,* 287-297.

Mieschke, P.E., Elliott, D., Helsen, W.F., Carson, R.G., & Coull, J.A. (2001). Manual asymmetries in the preparation and control of goal-directed movements. *Brain and Cognition, 45,* 129-140.

Nudo, R.J., Milliken, G.W., Jenkins, W.M., & Merzenich, M.M. (1996). Use-dependent alterations of movement representations in primary motor cortex of adult squirrel monkeys. *Journal of Neuroscience, 16,* 785-807.

Perelle, I.B., & Ehrman, L. (1983). The development of laterality. *Behavioral Science, 28,* 284-297.

Perelle, I.B., & Ehrman, L. (1994). An international study of human handedness: The data. *Behavioral Genetics, 24,* 217-227.

Perelle, I.B., & Ehrman, L. (2005). On the other hand. *Behavioral Genetics, 35,* 343-350.

Plamondon, R., & Alimi, A.M. (1997). Speed/accuracy trade-offs in target-directed movements. *Behavioral and Brain Sciences, 20,* 279-303.

Prestopnik, J., Haaland, K., Knight, R., & Lee, R. (2003). Hemispheric dominance in the parietal lobe for open and closed loop movements. *Journal of the International Neuropsychological Society, 9,* 1-2.

Prochazka, A. (1981). Muscle spindle function during normal movement. *International Review of Physiology, 25,* 47-90.

Pujol, J., Deus, J., Losilla, J.M., & Capdevila, A. (1999). Cerebral lateralization of language in normal left-handed people studied by functional MRI. *Neurology, 52,* 1038-1043.

Recanzone, G.H., Merzenich, M.M., Jenkins, W.M., Grajski, K.A., & Dinse, H.R. (1992). Topographic reorganization of the hand representation in cortical area 3b owl monkeys trained in a frequency-discrimination task. *Journal of Neurophysiology, 67,* 1031-1056.

Reeves, W.H. (1985). Concept formation, problem-solving and the right hemisphere. *International Journal of Neuroscience, 28,* 291-295.

Rogers, L., & Andrew, R. (2002). *Comparative vertebrate lateralization.* Cambridge, UK The Edinburgh Building, Cambridge CB2 2RU, UK): Cambridge University Press.

Roy, E.A., & Elliott, D. (1986). Manual asymmetries in visually directed aiming. *Canadian Journal of Psychology, 40,* 109-121.

Roy, E.A., Kalbfleisch, L., & Elliott, D. (1994). Kinematic analyses of manual asymmetries in visual aiming movements. *Brain and Cognition, 24,* 289-295.

Sainburg, R.L. (2002). Evidence for a dynamic-dominance hypothesis of handedness. *Experimental Brain Research, 142,* 241-258.

Sainburg, R.L. (2005). Handedness: Differential specializations for control of trajectory and position. *Exercise and Sport Sciences Reviews, 33,* 206-213.

Sainburg, R.L., Ghez, C., & Kalakanis, D. (1999). Intersegmental dynamics are controlled by sequential anticipatory, error correction, and postural mechanisms. *Journal of Neurophysiology, 81,* 1045-1056.

Sainburg, R.L., Ghilardi, M.F., Poizner, H., & Ghez, C. (1995). Control of limb dynamics in normal subjects and patients without proprioception. *Journal of Neurophysiology, 73,* 820-835.

Sainburg, R.L., & Kalakanis, D. (2000). Differences in control of limb dynamics during dominant and nondominant arm reaching. *Journal of Neurophysiology, 83,* 2661-2675.

Sainburg, R.L., Poizner, H., & Ghez, C. (1993). Loss of proprioception produces deficits in interjoint coordination. *Journal of Neurophysiology, 70,* 2136-2147.

Sainburg, R.L., & Schaefer, S.Y. (2004). Interlimb differences in control of movement extent. *Journal of Neurophysiology, 92,* 1374-1383.

Salmelin, R., Forss, N., Knuutila, J., & Hari, R. (1995). Bilateral activation of the human somatomotor cortex by distal hand movements. *Electroencephalography and Clinical Neurophysiology, 95,* 444-452.

Schabowsky, C.N., Hidler, J.M., & Lum, P.S. (2007). Greater reliance on impedance control in the nondominant arm compared with the dominant arm when adapting to a novel dynamic environment. *Experimental Brain Research, 182,* 567-577.

Schaefer, S.Y., Haaland, K.Y., & Sainburg, R.L. (2007). Ipsilesional motor deficits following stroke reflect hemispheric specializations for movement control. *Brain, 130*(Pt. 8), 2146-2158.

Scott, S.H. (2002). Optimal strategies for movement: Success with variability. *Nature Neuroscience, 5,* 1110-1111.

Scott, S.H. (2004). Optimal feedback control and the neural basis of volitional motor control. *Nature Reviews Neuroscience, 5,* 532-546.

Snyder, P.J., Bilder, R.M., Wu, H., Bogerts, B., & Lieberman, J.A. (1995). Cerebellar volume asymmetries are related to handedness: A quantitative MRI study. *Neuropsychologia, 33,* 407-419.

Sunderland, A. (2000). Recovery of ipsilateral dexterity after stroke. *Stroke, 31,* 430-433.

Swinnen, S.P., Jardin, K., Verschueren, S., Meulenbroek, R., Franz, L., Dounskaia, N., & Walter, C.B. (1998). Exploring interlimb constraints during bimanual graphic performance: Effects of muscle grouping and direction. *Behavioral Brain Research, 90,* 79-87.

Taniguchi, M., Yoshimine, T., Cheyne, D., Kato, A., Kihara, T., Ninomiya, H., Hirata M., Hirabuki, N., Nakamura, H., & Hayakawa, T. (1998). Neuromagnetic fields preceding unilateral movements in dextrals and sinistrals. *Neuroreport, 9,* 1497-1502.

Tanji, J., Okano, K., & Sato, K.C. (1988). Neuronal activity in cortical motor areas related to ipsilateral, contralateral, and bilateral digit movements of the monkey. *Journal of Neurophysiology, 60,* 325-343.

Todor, J.I., & Cisneros, J. (1985). Accommodation to increased accuracy demands by the right and left hands. *Journal of Motor Behavior, 17,* 355-372.

Todor, J.I., & Doane, T. (1977). Handedness classification: Preference versus proficiency. *Perceptual and Motor Skills, 45,* 1041-1042.

Todor, J.I., & Kyprie, P.M. (1980). Hand differences in the rate and variability of rapid tapping. *Journal of Motor Behavior, 12,* 57-62.

Todor, J.I., & Smiley-Oyen, A.L. (1987). Force modulation as a source of hand differences in rapid finger tapping. *Acta Psychologica, 65,* 65-73.

Todorov, E. (2004). Optimality principles in sensorimotor control. *Nature Neuroscience, 7,* 907-915.

Todorov, E., & Jordan, M.I. (2002). Optimal feedback control as a theory of motor coordination. *Nature Neuroscience, 5,* 1226-1235.

Todorov, E., Li, W.W., & Pan, X.C. (2005). From task parameters to motor synergies: A hierarchical framework for approximately optimal control of redundant manipulators. *Journal of Robotic Systems, 22,* 691-710.

Tompkins, C.A., & Flowers, C.R. (1985). Perception of emotional intonation by brain-damaged adults: The influence of task processing levels. *Journal of Speech and Hearing Research, 28,* 527-538.

Treffner, P.J., & Turvey, M.T. (1996). Symmetry, broken symmetry, and handedness in bimanual coordination dynamics. *Experimental Brain Research, 107,* 463-478.

Vallortigara, G., & Rogers, L.J. (2005). Survival with an asymmetrical brain: Advantages and disadvantages of cerebral lateralization. *Behavioral and Brain Sciences, 28,* 575-589.

Vauclair, J., Meguerditchian, A., & Hopkins, W.D. (2005). Hand preferences for unimanual and coordinated bimanual tasks in baboons (Papio anubis). *Brain Research. Cognitive Brain Research, 25,* 210-216.

Vergara-Aragon, P., Gonzalez, C.L., & Whishaw, I.Q. (2003). A novel skilled-reaching impairment in paw supination on the "good" side of the hemi-Parkinson rat improved with rehabilitation. *Journal of Neuroscience, 23,* 579-586.

Viviani, P., Perani, D., Grassi, F., Bettinardi, V., & Fazio, F. (1998). Hemispheric asymmetries and bimanual asynchrony in left- and right-handers. *Experimental Brain Research, 120,* 531-536.

Westergaard, G.C. (1993). Hand preference in the use of tools by infant baboons (Papio cynocephalus anubis). *Perceptual and Motor Skills, 76,* 447-450.

Wetter, S., Poole, J.L., & Haaland, K.Y. (2005). Functional implications of ipsilesional motor deficits after unilateral stroke. *Archives of Physical Medicine and Rehabilitation, 86,* 776-781.

Whitall, J., McCombe Waller, S., Silver, K.H., & Macko, R.F. (2000). Repetitive bilateral arm training with rhythmic auditory cueing improves motor function in chronic hemiparetic stroke. *Stroke, 31,* 2390-2395.

Winstein, C.J., & Pohl, P.S. (1995). Effects of unilateral brain damage on the control of goal-directed hand movements. *Experimental Brain Research, 105,* 163-174.

Wolman, D. (2005). *A left hand turn around the world.* Cambridge: Da Capo Press.

Woodworth, R.S. (1899). The accuracy of voluntary movement. *Psychological Review, Monograph Supplements, 3*(13), 1-119.

Wyke, M. (1967). Effect of brain lesions on the rapidity of arm movement. *Neurology, 17,* 1113-1120.

Yamamoto, C., & Ohtsuki, T. (1989). Modulation of stretch reflex by anticipation of the stimulus through visual information. *Experimental Brain Research, 77,* 12-22.

Yarosh, C.A., Hoffman, D.S., & Strick, P.L. (2004). Deficits in movements of the wrist ipsilateral to a stroke in hemiparetic subjects. *Journal of Neurophysiology, 92,* 3276-3285.

CHAPTER 13

Aglioti, S., DeSouza, J.F., & Goodale, M.A. (1995). Size-contrast illusions deceive the eye but not the hand. *Current Biology, 5,* 679-685.

Amazeen, E.L., & DaSilva, F. (2005). Psychophysical test for the independence of perception and action. *Journal of Experimental Psychology, 31,* 170-182.

Bernardis, P., Knox, P., & Bruno, N. (2005). How does action resist visual illusion? Uncorrected oculomotor information does not account for accurate pointing in peripersonal space. *Experimental Brain Research, 163,* 133-144.

Binsted, G., Chua, R., Helsen, W., & Elliott, D. (2001). Eye-hand coordination in goal-directed aiming. *Human Movement Science, 20,* 563-585.

Binsted, G., & Elliott, D. (1999). Ocular perturbations and retinal/extraretinal information: The coordination of saccadic and manual movements. *Experimental Brain Research, 127,* 193-206.

Bradshaw, M.F., Elliott, K.M., Watt, S.J., Hibbard, P.B., Davies, I.R., & Simpson, P.J. (2004). Binocular cues and the control of prehension. *Spatial Vision, 17,* 95-110.

Bridgeman, B., Aiken, W., Allen, J., & Maresh, T.C. (1997). Influence of acoustic context on sound localization: An auditory Roelofs effect. *Psychological Research, 60,* 238-243.

Bridgeman, B., Peery, S., & Anand, S. (1997). Interaction of cognitive and sensorimotor maps of visual space. *Perception & Psychophysics, 59,* 456-469.

Bruno, N., Bernardis, P., & Gentilucci, M. (2008). Visually guided pointing, the Müller-Lyer illusion, and the functional interpretation of the dorsal-ventral split: Conclusions from 33 independent studies. *Neuroscience and Biobehavioral Reviews, 32,* 423-437.

Bruno, N., & Bernardis, P. (2002). Dissociating perception and action in Kanizsa's compression illusion. *Psychonomic Bulletin & Review, 9,* 723-730.

Carey, D.P. (2001). Do action systems resist visual illusions? *Trends in Cognitive Science, 5,* 109-113.

Castiello, U. (1996). Grasping a fruit: Selection for action. *Journal of Experimental Psychology: Human Perception and Performance, 22,* 582-603.

Coello, Y., Danckert, J., Blangero, A., & Rossetti, Y. (2007). Do visual illusions probe the visual brain? Illusions in action without a dorsal stream. *Neuropsychologia, 45,* 1849-1858.

Coren, S., & Girgus, J.S. (1972). A comparison of five methods of illusion measurement. *Behavior Research Methods and Instrumentation, 4,* 240-244.

Coren, S., & Porac, C. (1984). Structural and cognitive components in the Müller-Lyer illusion assessed via Cyclopean presentation. *Perception & Psychophysics, 35,* 313-318.

Danckert, J.A., Sharif, N., Haffenden, A.M., Schiff, K.C., & Goodale, M.A. (2002). A temporal analysis of grasping in the Ebbinghaus illusion: Planning versus online control. *Experimental Brain Research, 144,* 275-280.

Daprati, E., & Gentilucci, M. (1997). Grasping an illusion. *Neuropsychologia, 35,* 1577-1582.

Dijkerman, H.C., Milner, A.D., & Carey, D.P. (1996). The perception and prehension of objects oriented in the depth plane. I. Effects of visual form agnosia. *Experimental Brain Research, 112,* 442-451.

Dyde, R.T., & Milner, A.D. (2001). Two illusions of perceived orientation: One fools all of the people some of the time; the other fools all of the people all of the time. *Experimental Brain Research, 144,* 518-527.

Elliott, D., Helsen, W.F., & Chua, R. (2001). A century later: Woodworth's (1899) two-component model of goal-directed aiming. *Psychological Bulletin, 127,* 342-357.

Elliott, D., & Lee, T.D. (1995). The role of target information on manual-aiming bias. *Psychological Research, 58,* 2-9.

Elliott, D., & Madalena, J. (1987). The influence of premovement visual information on manual aiming. *Quarterly Journal of Experimental Psychology, 39,* 541-559.

Franz, V.H. (2001). Action does not resist visual illusions. *Trends in Cognitive Science, 5,* 457-459.

Franz, V.H. (2003). Manual size estimation: A neuropsychological measure of perception? *Experimental Brain Research, 151,* 471-477.

Franz, V.H., Bülthoff, H.H., & Fahle, M. (2003). Grasp effects of the Ebbinghaus illusion: Obstacle avoidance is not the explanation. *Experimental Brain Research, 149,* 470-477.

Franz, V.H., Fahle, M., Bülthoff, H.H., & Gegenfurtner, K.R. (2001). Effects of visual illusions on grasping. *Journal of Experimental Psychology: Human Perception and Performance, 27,* 1124-1144.

Franz, V.H., Gegenfurtner, K.R., Bülthoff, H.H., & Fahle, M. (2000). Grasping visual illusions: No evidence for a dissociation between perception and action. *Psychological Science, 11,* 20-25.

Franz, V.H., Scharnowski, F., & Gegenfurtner, K.R. (2005). Illusion effects on grasping are temporally constant not dynamic. *Journal of Experimental Psychology: Human Perception and Performance, 31,* 1359-1378.

Jeannerod, M. (1986). The formation of finger grip during prehension. A cortically mediated visuomotor pattern. *Behavioral Brain Research, 19,* 99-116.

Flanagan, J.R., & Beltzner, M.A. (2000). Independence of perceptual and sensorimotor predictions in the size-weight illusion. *Nature Neuroscience, 3,* 737-741.

Gentilucci, M., Chieffi, S., Daprati, E., Saetti, M.C., & Toni, I. (1996). Visual illusion and action. *Neuropsychologia, 34,* 369-376.

Glazebrook, C.M., Dhillon, V.P., Keetch, K.M., Lyons, J., Amazeen, E., Weeks, D.J., & Elliott, D. (2005). Perception-action and the Müller-Lyer illusion: Amplitude or endpoint bias? *Experimental Brain Research, 160,* 71-78.

Glover, S. (2004). Separate visual representations in the planning and control of action. *Behavioral Brain Research, 27,* 3-78.

Glover, S., & Dixon, P. (2001a). Motor adaptation to an optical illusion. *Experimental Brain Research, 137,* 254-258.

Glover, S.R., & Dixon, P. (2001b). Dynamic illusion effects in a reaching task: Evidence for separate visual representations in the planning and control of reaching. *Journal of Experimental Psychology: Human Perception and Performance, 27,* 560-572.

Glover, S., & Dixon, P. (2004). A step and a hop on the Muller-Lyer: Illusion effects on lower-limb movements. *Experimental Brain Research, 154,* 504-512.

Goodale, M.A., & Humphrey, G.K. (1998). The objects of action and perception. *Cognition, 67,* 181-207.

Goodale, M.A., Jakobson, L.S., & Keillor, J.M. (1994). Differences in the visual control of pantomimed and natural grasping movements. *Neuropsychologia, 32,* 1159-1178.

Goodale, M.A., Meenan, J.P., Bülthoff, H.H., Nicolle, D.A., Murphy, K.J., & Racicot, C.I. (1994). Separate neural pathways for the visual analysis of object shape in perception and prehension. *Current Biology, 4,* 604-610.

Goodale, M.A., & Milner, A.D. (1992). Separate visual pathways for perception and action. *Trends in Neuroscience, 15,* 20-25.

Goodale, M.A., Milner, A.D., Jakobson, L.S., & Carey, D.P. (1991). A neurological dissociation between perceiving objects and grasping them. *Nature, 349,* 154-156.

Goodale, M.A., Pelisson, D., & Prablanc, C. (1986). Large adjustments in visually guided reaching do not depend on vision of the hand or perception of target displacement. *Nature, 320,* 748-750.

Grandy, M.S., & Westwood, D.A. (2006). Opposite perceptual and sensorimotor responses to a size-weight illusion. *Journal of Neurophysiology, 95,* 3887-3892.

Haffenden, A.M., & Goodale, M.A. (1998). The effect of pictorial illusion on prehension and perception. *Journal of Cognitive Neuroscience, 10,* 122-136.

Haffenden, A.M., Schiff, K.C., & Goodale, M.A. (2001). The dissociation between perception and action in the Ebbinghaus illusion: Nonillusory effects of pictorial cues on grasp. *Current Biology, 11,* 177-181.

Harris, J., Weiler, J., & Westwood, D.A. (2009). *Accurate stepping movements over objects in a 3D size-contrast illusion.* Manuscript in preparation.

Harvey, M.D., & Westwood, D.A. (2009). *Increased effect of a size-contrast illusion on grasping in monocular versus binocular viewing conditions.* Manuscript in preparation.

Heath, M., Rival, C., & Neely, K. (2006). Visual feedback schedules influence visuomotor resistance to the Müller-Lyer figures. *Experimental Brain Research, 168,* 348-356.

Heath, M., Rival, C., Westwood, D.A., & Neely, K. (2005). Time course analysis of closed- and open-loop grasping of the Müller-Lyer illusion. *Journal of Motor Behavior, 37,* 179-185.

Hu, Y., & Goodale, M.A. (2000). Grasping after a delay shifts size-scaling from absolute to relative metrics. *Journal of Cognitive Neuroscience, 12,* 856-868.

Khan, M.A., Elliott, D., Coull, J., Chua, R., & Lyons, J. (2002). Optimal control strategies under different feedback schedules: Kinematic evidence. *Journal of Motor Behavior, 34,* 45-57.

Lee, J.H., & van Donkelaar, P. (2002). Dorsal and ventral visual stream contributions to perception-action interactions during pointing. *Experimental Brain Research, 143,* 440-446.

Mack, A., Heuer, F., Villardi, K., & Chambers, D. (1985). The dissociation of position and extent in Müller-Lyer figures. *Perception & Psychophysics, 37,* 335-344.

Marotta, J.J., DeSouza, J.F., Haffenden, A.M., & Goodale, M.A. (1998). Does a monocularly presented size-contrast illusion influence grip aperture? *Neuropsychologia, 36,* 491-497.

McCarville, E.M., & Westwood, D.A. (2006). The visual control of stepping operates in real time: Evidence from a pictorial illusion. *Experimental Brain Research, 171,* 405-410.

Mendoza, J.E., Elliott, D., Meegan, D.V., Lyons, J.L., & Welsh, T.N. (2006). The effect of the Müller-Lyer illusion on the planning and control of manual aiming movements. *Journal of Experimental Psychology: Human Perception and Human Performance, 32,* 413-422.

Milner, A.D., Perrett, D.I., Johnston, R.S., Benson, P.J., Jordan, T.R., Heeley, D.W., Bettucci, D., Mortara, F., Mutani, R., Terazzi, E., & Davidson, D.L.W. (1991). Perception and action in 'visual form agnosia.' *Brain, 114,* 405-428.

Milner, A.D., & Goodale, M.A. (1995). *The visual brain in action.* New York: Oxford University Press.

Murray, D.J., Ellis, R.R., & Bandomir, C.A. (1999). Charpentier (1891) on the size-weight illusion. *Perception & Psychophysics, 61,* 1681-1685.

Otto-de Haart, E.G., Carey, D.P., & Milne, A.B. (1999). More thoughts on perceiving and grasping the Müller-Lyer illusion. *Neuropsychologia, 37,* 1437-1444.

Perenin, M.T., & Vighetto, A. (1988). Optic ataxia: A specific disruption in visuomotor mechanisms. I. Different aspects of the deficit in reaching for objects. *Brain, 111,* 643-674.

Rival, C., Olivier, I., Ceyte, H., & Ferrel, C. (2003). Age-related differences in a delayed pointing of a Müller-Lyer illusion. *Experimental Brain Research, 153,* 378-381.

Sengpiel, F., Sen, A., & Blakemore, C. (1997). Characteristics of surround inhibition in cat area 17. *Experimental Brain Research, 116,* 216-228.

Servos, P., & Goodale, M.A. (1994). Binocular vision and the on-line control of human prehension. *Experimental Brain Research, 98,* 119-127.

Servos, P., Goodale, M.A., & Jakobson, L.S. (1992). The role of binocular vision in prehension: A kinematic analysis. *Vision Research, 32,* 1513-1521.

Sincich, L.C., & Horton, J.C. (2005). The circuitry of V1 and V2: Integration of color, form, and motion. *Annual Review of Neuroscience, 28,* 303-326.

Smeets, J.B., & Brenner, E. (1999). A new view on grasping. *Motor Control, 3,* 237-271.

Smeets, J.B.J., & Brenner, E. (2006). 10 years of illusions. *Journal of Experimental Psychology: Human Perception and Performance, 32,* 1501-1504.

Thompson, A.A., & Westwood, D.A. (2007). The hand knows something that the eye does not: Reaching movements resist the Müller-Lyer illusion whether or not the target is foveated. *Neuroscience Letters, 426,* 111-116.

Tipper, S.P., Howard, L.A., & Jackson, S.R. (1997). Selective reaching to grasp: Evidence for distractor interference effects. *Visual Cognition, 4,* 1-48.

van Donkelaar, P. (1999). Pointing movements are affected by size-contrast illusions. *Experimental Brain Research, 125,* 517.

Vishton, P.M., Rea, J.G., Cutting, J.E., & Nuñez, L.N. (1999). Comparing effects of the horizontal-vertical illusion on grip scaling and judgment: Relative versus absolute, not perception versus action. *Journal of Experimental Psychology: Human Perception and Performance, 25,* 1659-1672.

Weiskrantz, L., Warrington, E.K., Sanders, M.D., & Marshall, J. (1974). Visual capacity in the hemianopic field following a restricted occipital ablation. *Brain, 97,* 709-728.

Welsh, T.N., Elliott, D., & Weeks, D.J. (1999). Hand deviations toward distractors: Evidence for response competition. *Experimental Brain Research, 127,* 207-212.

Westwood, D.A., Chapman, C.D., & Roy, E.A. (2000). Pantomimed actions may be controlled by the ventral visual stream. *Experimental Brain Research, 130,* 545-548.

Westwood, D.A., & Goodale, M.A. (2003a). A haptic size-contrast illusion affects size perception but not grasping. *Experimental Brain Research, 153,* 253-259.

Westwood, D.A., & Goodale, M.A. (2003b). Perceptual illusion and the real-time control of action. *Spatial Vision, 16,* 243-254.

Westwood, D.A., Heath, M., & Roy, E.A. (2000). The effect of a pictorial illusion on closed-loop and open-loop prehension. *Experimental Brain Research, 134,* 456-463.

Westwood, D.A., Heath, M., & Roy, E.A. (2001). The accuracy of reaching movements in brief delay conditions. *Canadian Journal of Experimental Psychology, 55,* 304-310.

Westwood, D.A., McEachern, T., & Roy, E.A. (2001). Delayed grasping of a Müller-Lyer figure. *Experimental Brain Research, 141,* 166-173.

Westwood, D.A., Pavlovic-King, J., & Christensen, B. (2009). *Perceptual effects of a size-contrast illusion are not correlated with grip aperture early or late in a grasping movement.* Manuscript submitted for publication.

White, J., & Westwood, D.A. (2009). *Prior learning of material density does not eliminate the perceptual size-weight illusion: Evidence against an expectation-mismatch model.* Manuscript in preparation.

Witkin, H.A., & Asch, S.E. (1947). Studies in space orientation. IV. Further experiments on perception of the upright with displaced visual fields. *Journal of Experimental Psychology, 38,* 762-782.

Wong, E., & Mack, A. (1981). Saccadic programming and perceived location. *Acta Psychologica, 48,* 123-131.

Woodworth, R.S. (1899). The accuracy of voluntary movement. *Psychological Review, Monograph Supplements, 3*(13), 1-119.

Wraga, M., Creem, S.H., & Proffitt, D.R. (2000). Perception-action dissociations of a walkable Müller-Lyer configuration. *Psychological Science, 11,* 239-243.

Yamagishi, N., Anderson, S.J., & Ashida, H. (2001). Evidence for dissociation between the perceptual and visuomotor systems in humans. *Proceedings of the Royal Society of London. Series B, Biological Sciences, 268,* 973-977.

Zelaznik, H.N., Hawkins, B., & Kisselburgh, L. (1983). Rapid visual feedback processing in single-aiming movements. *Journal of Motor Behavior, 15,* 217-236.

CHAPTER 14

Andersen, R.A., Snyder, L.H., Batista, A.P., Bueno, C.A., & Cohen, Y.E. (1998). Posterior parietal areas specialized for eye movements (LIP) and reach (PRR) using a common coordinate frame.

In G.R. Bock & J.A. Goode (Eds.), *The sensory guidance of movement* (pp. 109-122). Chichester, UK: Wiley.

Biegstraaten, M., de Grave, D.D.J., Smeets, J.B.J., & Brenner, E. (2007). Grasping the Müller-Lyer illusion: not a change in length. *Experimental Brain Research, 176,* 497–503.

Benson, D.F., & Greenberg, J.P. (1969). Visual form agnosia: A specific defect in visual discrimination. *Archives of Neurology, 20,* 82-89.

Blangero, A., Otac, H., Delporte, L., Revol, P., Vindras, P., Rode, G., Boisson, D., Vighetto, A., Rossetti, Y., & Pisella., L. (2007). Optic ataxia is not only 'optic': Impaired spatial integration of proprioceptive information. *NeuroImage, 36,* T61-T68.

Boussaoud, D., Ungerleider, L.G., & Desimone, R. (1990). Pathways for motion analysis: Cortical connections of the medial superior temporal and fundus of the superior temporal visual areas in the macaque. *Journal of Comparative Neurology, 296,* 462-495.

Boussaoud, D., Desimone, R., & Ungerleider, L.G. (1992). Subcortical connections of visual areas MST and FST in macaques. *Visual Neuroscience, 9,* 291-302.

Buxbaum, L.J., & Coslett, H.B. (1997). Subtypes of optic ataxia: Reframing the disconnectionist account. *Neurocase, 3,* 159-166.

Buxbaum, L.J., & Coslett, H.B. (1998). Spatio-motor representations in reaching: Evidence for subtypes of optic ataxia. *Cognitive Neuropsychology, 15,* 279-312.

Carey, D. P. (2001). Do action systems resist visual illusions? *Trends in Cognitive Sciences, 5,* 109–113.

Carey, D.P. (2004). Neuropsychological perspectives on sensorimotor integration. In N. Kanwisher, J. Duncan, & C. Umlita (Eds.), *Functional brain imaging of visual cognition (Attention and performance XX)* (pp. 481-502). Cambridge, MA: MIT Press.

Carey, D.P., Coleman, R.J., & Della Sala, S. (1997). Magnetic misreaching. *Cortex, 33,* 639-652.

Carey, D.P. Harvey M. & Milner A.D. (1996). Visuomotor sensitivity for shape and orientation in a patient with visual form agnosia. *Neuropsychologia, 34,* 329-337.

Carey, D.P., Ietswaart, M. & Della Sala, D. (2002). Neuropsychological perspectives on eye-hand coordination in visually-guided reaching. *Progress in Brain Research, 140,* 311-327.

Catani, M., Jones, D.K., Donato, R., & ffytche, D.H. (2003). Occipito-temporal connections in the human brain. *Brain, 126,* 2093-2107.

Chang, S.W.C., Dickinson, A.R., & Snyder, L.H. (2008). Limb-specific representation for reaching in the posterior parietal cortex. *Journal of Neuroscience, 28,* 6128-6140.

Clavagnier, S., Prado, J., Kennedy, H., & Perenin, M.-T. (2007). How humans reach: Distinct cortical systems for central and peripheral vision. *Neuroscientist, 13,* 22-27.

Crawford, J.R., & Garthwaite, P.H. (2005). Testing for suspected impairments and dissociations in single-case studies in neuropsychology: Evaluation of alternatives using Monte Carlo simulations and revised tests for dissociations. *Neuropsychology, 19,* 318-331.

Culham, J.C., Gallivan, J., Cavina-Pratesi, C., & Quinlan, D.J. (2008). fMRI investigations of reaching and ego space in human superior parieto-occipital cortex. In R.L. Klatzky, M. Behrmann, & B. MacWhinney (Eds.), *Embodiment, ego-space and action* (pp. 247-274). Madwah, NJ: Erlbaum.

Culham, J.C., Cavina-Pratesi, C., & Singhal, A. (2006). The role of parietal cortex in visuomotor control: What have we learned from neuroimaging? *Neuropsychologia, 44,* 2668-2684.

De Renzi, E. (1982). *Disorders of space exploration and cognition.* New York: Wiley.

Dijkerman, H.C., Lê, S., Démonet, J.-F., & Milner, A.D. (2004). Visuomotor performance in a case of visual form agnosia due to early brain damage. *Cognitive Brain Research, 20,* 12-25.

Dijkerman, H.C., McIntosh, R.D., Anema, H.A., de Haan, E.H.F., Kappelle, L.J., & Milner, A.D. (2006). Reaching errors in optic ataxia are linked to eye position rather than head or body position. *Neuropsychologia, 44,* 2766-2773.

Dunn, J.C., & Kirsner, K. (2003). What can we infer from double dissociations? *Cortex, 39,* 1-7.

Felleman, D.J., Xiao, Y., & McClendon, E. (1997). Modular organization of occipito-temporal pathways: Cortical connections between visual area 4 and visual area 2 and posterior inferotemporal ventral area in macaque monkeys. *Journal of Neuroscience, 17,* 3185-3200.

Galletti, C., Gamberini, M., Kutz, D.F., Fattori, P., Luppino, G., & Matelli, M. (2001). The cortical connections of area V6: An occipito-parietal network processing visual information. *European Journal of Neuroscience, 13,* 1572-1588.

Glickstein, M., May III, J.G., & Mercier, B.E. (1985). Corticopontine projection in the macaque: The distribution of labelled cortical cells after large injections of horseradish peroxidise in the pontine nuclei. *Journal of Comparative Neurology, 235,* 343-359.

Glover, S. (2004). Separate visual representations in the planning and control of action. *Behavioral and Brain Sciences, 27,* 3-24.

Glover, S., & Dixon, P. (2001). Dynamic illusion effects in a reaching task: Evidence for separate visual representations in the planning and control of reaching. *Journal of Experimental Psychology: Human Perception and Performance, 27,* 560-572.

Goodale, M.A. (1983).Vision as a sensorimotor system. In T.E. Robinson (Ed.), *Behavioral approaches to brain research* (pp. 41-61). New York: Oxford University Press.

Goodale, M.A., Jakobson, L.S., & Keillor, J.M. (1994). Differences in the visual control of pantomimed and natural grasping movements. *Neuropsychologia, 32,* 1159-1178.

Goodale, M.A., Meenan, J.P., Bülthoff, H.H., Nicolle, D.A., Murphy, K.J., & Racicot, C.I. (1994). Separate neural pathways for the visual analysis of object shape in perception and prehension. *Current Biology, 4,* 604-610.

Goodale, M.A., & Milner, A.D. (1992). Separate visual pathways for perception and action. *Trends in Neurosciences, 15,* 20-25.

Goodale, M.A., Milner, A.D., Jakobson, L.S., & Carey, D.P. (1991). A neurological dissociation between perceiving objects and grasping them. *Nature, 349,* 154-156.

Goodale, M.A., Westwood, D.A., & Milner, A.D. (2004). Two distinct modes of control for object-directed action. *Progress in Brain Research, 144,* 131-144.

Goodale, M. A., Wolf, M. E., Whitwell, R. L., Brown, L. E., Cant, J. S., Chapman, C. S., Witt, J. K., Arnott, S. R., Khan, S. A., Chouinard, P. A., Culham, J. C., & Dutton, G. N. (2008). Preserved motion processing and visuomotor control in a patient with large bilateral lesions of occipitotemporal cortex [Abstract]. *Journal of Vision,* 8, 371, 371a, http://journalofvision.org/8/6/371/, doi:10.1167/8.6.371.

Grol, M.J., Majdandzic, J., Stephan, K.E., Verhagen, L., Dijkerman, H.-C., Bekkering, H., Verstraten, F.A.J., & Toni, I. (2007). Parieto-frontal connectivity during visually guided grasping. *Journal of Neuroscience, 27,* 11877-11887.

Grüsser, O.-J., & Landis, T. (1991). *Visual agnosias and other disturbances.* London: Macmillan.

Himmelbach, M., & Karnath, H.-O. (2005). Dorsal and ventral stream interaction: Contributions from optic ataxia. *Journal of Cognitive Neuroscience, 17,* 632-640.

Himmelbach, M., Karnath, H.-O., Perenin, M.-T., Franz, V.H., & Stockmeier, K. (2006). A general deficit of the 'automatic pilot' with posterior parietal cortex lesions? *Neuropsychologia, 44,* 2749-2756.

Husain, M., & Stein, J. (1988). Rezso Balint and his most celebrated case. *Archives of Neurology, 45,* 89-93.

Jackson, S., Newport, R., Mort, D., & Husain, M. (2005). Where the eye looks, the hand follows: Limb-dependent magnetic misreaching in optic ataxia. *Current Biology, 15,* 42-46.

Jakobson, L.S., Archibald, Y.M., Carey, D.P., & Goodale, M.A. (1991). A kinematic analysis of reaching and grasping movements in a patient recovering from optic ataxia. *Neuropsychologia, 29,* 803–809.

James, T.W., Culham, J., Humphrey, G.K., Milner, A.D., & Goodale, M.A. (2003). Ventral occipital lesions impair object recognition but not object-directed grasping: An fMRI study. *Brain, 126,* 2463-2475.

Jeannerod, M. (1994). The representing brain: Neural correlates of motor intention and imagery. *Behavioral and Brain Sciences, 17,* 187-245.

Jeannerod, M., Decety, J., & Michel, F. (1994). Impairment of grasping movements following a bilateral posterior parietal lesion. *Neuropsychologia, 32,* 369-380.

Karnath, H.-O., & Perenin, M.T. (2005). Cortical control of visually guided reaching: Evidence from patients with optic ataxia. *Cerebral Cortex, 15,* 1561-1569.

Karnath, H.-O., Rüter, J., Mandler, A., & Himmelbach, M. (2009). The anatomy of object recognition—visual form agnosia caused by medial occipitotemporal stroke. *Journal of Neuroscience*, *29*, 5854 –5862.

Kentridge, R.W., Heywood, C.A., & Milner, A.D. (2004). Covert processing of visual form in the absence of area LO. *Neuropsychologia*, *42*, 1488-1495.

Khan, A.Z., Crawford, J.D., Blohm, G., Urquizar, C., Rossetti, Y., & Pisella, L. (2007). Influence of initial hand and target position on reach errors in optic ataxic and normal subjects. *Journal of Vision*, *7*, 1-16.

Konen, C., & Kastner, S. (2008). Two hierarchically organized neural systems for object information in human visual cortex. *Nature Neuroscience*, *11*, 224-231.

Kourtzi, Z., Erb, M., Grodd, W., & Bülthoff, H. (2003). Representation of the perceived 3-D object shape in the human lateral occipital complex. *Cerebral Cortex*, *13*, 911-920.

Lê, S., Cardebat, D., Boulanouar, K., Hénaff, M.-A., Michel, F., Milner, A.D., Dijkerman, C., Puel, M., & Démonet, J.-F. (2002). Seeing, since childhood, without ventral stream: a behavioural study. *Brain*, *125*, 58–74

McIntosh, R.D., McClements, K.I., Dijkerman, H.C., Birchall, D., & Milner, A.D. (2004). Preserved obstacle avoidance during reaching in patients with left visual neglect. *Neuropsychologia*, *42*, 1107-1117

Milner, A.D., Dijkerman, H.C., & Carey, D.P. (1998). Visuospatial processing in a pure case of visual-form agnosia. In N. Burgess, K. Jeffery, & J. O'Keefe (Eds.), *Spatial functions of the hippocampal formation and the parietal cortex* (pp.443-456). Oxford, U.K : Oxford University Press.

Milner, A.D., Dijkerman, H.C., McIntosh, R.D., Pisella, L., & Rossetti, Y. (2003). Delayed reaching and grasping in patients with optic ataxia. *Progress in Brain Research*, *142*, 225-242.

Milner, A.D., Dijkerman, H.C., Pisella, L., McIntosh, R.D., Tilikete, C., Vighetto, A., & Rossetti, Y. (2001). Grasping the past: Delay can improve visuomotor performance. *Current Biology*, *11*, 1896-1901.

Milner, A.D., & Goodale, M.A. (2008). Two visual systems re-viewed *Neuropsychologia*, *46*, 774-785.

Milner, A.D., & McIntosh, R.D. (2004). Reaching between obstacles in spatial neglect and visual extinction. *Progress in Brain Research*, *144*, 213-226.

Milner, A.D., Dijkerman, H.C., McIntosh, R.D., Rossetti, Y., & Pisella, L. (2003). Delayed reaching and grasping in patients with optic ataxia. *Progress in Brain Research*, *142*, 225-242.

Milner, A.D., Paulignan, Y., Dijkerman, H.C., Michel, F., & Jeannerod, M. (1999). A paradoxical improvement of optic ataxia with delay: New evidence for two separate neural systems for visual localization. *Proceedings of the Royal Society of London. Series B, Biological Sciences*, *266*, 2225-2230.

Milner, A.D., & Goodale, M.A. (1995). *The visual brain in action*. Oxford, U.K.: Oxford University Press.

Ratcliff, G., & Davies-Jones, G.A.B. (1972). Defective visual localization in focal brain wounds. *Brain*, *95*, 49-60.

Rice, N.J., McIntosh, R.D., Schindler, I., Mon-Williams, M., Démonet, J.-F., & Milner, A.D. (2006). Intact automatic avoidance of obstacles in patients with visual form agnosia. *Experimental Brain Research*, *174*, 176-188.

Rice, N.J., Edwards, M.G., Schindler, I., Punt, T.D., McIntosh, R.D., Humphreys, G.W., Lestou, V., & Milner, A.D. (2008). Delay abolishes the obstacle avoidance deficit in unilateral optic ataxia. *Neuropsychologia*, *46*, 1549-1557.

Riddoch, M.J., & Humphreys, G.W. (1993). BORB: Birmingham Object Recognition Battery. Hove, UK: Erlbaum.

Rondot, P., De Recondo, J., & Ribadeau Dumas, J.L. (1977). Visuomotor ataxia. *Brain*, *100*, 355-376.

Rorden, C., & Brett, M. (2001). Stereotaxic display of brain lesions. *Behavioral Neurology*, *12*, 191-200.

Rossetti, Y., McIntosh, R.D., Revol, P., Pisella, L., Rode, G., Danckert, J., Tilikete, C., Dijkerman, H.C., Boisson, D., Vighetto, A., Michel, F., & Milner, A.D. (2005). Visually guided reaching: Posterior parietal lesions cause a switch from visuomotor to cognitive control. *Neuropsychologia*, *42*, 162-177.

Petrides, M., & Pandya, D.N. (2007). Efferent association pathways from the rostral prefrontal cortex in the macaque monkey. *Journal of Neuroscience*, *27*, 11573-11586.

Pisella, L., Binkofski, F., Lasek, K., Toni, I., & Rossetti, Y. (2006). No double-dissociation between optic ataxia and visual agnosia: Multiple sub-streams for multiple visuo-manual integrations. *Neuropsychologia, 44,* 2734-2748.

Scannell, J.W., Blakemore, C., & Young, M.P. (1995). Analysis of connectivity in the cat cerebral cortex. *Journal of Neuroscience, 15,* 1463-1483.

Schenk, T., Ellison, A., Rice, N., & Milner, A.D. (2005). The role of V5/MT+ in the control of catching movements: A rTMS study. *Neuropsychologia, 43,* 189-198.

Schenk, T., Schindler, I., McIntosh, R.D., & Milner, A.D. (2005). The use of visual feedback is independent of visual awareness: Evidence from visual extinction. *Experimental Brain Research, 167,* 95-102.

Scherberger, H., Goodale, M.A., & Andersen, R.A. (2003). Target selection for reaching and saccades share a similar behavioral reference frame in the macaque. *Journal of Neurophysiolology, 89,* 1456-1466.

Schindler, I., Rice, N.J., McIntosh, R.D., Rossetti, Y., Vighetto, A., & Milner, A.D. (2004). Automatic avoidance of obstacles is a dorsal stream function: Evidence from optic ataxia. *Nature Neuroscience, 7,* 779-784.

Shipp, S., Blanton, M., & Zeki, S. (1998). A visuo-somatomotor pathway through superior parietal cortex in the macaque monkey: Cortical connections of areas V6 and V6A. *European Journal of Neuroscience, 10,* 3171-3193.

Snodgrass, J.G., & Vanderwart, M. (1980). A standardized set of 260 pictures: Norms for name agreement, image agreement, familiarity, and visual complexity. *Journal of Experimental Psychology: Human Learning and Memory, 6,* 174-215.

Steeves, J.K.E., Humphrey, G.K., Culham, J.C., Menon, R.S., Milner, A.D., & Goodale, M.A. (2004). Behavioral and neuroimaging evidence for a contribution of color and texture information to scene classification in a patient with visual form agnosia. *Journal of Cognitive Neuroscience, 16,* 955-965.

Toraldo, A., McIntosh, R.D., Dijkerman, H.C., & Milner, A.D. (2004). A revised method for analysing the landmark task. *Cortex, 40,* 415-431.

Tomassini, V., Jbabdi, S., Klein, J.C., Behrens, T.E.J., Pozzilli, C., Matthews, P.M., Rushworth, M.F.S., & Johansen-Berg, H. (2007). Diffusion-weighted imaging tractography-based parcellation of the human lateral premotor cortex identifies dorsal and ventral subregions with anatomical and functional specializations. *Journal of Neuroscience, 27,* 10259-10269.

Ungerleider, L.G. & Haxby, J.V. (1994) 'What' and 'where' in the human brain. *Current Opinion in Neurobiology, 4,* 157-165.

Ungerleider, L.G., & Mishkin, M. (1982). Two cortical visual systems. In D.J. Ingle, M.A. Goodale, & R.J.W. Mansfield (Eds.), *Analysis of visual behaviour* (pp. 549-586). Cambridge, MA: MIT Press.

van Donkelaar, P., & Adams, J. (2005). Gaze-dependent deviation in pointing induced by transcranial magnetic stimulation over the human posterior parietal cortex. *Journal of Motor Behavior, 37,* 157-163.

Verhagen, L., Dijkerman, H.-C., Grol, M.J., & Toni, I. (2008). Perceptuo-motor interactions during prehension movements. *Journal of Neuroscience, 28,* 4726-4735.

Warrington, E.K., & James, M. (1991). *VOSP: The visual object and space perception battery.* Bury St Edmunds, UK: Thames Valley Test Company.

Wolf, M. E., Whitwell, R. L., Brown, L. E., Cant, J. S., Chapman, C., Witt, J. K., Arnott, S. R., Khan, S. A., Chouinard, P. A., Culham, J. C., Dutton, G. N., & Goodale, M. A. (2008). Preserved visual abilities following large bilateral lesions of the occipitotemporal cortex [Abstract]. Journal of Vision, 8, 624, 624a, http://journalofvision.org/8/6/624/, doi:10.1167/8.6.624.

Yang, J., Wu, M., & Shen, Z. (2006). Preserved implicit form perception and orientation adaptation in visual form agnosia. *Neuropsychologia, 44,* 1833-1842.

Young, M.P. (1992). Objective analysis of the topological organization of the primate cortical visual system. *Nature, 358,* 152-155.

CHAPTER 15

Adams, J.A., Goetz, E.T., & Marshall, P.H. (1972). Response feedback and motor learning. *Journal of Experimental Psychology, 92,* 391-397.

Adams, J.A., Gopher, D., & Lintern, G. (1977). Effects of visual and proprioceptive feedback on motor learning. *Journal of Motor Behavior, 9,* 11-22.

Beggs, W.D.A., & Howarth, C.I. (1970). Movement control in a repetitive motor task. *Nature, 225,* 752-753.

Bennett, S.J., & Davids, K. (1995). The manipulation of vision during the powerlift squat: Exploring the boundaries of the specificity of practice hypothesis. *Research Quarterly for Exercise and Sport, 66,* 210-218.

Bullock, D., Cisek, P., & Grossberg, S. (1998). Cortical networks for control of voluntary arm movements under variable force conditions. *Cerebral Cortex, 8,* 48-62.

Carlton, L.G. (1992). Visual processing time and the control of movement. In L. Proteau & D. Elliott (Eds.), *Vision and motor control* (pp. 3-31). Amsterdam: Elsevier.

Chua, R., & Elliott, D. (1993). Visual regulation of manual aiming. *Human Movement Science, 12,* 365-401.

Cisek, P., Grossberg, S., & Bullock, D. (1998). A cortico-spinal model of reaching and proprioception under multiple task constraints. *Journal of Cognitive Neuroscience, 10,* 425-444.

Coull, J., Tremblay, L., & Elliott, D. (2001). Examining the specificity of practice hypothesis: Is learning modality specific? *Research Quarterly for Exercise and Sport, 72,* 345-354.

Crossman, E.R.F.W. (1959). A theory of acquisition of speed skills. *Ergonomics, 2,* 153-166.

Elliott, D., Carson, R.G., Goodman, D., & Chua, R. (1991). Discrete vs. continuous visual control of manual aiming. *Human Movement Science, 10,* 393-418.

Elliott, D., Helsen, W.F., & Chua, R. (2001). A century later: Woodworth's (1899) two-component model of goal-directed aiming. *Psychological Bulletin, 127,* 342-357.

Elliott, D., Hansen, S., Mendoza, J., & Tremblay, L. (2004). Learning to optimize speed, accuracy, and energy expenditure: A framework for understanding speed-accuracy relations in goal-directed aiming. *Journal of Motor Behavior, 36,* 339-351.

Ernst, M.O., & Bülthoff, H.H. (2004). Merging the senses into a robust percept. *Trends in Cognitive Sciences, 8,* 162-169.

Grush, R. (2004). The emulation theory of representation: Motor control, imagery, and perception. *Behavioral and Brain Sciences, 27,* 377-342.

Hansen, S., Cullen, J.D., & Elliott, D. (2005). Self-selected visual information during discrete manual aiming. *Journal of Motor Behavior, 37,* 343-347.

Hansen, S., Elliott, D., & Tremblay, L. (2007). Online control of discrete action following visual perturbation. *Perception, 36,* 268-287.

Jeannerod, M. (2006). *Motor cognition: What the actions tell to the self.* New York: Oxford University Press.

Karni, A., Meyer, G., Jezzard, P., Adams, M.M., Turner, R., & Ungerleider, L.G. (1995). Functional MRI evidence for adult motor cortex plasticity during motor skill learning. *Nature, 377,* 155-158.

Khan, M.A., Franks, I.M., & Goodman, D. (1998). The effect of practice on the control of rapid aiming movements: Evidence for an interdependency between programming and feedback processing. *Quarterly Journal of Experimental Psychology A: Human Experimental Psychology, 51,* 425-444.

Kimura, D. (1996). Sex, sexual orientation and sex hormones influence human cognitive function. *Current Opinion in Neurobiology, 6,* 259-263.

Kimura, D. (2000). *Sex and cognition.* Cambridge, MA: MIT Press.

Krigolson, O., Van Gyn, G., Tremblay, L., & Heath, M. (2006). Is there "feedback" during visual imagery? Evidence from a specificity of practice paradigm. *Canadian Journal of Experimental Psychology, 60,* 24-32.

Lashley, K.S. (1917). The accuracy of movement in the absence of excitation from the moving organ. *American Journal of Physiology, 43,* 169-194.

Laszlo, J.I., Bairstow, P.J., Ward, G.R., & Bancroft, H. (1980). Distracting information, motor performance and sex differences. *Nature, 283,* 377-378.

Mackrous, I., & Proteau, L. (2007). Specificity of practice results from differences in movement planning strategies. *Experimental Brain Research, 183,* 181-193.

Maquet, P. (2001). The role of sleep in learning and memory. *Science, 294,* 1048-1052.

Meredith, M.A., & Stein, B.E. (1986). Visual, auditory and somatosensory convergence on cells in superior colliculus results in multisensory integration. *Journal of Neurophysiology, 56,* 640-662.

Plamondon, R., & Alimi, A.M. (1997). Speed/accuracy trade-offs in target-directed movements. *Behavioral and Brain Sciences, 20,* 279-349.

Proteau, L. (1992). On the specificity of learning and the role of visual information for movement control. In L. Proteau & D. Elliott (Eds.), *Vision and motor control* (pp. 67-103). Amsterdam: North-Holland.

Proteau, L., Marteniuk, R.G., Girouard, Y., & Dugas, C. (1987). On the type of information used to control and learn an aiming movement after moderate and extensive training. *Human Movement Science, 6,* 181-199.

Proteau, L., Marteniuk, R.G., & Lévesque, L. (1992). A sensorimotor basis for motor learning: Evidence indicating specificity of practice. *Quarterly Journal of Experimental Psychology A: Human Experimental Psychology, 44,* 557-575.

Proteau, L., Tremblay, L., & DeJaeger, D. (1998). Practice does not diminish the role of visual information in on-line control of a precision walking task: Support for the specificity of practice hypothesis. *Journal of Motor Behavior, 30,* 143-150.

Reinking, R., Goldstein, G., & Houston, B.K. (1974). Cognitive style, proprioceptive skills, task set, stress, and the rod-and-frame test of field orientation. *Journal of Personality and Social Psychology, 30,* 807-811.

Robertson, S., Collins, J., Elliott, D., & Starkes, J. (1994). The influence of skill and intermittent vision on dynamic balance. *Journal of Motor Behavior, 26,* 333-339.

Robertson, S.D., Tremblay, L., Anson, J.G., & Elliott, D. (2002). Learning to cross a balance beam: Implications for teachers, coaches and therapists. In K. Davids, G. Savelsbergh, S. Bennett, & J. van der Kamp (Eds.), *Dynamic interceptive actions in sport: Current research and practical applications* (pp. 109-125). London: E & FN Spon.

Sato, H., Sando, I., & Takahashi, H. (1992). Computer-aided three-dimensional measurement of the human vestibular apparatus. *Otolaryngology: Head and Neck Surgery, 107,* 405-409.

Schmidt, R.A., & Lee, T.D. (2005). *Motor control and learning: A behavioral emphasis.* Champaign, IL: Human Kinetics.

Snoddy, G.S. (1926). Learning and stability: A psychophysical analysis of a case of motor learning with clinical applications. *Journal of Applied Psychology, 10,* 1-36.

Stein, B.E., & Stanford, T.R. (2008). Multisensory integration: Current issues from the perspective of the single neuron. *Nature Reviews Neuroscience, 9,* 255-266.

Tremblay, L., Elliott, D., & Starkes, J.L. (2004). Gender differences in the perception of self-orientation: Software or hardware? *Perception, 33,* 329-337.

Tremblay, L., & Proteau, L. (1998). Specificity of practice: The case of powerlifting. *Research Quarterly for Exercise and Sport, 69,* 284-289.

Tremblay, L., & Proteau, L. (2001). Specificity of practice in a ball interception task: Performance is specific to known ball trajectories not vision of the hand. *Canadian Journal of Experimental Psychology, 55,* 207-218.

Weiss, P. (1941). Self-differentiation of the basic patterns of coordination. *Comparative Psychology Monographs, 17,* 1-96.

Welch, R. (1978). *Perceptual modification: Adapting to altered sensory environments.* New York: Academic Press.

Whiting, H.T.A., Savelsbergh, G.J.P., & Pijpers, J.R. (1995). Specificity of motor learning does not deny flexibility. *Applied Psychology: An International Review, 44,* 315-332.

Witkin, H.A., & Asch, S.E. (1948). Studies in space orientation: IV. Further experiments on perception of the upright with displaced visual fields. *Journal of Experimental Psychology, 38,* 603-614.

Witkin, H.A., Lewis, H.B., Hertzman, M., Machover, K., Bretnall Meissner, P., & Wapner, S. (1977). *Personality through perception.* Westport, CT: Greenwood Press.

Woodworth, R.S. (1899). The accuracy of voluntary movement. *Psychological Review, Monograph Supplements, 3*(13), 1-119.

Wulf, G., & Prinz, W. (2001). Directing attention to movement effects enhances learning: A review. *Psychonomic Bulletin & Review, 8,* 648-660.

CHAPTER 16

Aglioti, S., Goodale, M.A., & DeSouza, J.F.X. (1993). Size contrast deceives the eye but not the hand. *Current Biology, 5,* 679-685.

Aslin, R.N., & Shea, S.L. (1990). Velocity thresholds in human infants—implications for the perception of motion. *Developmental Psychology, 2,* 589-598.

Atkinson, J. (2000). *The developing visual brain.* Oxford, UK: Oxford University Press.

Atkinson, J., & Braddick, O. (2003) Neurobiological models of normal and abnormal visual development. In M. de Haan & M.H. Johnson (Eds.), *The cognitive neuroscience of development* (pp. 43-71). Hove, UK: Psychology Press.

Atkinson, J., Braddick, O., Anker, S., Curran, W., Andrew, R., Wattam-Bell, J., & Braddick, F. (2003). Neurobiological models of visuospatial cognition in children with Williams syndrome: Measures of dorsal-stream and frontal function. *Developmental Neuropsychology, 23,* 139-172.

Atkinson, J., Braddick, O., Rose, F.E., Searcy, Y.M., Wattam-Bell, J., & Bellugi, U. (2006). Dorsal-stream motion processing deficits persist into adulthood in Williams syndrome. *Neuropsychologia, 44,* 828-833.

Atkinson, J., King, J., Braddick, O., Nokes, L., Anker, S., & Braddick, F. (1997). A specific deficit of dorsal stream function in Williams' syndrome. *Cognitive Neuroscience and Neuropsychology, 8,* 1919-1922.

Banton, T., Dobkins, K., & Bertenthal, B.I. (2001). Infant direction discrimination thresholds. *Vision Research, 41,* 1049-1056.

Bertenthal, B.I. (1996). Origins and early development of perception, action, and representation. *Annual Review of Psychology, 47,* 431-459.

Bertenthal, B.I., & Bradburry, A. (1992). Infants' detection of shearing motion in random-dot displays. *Developmental Psychology, 28,* 1056-1066.

Bower, T.G.R., & Wishart, J. (1972). The effects of motor skill on object permanence. *Cognition, 1,* 165-172.

Braddick, O., Atkinson, J., & Wattam-Bell, J. (2003). Normal and anomalous development of visual motion processing: Motion coherence and 'dorsal-stream vulnerability.' *Neuropsychologia, 41,* 1769-1784.

Clifton, R.K., Muir, D.W., Ashmead, D.H., & Clarkson, M.G. (1993). Is visually guided reaching in early infancy a myth? *Child Development, 64,* 1099-1110.

Clifton, R., Perris, E., & Bullinger, A. (1991). Infants' perception of auditory space. *Developmental Psychology, 27,* 187-197.

Clifton, R.K., Rochat, P., Robin, D.J., & Berthier, N.E. (1994). Multimodal perception in the control of infant reaching. *Journal of Experimental Psychology: Human Perception and Performance, 20,* 876-886.

Dannemiller, J.L., & Freedland, R.L. (1989). The detection of slow stimulus movement in 2- to 5-month-olds. *Journal of Experimental Child Psychology, 47,* 337-355.

Dannemiller, J.L., & Freedland, R.L. (1991). Detection of relative motion by human infants. *Developmental Pschology, 27,* 67-78.

Elliott, D. (1990). Intermittent visual pickup and goal directed movement: A review. *Human Movement Science, 9,* 531-548.

Elliott, D., Welsh, T.N., Lyons, J., Hansen, S., & Wu, M. (2006). The visual regulation of goal directed reaching movements in adults with Williams syndrome, Down syndrome and other developmental delays. *Motor Control, 10,* 34-54.

Gibson, E.J., & Pick, A.D. (2000). *An ecological approach to perceptual learning and development.* New York: Oxford University Press.

Gibson, J.J. (1986). *The ecological approach to visual perception.* Hillsdale, NJ: Erlbaum. (Original work published 1979)

Gilmore, R.O., & Johnson, M.H. (1997). Egocentric action in early infancy: Spatial frames of reference for saccades. *Psychological Science, 8,* 224-230.

Gilmore, R.O., & Johnson, M.H. (1998). Learning what is where: Oculomotor contributions to the development of spatial cognition. In F. Simion & G. Butterworth (Eds.), *The development of sensory, motor, and cognitive capacities in early infancy: From perception to cognition* (pp. 25-47). East Sussex, UK: Psychology Press.

Goodale, M.A., & Humphrey, G.K. (1998). The objects of action and perception. *Cognition, 67,* 181-207.

Goodale, M.A., Jakobson, L.S., Milner, A.D., Perrett, D.I., Benson, P.J., & Hietanen, J.K. (1994). The nature and limits of orientation and pattern processing supporting visuomotor control in a visual form agnosic. *Journal of Cognitive Neurosciences, 6,* 46-56.

Goodale, M.A., & Milner, A.D. (1992). Separate visual pathways for perception and action. *Trends in Neuroscience, 15,* 20-25.

Goodale, M.A., & Milner, A.D. (2004). *Sight unseen: An exploration of conscious and unconscious vision.* New York: Oxford University Press.

Goodale, M.A., Milner, A.D., Jakobson, L.S., & Carey, D.P. (1991). A neurological dissociation between perceiving objects and grasping them. *Nature, 349,* 154-156.

Gopnik, A., & Meltzoff, A.N. (1996). *Words, thoughts, and theories.* Cambridge, MA: MIT Press.

Handlovsky, I., Hansen, S., Lee, T.D., & Elliott, D. (2004). The Ebbinghaus illusion affects on-line movement control. *Neuroscience Letters, 366,* 308-311.

Held, R. (1965). Plasticity in sensory-motor systems. *Scientific American, 213,* 84-94.

Hood, B., & Willats, P. (1986). Reaching in the dark to an object's remembered position: Evidence for object permanence in 5-month-old infants. *British Journal of Developmental Psychology, 4,* 57-65.

Hu, Y., Eagleson, R., & Goodale, M.A. (1999). The effects of delay on the kinematics of grasping. *Experimental Brian Research, 126,* 109-116.

Johnson, S.P. (2004). Development of perceptual completion in infancy. *Psychological Science, 15,* 769-775.

Johnson, S.P., Bremner, G., Slater, A., Mason, U., Foster, K., & Cheshire, A. (2003). Infants' perception of object trajectories. *Child Development, 74,* 94-108.

Jonsson, S.P., & von Hofsten, C. (2003). Infants' ability to track and reach for temporarily occluded objects. *Developmental Science, 6,* 86-99.

Kaufmann, F., Stucki, M., & Kaufmann-Hayoz, R. (1985). Development of infants' sensitivity for slow and rapid motions. *Infant Behavior & Development, 8,* 89-95.

Kayed, N.S., & van der Meer, A. (2000). Timing strategies used in defensive blinking to optical collisions in 5- to 7-month-old infants. *Infant Behavior & Development, 23,* 253-270.

Kayed, N.S., & van der Meer, A. (2007). Infants' timing strategies to optical collisions: A longitudinal study. *Infant Behavior & Development, 30,* 50-59.

Kellman, P.J., & Arterberry, M.E. (1998). *The cradle of knowledge: Development of perception in infancy.* Cambridge, MA: MIT Press.

Lee, D.N. (1976). A theory of visual control of braking based on information about time-to-collision. *Perception, 5,* 437-459.

Mason, A.J.S., Braddick, O.J., & Wattam-Bell, J. (2003). Motion corherence thresholds in infants—different tasks identify at least two distinct motion systems. *Vision Research, 43,* 1149-1157.

McCarty, M.E., & Ashmead, D.H. (1999). Visual control of reaching and grasping in infants. *Developmental Psychology, 35,* 620-631.

McCarty, M.E., Clifton, R.K., Ashmead, D.H., Lee, P., & Goubet, N. (2001). How infants use vision for grasping objects. *Child Development, 72,* 973-987.

Mendoza, J., Hansen, S., Glazebrook, C.M., Keetch, K.M., & Elliott, D. (2005). Visual illusions affect both movement planning and on-line control: A multiple cue position on bias and goal-directed action. *Human Movement Science, 24,* 760-773.

Michaels, C.F. (2000). Information, perception, and action: What should ecological psychologists learn from Milner and Goodale (1995)? *Ecological Psychology, 12,* 241-258.

Milner, A.D., & Goodale, M.A. (1995). *The visual brain in action.* Oxford, UK: Oxford University Press.

Milner, A.D., & Goodale, M.A. (2008). Two visual systems re-viewed. *Neuropsychologia, 46,* 774-785.

Munakata, Y., Jonsson, B., Spelke, E.S., & von Hofsten, C. (1996, April). *When it helps to occlude and obscure: 6-month-olds' predictive tracking of moving toys.* Poster presented at the Tenth International Conference on Infants Studies, Providence, RI.

Netelenbos, J.B. (2000). *Motorische ontwikkeling van kinderen. Handboek 2: Theorie.* Amsterdam: Boom.

Perenin, M.T., & Vighetto, A. (1983). Optic ataxia: A specific disorder in visuomotor coordination. In A. Hein & M. Jeannerod (Eds.), *Spatially oriented behavior* (pp. 305-326). New York: Springer-Verlag.

Perenin, M.T., & Vighetto, A. (1988). Optic ataxia: A specific disruption in visuomotor mechanisms. I. Different aspects of the deficit in reaching for objects. *Brain, 111,* 643-674.

Piaget, J. (1952). *The origins of intelligence in children.* New York: Basic Books.

Reed, E.S. (1996). *Encountering the world: Toward an ecological psychology.* New York: Oxford University Press.

Robin, D.J., Berthier, N.E., & Clifton, R.K. (1996). Infants' predictive reaching for moving objects in the dark. *Developmental Psychology, 32,* 824-835.

Rochat, P. (2001). *The infant's world.* Cambridge, MA: Harvard University Press.

Rosander, K., & von Hofsten, C. (2000). Visual-vestibular interaction in early infancy. *Experimental Brain Research, 133,* 321-333.

Rosander, K., & von Hofsten, C. (2002). Development of gaze tracking of small and large objects. *Experimental Brain Research, 146,* 257-264.

Rosander, K., & von Hofsten, C. (2004). Infants' emerging ability to represent occluded object motion. *Cognition, 91,* 1-22.

Rossetti, Y., & Pisella, L. (2002). Several 'vision for action' systems: A guide to dissociating and integrating dorsal and ventral functions. In W. Prinz & B. Hommel (Eds.), *Attention and performance XIX: Common mechanisms in perception and action* (pp. 62-119). New York: Oxford University Press.

Savelsbergh, G., Caljouw, S., van Hof, P., & van der Kamp, J. (2007). Visual constraints in the development of action. *Progress in Brain Research, 164,* 213-225.

Sitskoorn, M.M., & Smitsman, A.W. (1995). Infants' perception of dynamic relations between objects: Passing through or support? *Developmental Psychology, 31,* 437-447.

Smeets, J.B., & Brenner, E. (1995). Perception and action are based on the same visual information: Distinction between position and velocity. *Journal of Experimental Psychology: Human Perception and Performance, 21,* 19-31.

Spelke, E.S., Katz, G., Purcell, S.E., Ehrlich, S.M., & Breinlinger, K. (1994). Early knowledge of object motion: Continuity and inertia. *Cognition, 51,* 131-176.

van der Kamp, J. (1999). *The information-based regulation of interceptive timing* (Doctoral dissertation, VU University). Nieuwegein, Netherlands: Digital Printing Partners Utrecht.

van der Kamp, J., Oudejans, R., & Savelsbergh, G.J.P. (2003). The development and learning of the visual control of movement: An ecological perspective. *Infant Behavior & Development, 26,* 495-515.

van der Kamp, J., Rivas, F., van Doorn, H., & Savelsbergh, G.J.P. (2008). Ventral and dorsal system contribution to visual anticipation in fast ball sports. *International Journal of Sport Psychology, 39,* 100-130.

van der Kamp, J., & Savelsbergh, G.J.P. (2000). Action and perception in infancy. *Infant Behavior & Development, 23,* 237-251.

van der Kamp, J., & Savelsbergh, G.J.P. (2002). On the development of the two visual systems. *Behavioral and Brain Sciences, 25,* 120.

van der Kamp, J., Savelsbergh, G.J.P., & Rosengren, K. (2001). The separation of action and perception, and the issue of affordances. *Ecological Psychology, 13,* 167-172.

van der Kamp, J., Savelsbergh, G.J.P., & Smeets, J. (1997). Multiple information sources in interceptive timing. *Human Movement Science, 16*, 787-821.

van der Meer, A.L.H., van der Weel, F.R., & Lee, D.N. (1994). Prospective control in catching by infants. *Perception, 23*, 287-302.

van Doorn, H., van der Kamp, J., & Savelsbergh, G.J.P. (2007). Grasping the Müller-Lyer illusion: The contribution of vision for perception in action. *Neuropsychologia, 45*, 1939-1947.

van Hof, P. (2005). *Perception-action couplings in early infancy* (Doctoral dissertation, VU University). Enschede, Netherlands: Febodruk BV.

van Hof, P., van der Kamp, J., & Savelsbergh, G.J.P. (2002). The relation of unimanual and bimanual reaching to crossing the midline. *Child Development, 73*, 1353-1362.

van Hof, P., van der Kamp, J., & Savelsbergh, G.J.P. (2006). Two- to eight-month-old infants' catching under monocular and binocular vision. *Human Movement Sciences, 25*, 18-36.

van Hof, P., van der Kamp, J., & Savelsbergh, G.J.P. (2008). The relation between infants' perception of catchableness and the control of catching. *Developmental Psychology, 44*, 182-194.

Volkmann, F.C., & Dobson, M.C. (1976). Infant responses of ocular fixation to moving visual stimuli. *Journal of Experimental Child Psychology, 22*, 86-99.

von Hofsten, C. (1980). Predictive reaching for moving objects. *Journal of Experimental Child Psychology, 30*, 369-382.

von Hofsten, C. (1983). Catching skills in infancy. *Journal of Experimental Psychology: Human Perception and Performance, 9*, 75-85.

von Hofsten, C. (2004). An action perspective on motor development. *Trends in Cognitive Sciences, 8*, 266-272.

von Hofsten, C., Kochukhova, O., & Rosander, K. (2007). Predictive tracking over occlusions by 4-month-old infants. *Developmental Science, 10*, 625-640.

von Hofsten, C., & Lindhagen, K. (1979). Observations on the development of reaching for moving objects. *Journal of Experimental Child Psychology, 28*, 158-173.

von Hofsten, C., & Rosander, K. (1996). The development of gaze control and predictive tracking in young infants. *Vision Research, 36*, 81-96.

von Hofsten, C., & Rosander, K. (1997). Development of smooth pursuit tracking in young infants. *Vision Research, 37*, 1799-1810.

von Hofsten, C., Vishton, P., Spelke, E.S., Feng, Q., & Rosander, K. (1998). Predictive action in infancy: Tracking and reaching for moving objects. *Cognition, 67*, 255-285.

Wattam-Bell, J. (1991). Development of motion-specific cortical responses in infancy. *Vision Research, 31*, 287-297.

Wattam-Bell, J. (1992). The development of maximum displacement limits for discrimination of motion direction in infancy. *Vision Research, 32*, 621-630.

Wattam-Bell, J. (1994). Coherence thresholds for discrimination of motion direction in infants. *Vision Research, 34*, 877-883.

Wattam-Bell, J. (1996a). Visual motion processing in one-month-old infants: Habituation experiments. *Vision Research, 36*, 1679-1685.

Wattam-Bell, J. (1996b). Visual motion processing in one-month-old infants: Preferential looking experiments. *Vision Research, 36*, 1671-1677.

Wattam-Bell, J. (1996c). Infants' discrimination of absolute direction of motion. *Investigative Ophthalmology and Visual Science, 37*, S137.

Westwood, D.A., Chapman, C.D., & Roy, E.A. (2000). Pantomimed actions may be controlled by the ventral visual stream. *Experimental Brain Research, 130*, 545-548.

Westwood, D.A., & Goodale, M.A. (2003). Perceptual illusion and the real-time control of action. *Spatial Vision, 16*, 243-254.

Westwood, D.A., McEachern, T., & Roy, E.A. (2001). Delayed grasping of a Müller-Lyer figure. *Experimental Brain Research, 141*, 166-173.

CHAPTER 17

Adams, J.A. (1986). Use of the model's knowledge of results to increase the observer's performance. *Journal of Human Movement Studies, 12,* 89-98.

Al-Abood, S.A., Davids, K., & Bennett, S.J. (2001). Specificity of task constraints and effects of visual demonstrations and verbal instructions in directing a learner's search during skill acquisition. *Journal of Motor Behavior, 33,* 295-305.

Al-Abood, S.A., Davids, K., Bennett, S.J., Ashford, D., & Martinez-Marin, M. (2001). Effects of manipulating relative and absolute motion information during observational learning of an aiming task. *Journal of Sports Sciences, 19,* 507-520.

Annett, J. (1996). On knowing how to do things: A theory of motor imagery. *Cognitive Brain Research, 3,* 65-69.

Anquetil, T., & Jeannerod, M. (2007). Simulated actions in the first and in the third person perspectives share common representations. *Brain Research, 1130,* 125-129.

Ashford, D., Bennett, S.J., & Davids, K. (2006). Observational modeling effects for movement dynamics and movement outcome measures across differing task constraints: A meta-analysis. *Journal of Motor Behavior, 38,* 185-205.

Ashford, D., Davids, K., & Bennett, S.J. (2007). Developmental effects influencing observational modeling: A meta-analysis. *Journal of Sports Sciences, 25,* 547-558.

Badets, A., & Blandin, Y. (2004). The role of knowledge of results frequency in learning through observation. *Journal of Motor Behavior, 36,* 62-70.

Badets, A., & Blandin, Y. (2005). Observational learning: Effects of bandwidth knowledge of results. *Journal of Motor Behavior, 37,* 211-216.

Badets, A., Blandin, Y., Bouquet, C.A., & Shea, C.H. (2006). The intention superiority effect in motor skill learning. *Journal of Experimental Psychology: Learning, Memory, and Cognition, 32,* 491-505.

Badets, A., Blandin, Y., & Shea, C.H. (2006). Intention in motor learning through observation. *Quarterly Journal of Experimental Psychology, 59,* 377-386.

Badets, A., Blandin, Y., Wright, D.L., & Shea, C.H. (2006). Error detection processes during observational learning. *Research Quarterly for Exercise and Sport, 77,* 177-184.

Bandura, A. (1965). Vicarious processes: A case of no-trial learning. In L. Berkowitz (Ed.), *Advances in experimental social psychology* (Vol. 2, pp. 1-55). New York: Academic Press.

Bandura, A. (1971). Analysis of modeling processes. In A. Bandura (Ed.), *Psychological modeling: Conflicting theories* (pp. 1-62). Chicago: Adline-Atherton.

Bandura, A. (1977). *Social learning theory.* New York: General Learning Press.

Bandura, A. (1986). *Social foundations of thought and action: A social cognitive theory.* Englewood Cliffs, NJ: Prentice Hall.

Bekkering, H., Wohlschlager, A., & Gattis, M. (2000). Imitation of gestures in children is goal-directed. *Quarterly Journal of Experimental Psychology A: Human Experimental Psychology, 53,* 153-164.

Berry, D.C., & Broadbent, D. (1988). On the relationship between task performance and associated task knowledge. *Quarterly Journal of Experimental Psychology A: Human Experimental Psychology, 36,* 209-231.

Bird, G., & Heyes, C. (2005). Effector-dependent learning by observation of a finger movement sequence. *Journal of Experimental Psychology: Human Perception and Performance, 31,* 262-275.

Bird, G., Brindley, R., Leighton, J., & Heyes, C. (2007). General processes, rather than "goals," explain imitation errors. *Journal of Experimental Psychology: Human Perception and Performance, 33,* 1158-1169.

Black, C.B., & Wright, D.L. (2000). Can observational practice facilitate error recognition and movement production? *Research Quarterly for Exercise and Sport, 71,* 331-339.

Black, C.B., Wright, D.L., Magnuson, C.E., & Brueckner, S. (2005). Learning to detect error in movement timing using physical and observational practice. *Research Quarterly for Exercise and Sport, 76,* 28-41.

Blandin, Y., & Proteau, L. (2000). On the cognitive basis of observational learning: Development of mechanisms for the detection and correction of errors. *Quarterly Journal of Experimental Psychology A: Human Experimental Psychology, 53,* 846-867.

Blandin, Y., Lhuisset, L., & Proteau, L. (1999). Cognitive processes underlying observational learning of motor skills. *Quarterly Journal of Experimental Psychology A: Human Experimental Psychology, 52,* 957-979.

Bouquet, C.A., Gaurier, V., Shipley, T., Toussaint, L., & Blandin, Y. (2007). Influence of the perception of biological or non-biological motion on movement execution. *Journal of Sports Sciences, 25,* 519-530.

Brass, M., & Heyes, C. (2005). Imitation: Is cognitive neuroscience solving the correspondence problem? *Trends in Cognitive Sciences, 9,* 489-495.

Brass, M., Bekkering, H., & Prinz, W. (2001). Movement observation affects movement execution in a simple response task. *Acta Psychologica, 106,* 3-22.

Brass, M., Bekkering, H., Wohlschlager, A., & Prinz, W. (2000). Compatibility between observed and executed finger movements: Comparing symbolic, spatial, and imitative cues. *Brain and Cognition, 44,* 124-143.

Breslin, G., Hodges, N.J., & Williams, A.M. (in press). Manipulating the timing of relative motion information to facilitate observational learning. *Research Quarterly for Exercise and Sport.*

Breslin, G., Hodges, N.J., Williams, A.M., Kremer, J., & Curran, W. (2005). Modelling relative motion to facilitate intra-limb coordination. *Human Movement Science, 24,* 446-463.

Breslin, G., Hodges, N.J., Williams, A.M., Kremer, J., & Curran, W. (2006). A comparison of intra- and inter-limb relative motion information in modelling a novel motor skill. *Human Movement Science, 25,* 753-766.

Buccino, G., Binkofski, F., Fink, G.R., Fadiga, L., Fogassi, G., Gallese, V., Seitz, R.J., Zilles, K., Rizzolatti, G., & Freund, H.-J. (2001). Action observation activates premotor and parietal areas in a somatotopic manner: An fMRI study. *European Journal of Neuroscience, 13,* 400-404.

Buccino G., Vogt, S., Ritzl, A., Fink, G.R., Zilles, K., Freund, H.J., & Rizzolatti, G. (2004). Neural circuits underlying imitation learning of hand actions: An event-related fMRI study. *Neuron, 42,* 323-334.

Buchanan, J.J., Ryu, Y.U., Zihlman, K.A., & Wright, D. (2008). Observational learning of relative but not absolute motion features in a single-limb multi-joint coordination task. *Experimental Brain Research, 191,* 157-169.

Calvo-Merino, B., Glaser, D.E., Grezes, J., Passingham, R.E., & Haggard, P. (2005). Action observation and acquired motor skills: An fMRI study with expert dancers. *Cerebral Cortex, 15,* 1243-1249.

Calvo-Merino, B., Grezes, J., Glaser, D.E., Passingham, R.E., & Haggard, P. (2006). Seeing or doing? Influence of visual and motor familiarity in action observation. *Current Biology, 16,* 1905-1910.

Candidi, M., Urgesi, C., Ionta, S., & Aglioti, S.M. (2007). Virtual lesion of ventral premotor cortex impairs visual perception of biomechanically possible but not impossible actions. *Social Neuroscience, 3,* 388-400.

Carroll, W.R., & Bandura, A. (1982). The role of visual monitoring in observational learning of action patterns: Making the unobservable observable. *Journal of Motor Behavior, 14,* 153-167.

Carroll, W.R., & Bandura, A. (1990). Representational guidance of action production in observational learning: A causal analysis. *Journal of Motor Behavior, 22,* 85-97.

Casile, A., & Giese, M.A. (2006). Nonvisual motor training influences biological motion perception. *Current Biology, 16,* 69-74.

Chaminade, T., Meltzoff, A.N., & Decety, J. (2002). Does the end justify the means? A PET exploration of imitation. *NeuroImage, 15,* 318-328.

Craighero, L., Bello, A., Fadiga, L., & Rizzolatti, G. (2002). Hand action preparation influences the responses to hand pictures. *Nueropsychologia, 40,* 492-502.

Cross, E.S., Hamilton, A., & Grafton, S.T. (2006). Building a motor simulation de novo: Observation of dance by dancers. *NeuroImage, 31,* 1257-1267.

d'Arripe-Longeuville, F., Gernigon, C., Huet, M.L., Cadopi, M., & Winnykamen, F. (2002). Peer tutoring in a physical education setting: Influence of tutor skill level on novice learners' motivation and performance. *Journal of Teaching in Physical Education, 22,* 105-123.

Decety, J., & Grezes, J. (1999). Neural mechanisms subserving the perception of human actions. *Trends in Cognitive Sciences, 5,* 172-178.

Decety, J., Grezes, J., Costes, N., Perani, D., Jeannerod, M., Procyk, E., Grassi, F., & Fazio, F. (1997). Brain activity during observation of actions: Influence of action content and subject's strategy. *Brain, 120,* 1763-1777.

Decety, J., Sjoholm, H., Ryding, E., Stenberg, G., & Ingvar, D.H. (1990). The cerebellum participates in mental activity: Tomographic measurements of regional cerebral blood flow. *Brain Research, 535,* 313-317.

Désy, M.C., & Théoret, H. (2007). Modulation of motor cortex excitability by physical similarity with an observed hand action. *PLoS, ONE, 10,* 1371.

di Pellegrino, G., Fadiga, L., Fogassi, L., Gallese, V., & Rizzolatti, G. (1992). Understanding motor events: A neurophysiological study. *Experimental Brain Research, 91,* 176-180.

Dowrick, P.W. (1999). A review of self-modeling and related interventions. *Applied and Preventative Psychology, 8,* 23-39.

Edwards, C., Cybucki, J., Balzer, W., Maolovat, D., Chua, K., & Hodges, N.J. (2008). Visual search and bimanual coordination: Searching for strategies of performance. *Journal of Sport & Exercise Psychology,* S75.

Elsner, B., & Hommel, B. (2001). Effect anticipation and action control. *Journal of Experimental Psychology: Human Perception and Performance, 27,* 229-240.

Fadiga, L., & Craighero, L. (2003). New insights on sensorimotor integration: From hand action to speech perception. *Brain and Cognition, 53,* 514-524.

Fadiga, L., & Craighero, L. (2004). Electrophysiology of action representation. *Journal of Clinical Neurophysiology, 21,* 157-169.

Fadiga, L., Fogassi, L., Pavesi, G., & Rizzolatti, G. (1995). Motor facilitation during action observation: A magnetic stimulation study. *Journal of Neurophysiology, 73,* 2608-2611.

Falck-Ytter, T., Gredebäck, G., & von Hofsten, C. (2006). Infants predict other people's action goals. *Nature Neuroscience, 9,* 878-879.

Flanagan, J.R., & Johansson, R.S. (2003). Action plans used in action observation. *Nature, 424,* 769-771.

Fogassi, L., Ferrari, P.F., Gesierich, B., Rozzi, S., Chersi, F., & Rizzolatti, G. (2005). Parietal lobe: From action organization to intention understanding. *Science, 308,* 662-667.

Ford, P., Hodges, N.J., Huys, R., & Williams, A.M. (2006). The role of external action-effects in the execution of a soccer kick: A comparison across skill-level. *Motor Control, 10,* 386-404.

Ford, P., Hodges, N.J., & Williams, A.M. (2005). On-line attentional-focus manipulations in a soccer dribbling task: Implications for the proceduralization of motor skills. *Journal of Motor Behavior, 37,* 386-394.

Gallese, V., Fadiga, L., Fogassi, L., & Rizzolatti, G. (1996). Action recognition in the premotor cortex. *Brain, 119,* 593-609.

Gazzola, V., Rizzolatti, G., Wicker, B., & Keysers, C. (2007). The anthropomorphic brain: The mirror neuron system responds to human and robotic actions. *NeuroImage, 35,* 1674-1684.

Gentile, A.M. (1972). A working model of skill acquisition to teaching. *Quest, 17,* 3-23.

Gergely, G., Bekkering, H., & Kiraly, I. (2002). Rational imitation in preverbal infants. *Nature, 415,* 755.

Gould, D.R., & Roberts, G.C. (1981). Modeling and motor skill acquisition. *Quest, 33,* 214-230.

Grafton, S.T., Arbib, M.A., Fadiga, L., & Rizzolatti, G. (1996). Localization of grasp representations in humans by positron emission tomography. *Experimental Brain Research, 112,* 103-111.

Green, T.D., & Flowers, J.H. (1991). Implicit versus explicit learning processes in a probabilistic, continuous fine-motor catching task. *Journal of Motor Behavior, 23,* 293-300.

Grezes, J., Armony, J.L., Rowe, J., & Passingham, R.E. (2003). Activations related to "mirror" and "canonical" neurons in the human brain: An fMRI study. *NeuroImage, 18,* 928-937.

Grezes, J., Costes, N., & Decety, J. (1998). Top-down effect of strategy on the perception of meaningless actions. *Brain, 122,* 1875-1887.

Griffin, K., & Meaney, K.S. (2000). Modeling and motor performance: An examination of model similarity and model type on children's motor performance. *Research Quarterly for Exercise and Sport, 71,* A-56, 67.

Hamilton, A., & Grafton, S.T. (2006). Goal representation in human anterior intraparietal sulcus. *Journal of Neuroscience, 26,* 1133-1137.

Haslinger, B., Erhard, P., Altenmuller, E., Schroeder, U., Boecker, H., & Ceballos-Baumann, O. (2005). Transmodal sensorimotor networks during action observation in professional pianist. *Journal of Cognitive Neuroscience, 17,* 282-293.

Hayes, S.J., Ashford, D., & Bennett, S.J. (2008). Goal-directed imitation: The means to an end. *Acta Psychologica, 127,* 407-415.

Hayes, S.J., Hodges, N.J., Huys, R., & Williams, A.M. (2007). End-point focus manipulations to determine what information is used during observational learning. *Acta Psychologica, 126,* 120-137.

Hayes, S.J., Hodges, N.J., Scott, M.A., Horn, R.R., & Williams, A.M. (2006). Scaling a motor skill through observation and practice. *Journal of Motor Behavior, 38,* 357-366.

Hayes, S.J., Hodges, N.J., Scott, M.A., Horn, R.R., & Williams, A.M. (2007). The efficacy of demonstrations in teaching children an unfamiliar movement skill: The effects of object-orientation and point-light demonstrations. *Journal of Sports Sciences, 25,* 559-575.

Hecht, H., Vogt, S., & Prinz, W. (2001). Motor learning enhances perceptual judgment: A case for action-perception transfer. *Psychological Research, 65,* 3-14.

Herbert, E.P., & Landin, D. (1994). Effects of a learning model and augmented feedback in tennis skill acquisition. *Research Quarterly for Exercise and Sport, 65,* 250-257.

Hesse, M.D., & Fink, G.R. (2007). End or means? Attentional modulation of the human mirror neuron system. *Clinical Neurophysiology, 118,* e46.

Heyes, C.M. (2002). Transformational and associative theories of imitation. In K. Dautenhahn & C. Nehaniv (Eds.), *Imitation in animals and artifacts* (pp. 501-523). Cambridge, MA: MIT Press.

Heyes, C., & Foster, C.L. (2002). Motor learning by observation: Evidence from a serial reaction time task. *Quarterly Journal of Experimental Psychology A: Human Experimental Psychology, 55,* 593-607.

Hodges, N.J., & Franks, I.M. (2000). Attention focusing instructions and coordination bias: Implications for learning a novel bimanual task. *Human Movement Science, 19,* 843-867.

Hodges, N.J., & Franks, I.M. (2001). Learning a coordination skill: Interactive effects of instruction and feedback. *Research Quarterly for Exercise and Sport, 72,* 132-142.

Hodges, N.J., & Franks, I.M. (2002a). Learning as a function of coordination bias: Building upon pre-practice behaviours. *Human Movement Science, 21,* 231-258.

Hodges, N.J., & Franks, I.M. (2002b). Modelling coaching practice: The role of instructions and demonstrations. *Journal of Sports Sciences, 20,* 1-19.

Hodges, N.J., Chua, R., & Franks, I.M. (2003). The role of video in facilitating perception and action of a novel coordination movement. *Journal of Motor Behavior, 35,* 247-260.

Hodges, N.J., Hayes, S., Breslin, G., & Williams, A.M. (2005). An evaluation of the minimal constraining information during movement observation and reproduction. *Acta Psychologica, 119,* 264-282.

Hodges, N.J., Hayes, S.J., Eaves, D., Horn, R., & Williams, A.M. (2006). End-point trajectory matching as a method for teaching kicking skills. *International Journal of Sport Psychology, 37,* 230-247.

Hodges, N.J., Williams, A.M., Hayes, S.J., & Breslin, G. (2007). What is modelled during observational learning? *Journal of Sports Sciences, 25,* 531-545.

Hommel, B., Musseler, J., Aschersleben, G., & Prinz, W. (2001). The theory of event coding (TEC): A framework for perception and action planning. *Behavioral and Brain Sciences, 24,* 849-878.

Horn, R.R., & Williams, A.M. (2004). Observational learning: Is it time we took another look? In A.M. Williams & N.J. Hodges (Eds.), *Skill acquisition in sport: Research, theory and practice* (pp. 175-206). New York: Routledge. Horn, R.R., Williams, A.M., & Scott, M.A. (2002). Learning from demonstrations: The role of visual search during observational learning from video and point-light models. *Journal of Sports Sciences, 20,* 253-269.

Horn, R.R., Williams, A.M., Scott, M.A., & Hodges, N.J. (2005). Visual search and coordination changes in response to video and point-light demonstrations without KR motion. *Journal of Motor Behavior, 37,* 265-275.

Howard, J.H., Jr., Mutter, S.A., & Howard, D.V. (1992). Direct and indirect measures of serial pattern learning by event observation. *Journal of Experimental Psychology: Learning, Memory, and Cognition, 18*, 1029-1039.

Hurley, S., & Chater, N. (Eds.). (2005). *Perspectives on imitation: From neuroscience to social science.* Cambridge, MA: MIT Press.

Iacoboni, M. (2005). Neural mechanisms of imitation. *Current Opinion in Neurobiology, 15*, 632-637.

Iacoboni, M., Molnar-Szakacs, I., Gallese, V., Buccino, G., Mazziotta, J.C., & Rizzolatti, G. (2005). Grasping the intentions of others with one's own mirror neuron system. *PLoS Biology, 3*(3), 529-535.

James, W. (1890). *The principles of psychology.* New York: HoltJanelle, C.M., Champenoy, J.D., Coombes, S.A., & Mousseau, M.B. (2003). Mechanisms of attentional cueing during observational learning to facilitate motor skill acquisition. *Journal of Sports Sciences, 21*, 825-838.

Jeannerod, M. (1994). The representing brain: Neural correlates of motor intention and imagery. *Behavioral and Brain Sciences, 17*, 197-245.

Jeannerod, M. (2001). Neural simulation of action: A unifying mechanism for motor cognition. *NeuroImage, 14*, S103-S109.

Jeannerod, M., & Frak, V. (1999). Mental imaging of motor activity in humans. *Current Opinion in Neurobiology, 9*, 735-739.

Johansson, G. (1971). *Visual motion perception: A model for visual motion and space perception from changing proximal stimulation* (Rep. No. 98). Uppsala, Sweden: Uppsala University, Department of Psychology.

Johansson, G. (1973). Visual perception of biological motion and a model for its analysis. *Perception & Psychophysics, 14*, 201-211.

Johansson, G. (1975). Visual motion perception. *Scientific American, 232*, 76-89.

Kelly, A.M., & Garavan, H. (2005). Human functional neuroimaging of brain changes associated with practice. *Cerebral Cortex, 15*, 1089-1102.

Kilner, J.M., Paulignan, Y., & Blackmore, S.J. (2003). An interference effect of observed biological movement on action. *Current Biology, 13*, 522-525.

Koch, I., Keller, P., & Prinz, W. (2004). The ideomotor approach to action control: Implications for skilled performance. *International Journal of Sport & Exercise Psychology, 2*, 362-375.

Kohl, R.M., & Shea, C.H. (1992). Observational learning: Influences on temporal response organization. *Human Performance, 5*, 235-244.

Kohler, E., Keysers, C., Umilta, M.A., Fogassi, L., Gallese, V., & Rizzolatti, G. (2002). Hearing sounds, understanding actions: Action representation in mirror neurons. *Science, 297*, 846-848.

Kugler, P.N., Kelso, J.A.S., & Turvey, M.T. (1980). On the concept of coordinative structures as dissipative structures: Theoretical lines of convergence. In G.E. Stelmach & J. Requin (Eds.), *Tutorials in motor behavior* (pp. 3-47). Amsterdam: North-Holland.

Kugler, P.N., Kelso, J.A.S., & Turvey, M.T. (1982). On the control and co-ordination of naturally developing systems. In J.A.S. Kelso & J.E. Clark (Eds.), *The development of movement control and co-ordination* (pp. 5-78). New York: Wiley.

Landers, D.M., & Landers, D.M. (1973). Teacher versus peer models: Effects of model's presence and performance level on motor behavior. *Journal of Motor Behavior, 5*, 129-139.

Lee, T.D., & White, M.A. (1990). Influence of an unskilled model's practice schedule on observational motor learning. *Human Movement Science, 9*, 349-367.

Lee, T.D., Swinnen, S.P., & Verschueren, S. (1995). Relative phase alterations during bimanual skill acquisition. *Journal of Motor Behavior, 27*, 263-274.

Magill, R.A., & Clark, R. (1997). Implicit versus explicit learning of pursuit-tracking patterns. *Journal of Exercise and Sport Psychology, 19*, S85.

Martens, R., Burwitz, L., & Zuckerman, J. (1976). Modeling effects on motor performance. *Research Quarterly, 47*, 277-291.

Maslovat, D., Hodges, N.J., Krigolson, O. & Handy, T (in review). Physical versus observational practice of a novel coordination skill: Behavioural and neurological changes. *Experimental Brain Research*

Mataric, M.J., & Pomplun, M. (1998). Fixation behavior in observation and imitation of human movement. *Cognitive Brain Research, 7,* 191-202.

Mather, G., Radford, K., & West, S. (1992). Low-level visual processing of biological motion. *Proceedings: Biological Sciences, 249,* 149-155.

Mattar, A.A.G., & Gribble, P.L. (2005). Motor learning by observing. *Neuron, 46,* 153-160.

McCullagh, P. (1986). Model status as a determinant of attention in observational learning and performance. *Journal of Sport Psychology, 8,* 319-331.

McCullagh, P., & Caird, J.K. (1990). Correct and learning models and the use of model knowledge of results in the acquisition and retention of a motor skill. *Journal of Human Movement Sciences, 18,* 107-116.

McCullagh, P., & Meyer, K.N. (1997). Learning versus correct models: Influence of model type on the learning of a free-weight squat lift. *Research Quarterly for Exercise and Sport, 68,* 56-61.

McCullagh, P., & Weiss, M.R. (2001). Modeling: Considerations for motor skill performance and psychological responses. In R.N. Singer, H.A. Hausenblaus, & C.M. Janelle (Eds.), *Handbook of sport psychology* (2nd ed., pp. 205-238). New York: Wiley.

Meegan, D., Aslin, R.N., & Jacobs, R.A. (2000). Motor timing learned without motor straining. *Nature Neuroscience, 3,* 860-862.

Meltzoff, A.N. (1993). Molyneux's babies: Cross-modal perception, imitation, and the mind of the preverbal infant. In N. Eilan, R. McCarthy, & B. Brewer (Eds.), *Spatial representation: Problems in philosophy and psychology* (pp. 219-235). Cambridge, MA: Blackwell.

Meltzoff, A.N. (2002). Elements of a developmental theory of imitation. In A.N. Meltzoff & W. Prinz (Eds.), *The imitative mind: Development, evolution and brain bases* (pp. 19-41). Cambridge: Cambridge University Press.

Meltzoff, A.N., & Moore, M.K. (1977). Imitation of facial and manual gestures by human neonates. *Science, 198,* 75-78.

Meltzoff, A.N., & Moore, M.K. (1983). Newborn infants imitate adult facial gestures. *Child Development, 54,* 702-709.

Meltzoff, A.N., & Moore, M.K. (1989). Imitation in newborn infants: Exploring the range of gestures imitated and the underlying mechanisms. *Developmental Psychology, 25,* 954-962.

Meltzoff, A.N., & Moore, M.K. (1997). Explaining facial imitation: A theoretical model. *Early Development and Parenting, 6,* 179-192.

Meltzoff, A.N., & Moore, M.K. (2002). Imitation, memory, and the representation of persons. *Infant Behavior & Development, 25,* 39-61.

Meltzoff, A.N., & Prinz, W. (Eds.). (2002). *The imitative mind: Development, evolution, and brain bases.* Cambridge: Cambridge University Press.

Miall, R.C., Stanley, J., Todhunter, S., Levick, C., Lindo, S., & Miall, J.D. (2006). Performing hand actions assists the visual discrimination of similar hand postures. *Neuropsychologia, 44,* 966-976.

Milton, J., Small, S.L., & Solodkin, A (2008). Imaging motor imagery: methodological issues related to expertise, *Methods, 45,* 336-341.

Molnar-Szakacs, I., Kaplan, J., Greenfield, P.M., & Iacoboni, M. (2006). Observing complex action sequences: The role of the fronto-partietal mirror neuron system. *NeuroImage, 33,* 923-935.

Mulder, T., Zijlstra, S., Zijlstra, W., & Hochstenbach, J. (2007). The role of motor imagery in learning a totally novel movement. *Experimental Brain Research, 154,* 211-217.

Newell, K.M. (1981). Skill learning. In D. Holding (Ed.), *Human skills* (pp. 203-226). New York: Wiley.

Newell, K.M. (1985). Coordination, control and skill. In D. Goodman, R.B. Wilberg, & I.M. Franks (Eds.), *Differing perspectives in motor learning, memory and control* (pp. 295-317). Amsterdam: Elsevier.

Newell, K.M., Morris, L.R., & Scully, D.M. (1985). Augmented information and the acquisition of skills in physical activity. In R.L. Terjung (Ed.), *Exercise and sport sciences reviews* (pp. 235-261). New York: Macmillan.

Perani, D., Fazio, F., Borghese, N.A., Tettamanti, M., Ferrari, S., Decety, J., & Gilardi, M.C. (2001). Different brain correlates for watching real and virtual hand actions. *NeuroImage, 14,* 749-758.

Pinto, J., & Shiffrar, M. (1999). Subconfigurations of the human form in the perception of biological motion displays. *Acta Psychologica, 102,* 293-318.

Pollock, B.J., & Lee, T.D. (1992). Effects of the model's skill level on observational motor learning. *Research Quarterly for Exercise and Sport, 63,* 25-29.

Porro, C.A., Facchin, P., Fusi, S., Dri, G., & Fadiga, L. (2007). Enhancement of force after action observation: Behavioural and neurophysiological studies. *Neuropsychologia, 45,* 3114-3121.

Press, C., Gillmeister, H., & Heyes, C. (2007). Sensorimotor experience enhances automatic imitation of robotic action. *Proceedings of the Royal Society of London. Series B, Biological Sciences, 274,* 2509-2514.

Prinz, W. (1997). Perception and action planning. *European Journal of Cognitive Psychology, 9,* 129-154.

Prinz, W. (2002). Experimental approaches to imitation. In A.N. Meltzoff & W. Prinz (Eds.), *The imitative mind: Development, evolution, and brain bases* (pp. 143-162). Cambridge: Cambridge University Press.

Prinz, W. (2005). An ideomotor approach to imitation. In S. Hurley & N. Chater (Eds.), *Perspectives on imitation: From neuroscience to social science* (Vol. 1, pp. 141-156). Cambridge, MA: MIT Press.

Prinz, W. (2006). What re-enactment earns us. *Cortex, 42,* 515-517.

Ram, N., Riggs, S.M., Skaling, S., Landers, D.M., & McCullagh, P. (2007). A comparison of modelling and imagery in the acquisition and retention of motor skills. *Journal of Sport Sciences, 25,* 587-597.

Reed, C.L., & Farah, M.J. (1995). The psychological reality of the body schema: A test with normal participants. *Journal of Experimental Psychology: Human Perception and Performance, 21,* 334-343.

Rizzolatti, G., & Craighero, L. (2004). The mirror-neuron system. *Annual Review of Neuroscience, 27,* 169-192.

Rizzolatti, G., Fadiga, L., Gallese, V., & Fogassi, L. (1996). Premotor cortex and the recognition of motor actions. *Cognitive Brain Research, 3,* 131-141.

Rizzolatti, G., Fogassi, L., & Gallese, V. (2001). Neurophysiological mechanisms underlying the understanding of imitation and action. *Nature Reviews Neuroscience, 2,* 661-670.

Romack, J.L. (1995). Information in visual event perception and its use in observational learning. In B.G. Bardy, R.J. Bootsma, & Y. Guiard (Eds.), *Studies in perception and action III* (pp. 289-294). Hillsdale, NJ: Erlbaum.

Rothstein, A.L., & Arnold, R.K. (1976). Bridging the gap: Application of research on videotape feedback and bowling. *Motor Skills: Theory Into Practice, 1,* 35-62.

Rotman, G., Troje, N.F., Johansson, R.S., & Flanagan, J.R. (2006). Eye movements when observing predictable and unpredictable actions. *Journal of Neurophysiology, 96,* 1358-1369.

Rumiati, R.I., & Bekkering, H. (2003). To imitate or not to imitate? How the brain can do it, that is the question! *Brain and Cognition, 53,* 479-482.

Rumiati, R.I., Weiss, P.H., Tessari, A., Assmus, A., Zilles, K., Herzog, H., & Fink, G.R. (2005). Common and differential neural mechanisms supporting imitation of meaningful and meaningless actions. *Journal of Cognitive Neuroscience, 17,* 1420-1431.

Scully, D.M., & Carnegie, E. (1998). Observational learning in motor skill acquisition: A look at demonstrations. *Irish Journal of Psychology, 19,* 472-485.

Scully, D.M., & Newell, K.M. (1985). Observational learning and the acquisition of motor skills: Toward a visual perception perspective. *Journal of Human Movement Studies, 11,* 169-186.

Shea, C.H., Wright, D.L., Wulf, G., & Whitacre, C. (2000). Physical and observational practices afford unique learning opportunities. *Journal of Motor Behavior, 32,* 27-36.

Sheffield, F.D. (1961). Theoretical considerations in the learning of complex sequential tasks from demonstration and practice. In A.A. Lumsdaine (Ed.), *Student response in programmed instructions: A symposium* (pp 13-52). Washington, DC: National Academy of Sciences, National Research Council.

Stanley, J., Gowen, E., & Miall, R.C. (2007). Effects of agency on movement interference during observation of a moving dot stimulus. *Journal of Experimental Psychology: Human Perception and Performance, 33,* 915-926.

Stevens, J.A., Fonlupt, P., Shiffrar, M., & Decety, J. (2000). New aspects of motion perception: Selective neural encoding of apparent human movements. *Neuroreport, 11,* 109-115.

Tai, Y.F., Scherfler, C., Brooks, D.J., Sawamoto, N., & Castiello, U. (2004). The human premotor cortex is 'mirror' only for biological actions. *Current Biology, 14,* 117-120.

Tessari, A., Bosanac, D., & Rumiati, R.I. (2006). Effect of learning on imitation of new actions: Implications for a memory model. *Experimental Brain Research, 173,* 507-513.

Tomasino, B., Werner, C.J., Weiss, P.H., & Fink, G.R. (2007). Stimulus properties matter more than perspective: An fMRI study of mental imagery and silent reading of action phrases. *NeuroImage, 36,* T128-T141.

Umilta, M.A., Kohler, E., Gallese, V., Fogassi, L., Fadiga, L., Keysers, C., & Rizzolatti, G. (2001). I know what you are doing: A neurophysiological study. *Neuron, 31,* 155-165.

van Schie, H.T., Mars, R.B., Coles, M.G.H., & Bekkering, H. (2004). Modulation of activity in medial frontal and motor cortices during error observation. *Nature Neuroscience, 7,* 549-554.

Vereijken, B. (1991). The dynamics of skill acquisition. Amsterdam: Free University of Amsterdam.

Vereijken, B., & Whiting, H.T.A. (1990). In defence of discovery learning. *Canadian Journal of Sports Sciences, 15,* 99-106.

Vogt, S. (1996). Imagery and perception-action mediation in imitative actions. *Cognitive Brain Research, 3,* 79-86.

Vogt, S. (2002). Visuomotor couplings in object-oriented and imitative actions. In A.N. Meltzoff & W. Prinz (Eds.), *The imitative mind: Development, evolution, and brain bases* (pp. 206-220). Cambridge: Cambridge University Press.

Vogt, S., & Thomaschke, R. (2007). From visuo-motor interactions to imitation learning: Behavioural and brain imaging studies. *Journal of Sports Sciences, 25,* 3-23.

Vogt, S., Buccino, G., Wohlschlager, A.M., Canessa, N., Jon Shah, N.J., Zilles, K., Eickhoff, S.B., Freund, H.J., Rizzolatti, G., & Fink, G.R. (2007). Prefrontal involvement in imitation learning of hand actions: Effects of practice and expertise. *NeuroImage, 37,* 1371-1383.

Vogt, S., Taylor, P., & Hopkins, B. (2003). Visuomotor priming by pictures of hand postures: Perspective matters. *Neuropsychologia, 41,* 941-951.

Weeks, D.L., & Anderson, L.P. (2000). The interaction of observational learning with overt practice: Effects on motor skill learning. *Acta Psychologica, 104,* 259-271.

Weir, P.L., & Leavitt, J.L. (1990). Effects of model's skill level and model's knowledge of results on the performance of a dart throwing task. *Human Movement Science, 9,* 369-383.

Whiting, H.T.A., & den Brinker, B.P.L.M. (1982). Image of the act. In J.P. Das, R.F. Mulcahy, & A.E. Wall (Eds.), *Theory and research in learning disabilities* (pp. 217-235). New York: Plenum Press.

Whiting, H.T.A., Bijlard, M.J., & den Brinker, B.P.L.M. (1987). The effect of the availability of a dynamic model on the acquisition of a complex cyclical action. *Quarterly Journal of Experimental Psychology A: Human Experimental Psychology, 39,* 43-59.

Williams, A.M., Davids, K., & Williams, J.G. (1999). *Visual perception and action in sport.* London: E & FN Spon.

Wilson, M., & Knoblich, G. (2005). The case for motor involvement in perceiving conspecifics. *Psychological Bulletin, 131,* 460-473.

Wohlschlager, A., Gattis, M., & Bekkering, H. (2003). Action generation and action perception in imitation: An instance of the ideomotor principle. *Philosophical Transactions of the Royal Society of London B: Biological Sciences 358,* 501-516.

Wright, D.L., Li, Y., & Coady, W. (1997). Cognitive processes related to contextual interference and observational learning: A replication of Blandin, Proteau and Alain. *Research Quarterly for Exercise and Sport, 68,* 106-109.

Zentgraf, K., Stark, R., Reiser, M., Kunzell, S., Schienle, A., Kirsch, P., Walter, B., Vaitl, D., & Munzert, J. (2005). Differential activation of pre-SMA and SMA proper during action observation: Effects of instructions. *NeuroImage, 26,* 662-672.

CHAPTER 18

Adler, R.E. (2002). *Science firsts: From the creation of science to the science of creation.* Hoboken, NJ: Wiley.

Anzola, G.P., Bertoloni, G., Buchtel, H.A., & Rizzolatti, G. (1977). Spatial compatibility and anatomical factors in simple and choice reaction time. *Neuropsychologia, 15*, 295-302.

Bryan, W.L., & Harter, N. (1899). Studies in the physiology and psychology of the telegraphic language. *Psychological Review, 4*, 345-375.

Chapanis, A. (1965). *Man-machine engineering*. Belmont, CA: Wadsworth Publishing.

Colavita, F.B. (1974). Human sensory dominance. *Perception & Psychophysics, 16*, 409-412.

Donders, F.C. (1969). On the speed of mental processes. In W.G. Koster (Ed. & Trans.), *Attention and performance II*. Amsterdam: North-Holland. (Original work published 1868)

Edwards, E. (1988). Introductory overview. In F.L. Wiener & D.C. Nagel (Eds.), *Human factors in aviation* (pp. 3-25). San Diego: Academic Press.

Fechner, G.T. (1966). *Elements of psychophysics* (Vol. 1, E.G. Boring & D.H. Howes, Eds., H.E. Adler, Trans.). New York: Holt, Rienhart & Winston. (Original work published 1860)

Fitts, P.M. (1947). Psychological research on equipment design in the AAF. *American Psychologist, 2*, 93-98.

Fitts, P.M. (1954). The information capacity of the human motor system in controlling the amplitude of movement. *Journal of Experimental Psychology, 47*, 381-391.

Fitts, P.M., & Jones, R.E. (1947). Reduction of pilot error by design of aircraft controls. *Technical Data Digest U.S. Air Force Air Materiel Command. Documents Division, 127-20*.

Fitts, P.M., & Crannell, C. (1950). *Location discrimination. II. Accuracy of reaching movements to twenty-four different areas*. USAF Air Materiel Command Tech. Rep. 5833.

Fitts, P.M., Jones, R.E., & Milton, J.L. (1950). Eye movements of aircraft pilots during instrument-landing approaches. *Aeronautical Engineering Review, 9*, 1-6.

Fitts, P.M., & Seeger, C.M. (1953). S-R compatibility: Spatial characteristics of stimulus and response codes. *Journal of Experimental Psychology, 46*, 199-210.

Graham, E.D., & MacKenzie, C.L. (1995). Pointing on a computer display. Proceedings of the Conference on Human Factors in Computing Systems CHI '95. *ACM Press*, 314-315.

Graham, E.D., & MacKenzie, C.L. (1996). Virtual pointing on a computer display: Non-linear control-display gain mappings. *Graphics Interface '96*, 39-46.

Hedge, A., & Marsh, N.W. (1975). The effect of irrelevant spatial correspondences on two-choice response-time. *Acta Psychologica, 39*, 427-439.

Heilman, K.M., & Valenstein, E. (1979). Mechanisms underlying hemispatial neglect. *Annals of Neurology, 5*, 166-170.

Heister, G., Ehrenstein, W.H., & Schroeder-Heister, P. (1986). Spatial S-R compatibility effects with unimanual two-finger choice reactions for prone and supine hand positions. *Perception & Psychophysics, 40*, 271-278.

Heister, G., Ehrenstein, W.H., & Schroeder-Heister, P. (1987). Spatial S-R compatibility with unimanual two-finger choice reactions: Effects of irrelevant stimulus location. *Perception & Psychophysics, 42*, 195-201.

Heister, G., & Schroeder-Heister, P. (1987). Evidence for stimulus-response compatibility effects in a divided visual field study of cerebral lateralization. *Acta Psychologica, 66*, 127-138.

Hick, W.E. (1951). Man as an element in a control system. *Research, 4*, 112-118.

Hick, W.E. (1952). On the rate of gain of information. *Quarterly Journal of Experimental Psychology, 4*, 11-26.

Hoffmann, E.R. (1992). Fitts' law with transmission delay. *Ergonomics, 35*, 37-48.

Hyman, R. (1953). Stimulus information as a determinant of reaction time. *Journal of Experimental Psychology, 45*, 188-196.

Kornblum, S., Hasbroucq, T., & Osman, A. (1990). Dimensional overlap: Cognitive basis for stimulus-response compatibility—a model and taxonomy. *Psychological Review, 97*, 253-270.

Ladavas, E. (1990). Selective spatial attention in patients with visual extinction. *Brain: A Journal of Neurology, 113*, 1527-1538.

Landsberger, H.A. (1958). *Hawthorne revisited*. Ithaca, NY: Cornell University Press.

Lyons, J. & Hansen, S.D. (submitted). Handheld and Head-Operated Computer Device Employment by Individuals with Spinal Cord Injury. Disability and Rehabilitation: Assistive Technology.

Mayo, E. (1933). *The human problems of an industrial civilization*. Manchester, NH: Ayer.

Merry, S., Weeks, D.J., & Chua, R. (2003). 3D spatial compatibility effects. *Journal of Human Movement Studies, 45*, 347-358.

Michaels, C.F. (1988). Stimulus-response compatibility between response position and destination of apparent motion: Evidence of the detection of affordances. *Journal of Experimental Psychology: Human Perception and Performance, 14*, 231-240.

Passmore, S.R, Burke, J., & Lyons, J. (2007). Older adults demonstrate reduced performance in a Fitts' task. *Adapted Physical Activity Quarterly, 24*, 352-363.

Proctor, R.W., & Van Zandt, T. (1994). Human factors in simple and complex systems. Boston: Allyn & Bacon.

Schmidt, R.A. (1976). Control processes in motor skills. *Exercise and Sport Sciences Reviews, 4*, 229-261.

Shannon, C.E. (1948). A mathematical theory of communication. *Bell System Technical Journal, 27*(July and October), 379-423, 623-656.

Shannon, C.E., & Weaver, W. (1949). *The mathematical theory of communication*. Champaign, IL: University of Illinois Press.

Simon, J.R. (1968). Effect of ear stimulated on reaction time and movement time. *Journal of Experimental Psychology, 78*, 344-346.

Simon, J. R. & Rudell, A. P. (1967). Auditory S-R compatibility: the effect of an irrelevant cue on information processing. *Journal of Applied Psychology, 51*, 300-304.

Simon, J.R., & Small, A.M. (1967). Auditory S-R compatibility: The effect of an irrelevant cue on information processing. *Journal of Applied Psychology, 51*, 300-304.

Simon, J.R., Sly, P.E., & Vilapakkam, S. (1981). Effect of compatibility of S-R mapping on reactions toward the stimulus source. *Acta Psychologica, 47*, 63-81.

So, R.H.Y., Chung, G.K.M., & Goonetilleke, R.S. (1999). Target-directed head movements in a head-coupled virtual environment: Predicting the effects of lags using Fitts' law. *Human Factors, 41*, 474-486.

Umilta, C., & Nicoletti, R. (1985). Attention and coding effects in stimulus-response compatibility due to irrelevant spatial cues. In M.I. Posner & O.S.M. Martin (Eds.), *Attention and performance XI* (pp. 457-471). Hillsdale, NJ: Erlbaum.

Wallace, R.J. (1971). S-R compatibility and the idea of a response code. *Journal of Experimental Psychology, 88*, 354-360.

Weber, E.H. (1978). Per tastsinn und das gemeingfuhl. In H.E. Ross & D.J. Murray (Eds., D.J. Murray, Trans.), *E.H. Weber: The sense of touch*. New York: Academic Press. (Original work published 1846)

Wickens, C.D., Lee, J.D., Liu, Y., & Gordon-Becker, S. (2004). *An introduction to human factors engineering* (2nd ed.). Upper Saddle River, NJ: Pearson Prentice Hall.

INDEX

ABOUT THE EDITORS

Digby Elliott, PhD, is a professor of motor control and behavioral neuroscience in the School of Sport and Exercise Sciences at Liverpool John Moores University (Liverpool, United Kingdom). Previously, he was the Canada research chair in motor control and special populations at McMaster University (Hamilton, Ontario), where he was also a professor emeritus. He has served as president of the Canadian Society for Psychomotor Learning and Sport Psychology (SCAPPS) and as president of the North American Society for the Psychology of Sport and Physical Activity (NASPSPA).

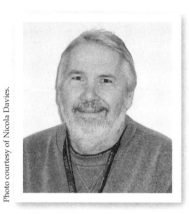

Photo courtesy of Nicola Davies.

Elliott has over 30 years of research experience in the area of motor control with over 200 peer-reviewed articles in publication. He has held visiting professorships at universities throughout the world, most recently at the University of Otago in New Zealand as a William Evans scholar in 2000 and at Katholieke Universiteit Leuven in Belgium as a senior research fellow in 1999. Elliott was awarded the Wood Award for Research Excellence in 2000 from the Down Syndrome Research Foundation.

Elliott and his wife, Elaine, reside in Bancroft, Ontario. In his free time, he enjoys hiking, snorkeling, and playing with his seven grandchildren.

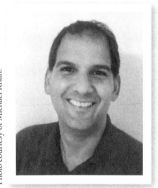

Photo courtesy of Michael Khan.

Michael Khan, PhD, is a professor of motor control and learning and head of the School of Sport, Health, and Exercise Sciences at Bangor University in Wales, United Kingdom.

He has more than 15 years of research experience in the area of motor control. Collaborating with researchers in the United Kingdom, Europe, and North America, Khan has focused his research on the investigation of cognitive processes underlying movement control. He has published more than 30 peer-reviewed articles, book chapters, and conference proceedings. Khan has presented his research as an invited lecturer in the United Kingdom, Europe, North America, and the Caribbean.

A sport enthusiast, especially in West Indian cricket, Kahn also enjoys playing and coaching squash. He was a former top national squash player for Trinidad and Tobago and is currently very active as a coach at the junior level. He and his wife, Martha, reside at Tregarth in Gwynedd, Wales.

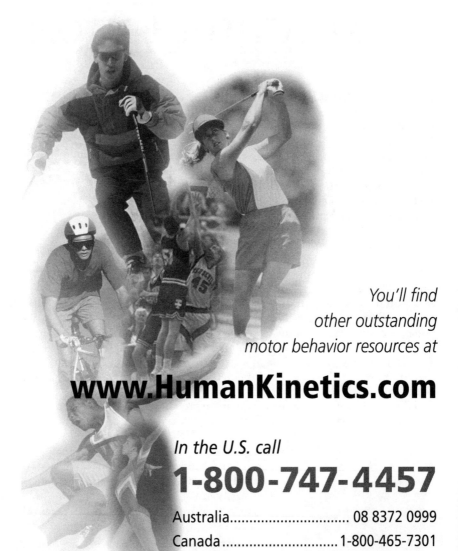